Conditioning for Outdoor Fitness

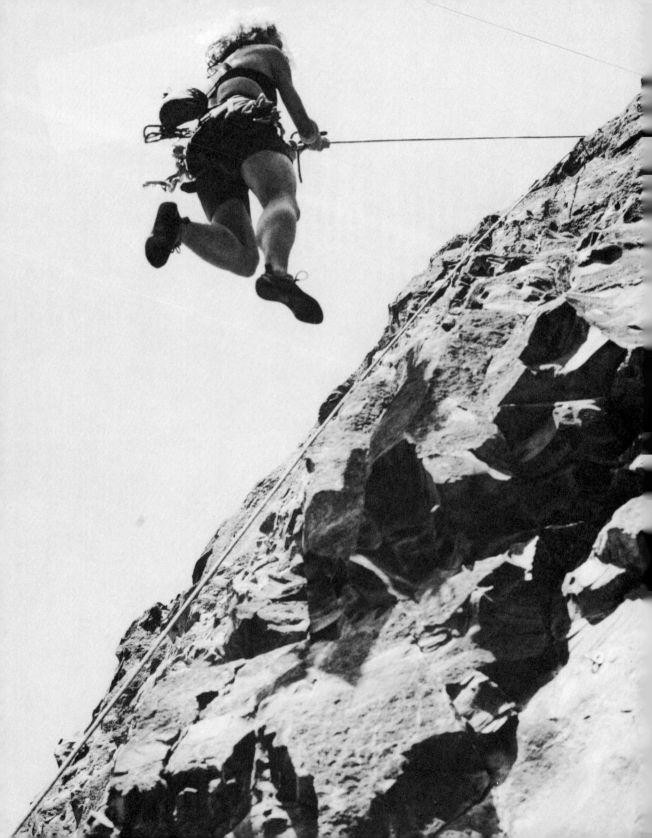

Conditioning for Outdoor Fitness

David Musnick, M.D.
and Mark Pierce, A.T.C.
with the assistance of
Sandra K. Elliott, P.T.

THE
MOUNTAINEERS

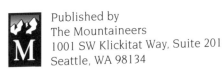

Published by
The Mountaineers
1001 SW Klickitat Way, Suite 201
Seattle, WA 98134

First edition, 1999

Published simultaneously in Great Britain by Cordee, 3a DeMontfort
Street, Leicester, England, LE1 7HD

Printed in Canada

Managing Editor: Cynthia Newman Bohn
Edited by Kris Fulsaas
Cover design by Jennifer Shontz
Book design and layout by Jennifer Shontz

Front cover photograph: *Running in the Teton Range, Targhee National
Forest, Wyoming* © Gregg Adams
Back cover photographs; *Ascending Mount Chiwawa, Glacier Peak Wilder-
ness, Washington* © Ken Lans (top); PhotoDisc, Inc. (middle, bottom)

Library of Congress Cataloging-in-Publication Data
Musnick, David, 1953–
    Conditioning for outdoor fitness / David Musnick and Mark
Pierce with the assistance of Sandra K. Elliott. — 1st ed.
        p.   cm.
    Includes bibliographical references and index.
    ISBN 0-89886-450-X (pbk.)
    1. Exercise. 2. Physical fitness. 3. Outdoor recreation. I.
Pierce, Mark. II. Elliott, Sandra K. III. Title.
    GV481 .M89 1999
    613.7'11—dc21
                                                            99-6365
                                                            CIP

To my father, Henry Musnick, M.D., who took me

on my first hike when I was in elementary school. My early

introduction to aerobic exercise was fast walking with him.

He set an example for me that persistence and hard work are

important in order to achieve life's important goals.

Contents

INTRODUCTION

This is an exercise guide for everyone. No matter what your sport or activity, whether you prefer indoor or outdoor activities, whether you are an experienced athlete or are just beginning to exercise and would like to develop a program tailored to your needs, this book is for you. There are many books about exercise, but no one book written for the layperson combines comprehensive information on functional strength training, basic exercise concepts, posture, movement patterns, balance, and agility with detailed discussions of exercises that embody the state-of-the-art thinking on these subjects. Written by specialists in sports medicine, nutrition, physical therapy, and fitness and athletic training, and designed to be the one volume you turn to for all your conditioning needs, this book

- can be used by people of all ages
- teaches basic concepts so that you will be able to better evaluate exercises, programs, and equipment
- contains many unique exercises
- focuses on functional conditioning so your muscles and your aerobic system are trained in ways that mimic how you actually use them in your indoor or outdoor activities
- uses a body-region approach designed to increase your knowledge of your musculoskeletal system and how it functions
- will help you develop awareness of muscle imbalances in your own body and how to correct them

- emphasizes safety and injury prevention
- emphasizes proper movement patterns and posture
- places particular emphasis on the important areas of the back and neck, both in terms of maintaining their health and strength and in exercising safely
- extensively details the health benefits of exercise
- will help you set fitness goals and plan your own conditioning program.
- devotes entire chapters to the specific exercises required to excel in particular sports

The structure and function of the musculoskeletal and cardiorespiratory systems have been extensively studied, but much of the research is unavailable to laypeople, or when it is available is written in language aimed at scientists or medical personnel. Because we feel strongly that knowing these basic concepts will enhance both your understanding of your body and of the hows and whys of exercising, this book is packed with the most up-to-date information, translated into terms that you can understand. In the more complex sections, you may find you need to read carefully, so take a deep breath and take it slow, but *do* take the time to understand this material. Doing so will benefit you far more than any recipe-list of generic exercises.

Many people find that they can get by with cars that they take to the shop for maintenance, without learning about the car's parts or how it functions. This approach might work fine for cars, but it does not work well for the human body, especially the musculoskeletal system. You can greatly improve your present and future health just by improving how you sit, stand, move, and condition the amazing machine that is your body.

Our bodies are physiological and biomechanical structures that change gradually with time. In order to optimize your time and health and to maximally enjoy your outdoor activities, you need to choose wisely from a wide range of choices for maintaining and conditioning your musculoskeletal and cardiovascular systems. It can be difficult to get advice on what type of conditioning will best achieve a particular goal or on how to devise an exercise program that is challenging, that is specific to and functionally supportive of your chosen activities, and that keeps you interested. Although you might employ the help of a health care or fitness professional along the way, ultimately you are in charge of your own conditioning program. The components of any conditioning program should address:

- basic aerobic fitness and endurance
- muscular strength (for tone and function)
- balance and agility
- flexibility
- activity-specific coordination and skill

In this book, we emphasize functional and activity-specific training not only because they are extremely important but also because they are overlooked in most books and fitness training programs. Functional conditioning is exercise in which your muscles and joints are deployed in positions similar to those of the particular sport or activity being pursued; in these exercises the muscles and joints have the same relationship to gravity and must meet the same, or similar, balance and coordination challenges as in the activity itself. We have also integrated into the exercises presented here the concepts of proper posture, safe movement patterns, and injury prevention.

HOW TO USE THIS BOOK

This book is organized into three parts: Part I covers the basic principles of conditioning; Part II discusses the anatomy of specific body regions and details appropriate exercises for each; and Part III focuses on conditioning for specific outdoor activities. The first two parts are intended for those who would like to learn more about their bodies and improve their fitness status. Each chapter begins by highlighting its objectives; you can get an overview of any chapter by reading its objectives as well as its brief introduction and the "practical point" pullouts found throughout.

The chapters in Part I, Basic Principles, cover exercise physiology, aerobic conditioning, nutrition, warm-up and stretching, strength and balance training, posture, planning your conditioning program, and training outdoors. Chapter 2, Aerobic Conditioning and Interval Training, chapter 4, Warm-up and Stretching, and chapter 5, Strength and Balance Training, lay the foundations for building endurance and strength and should be read before moving on to the activity-specific chapters. Chapter 6, Body Posture and Movement Patterns, will help you improve your posture and efficiency of movement. If you have a specific activity goal (climbing a mountain, biking a long ride, running a race, etc.), if you plan on a season of physically demanding activity such as skiing or climbing, or if you want to make progress in your conditioning program, chapter 7, Training Concepts, Conditioning Goals, and Program Planning, is helpful. Chapter 8, Creative Use of the Outdoors in Training, is excellent source of ideas on how to improve your agility and add diversity to your training.

Part II, Body Regions, educates you about

the anatomy, common muscle imbalances, movement faults, and preferred ways to functionally exercise your major body regions. It contains descriptions and pictures of particular exercises as well as recommendations on how to keep a particular body region in shape. Read Chapter 9, Anatomy, Muscle Balance, and Musculoskeletal Injury, for an overview, before reading about a specific body region. Chapters 10–16 present the most current and exciting information from the physical therapy and sports medicine fields. Much of this material is normally available to individuals only after they have been injured. Why wait for an injury?!

The exercises in Part II have been designed by physical therapists, athletic trainers, and sports medicine doctors, all of whom are experts in their fields. Safe positioning and movement patterns are emphasized and for many exercises additional variations are given as well as cross-references to further choices in other chapters. Chapter 10, The Abdominal Region, presents unique abdominal exercises and should be read by anyone seeking to improve tone, balance, or back health. Chapter 11, The Knee, Thigh, Hip, and Buttock Region, presents a very comprehensive set of functional lower-body exercises; it should be read by anyone doing a general conditioning program or performing any lower-body activity. Everyone should read chapter 14, The Neck and Mid and Low Back Region, and chapter 15, The Shoulder, Upper Torso, and Arm Region; the neck, back, shoulder, arm, and upper torso are common areas of injury and problems with them can keep you away from your activities for prolonged periods of time. These body regions are frequently neglected when it comes to safety and muscle balance.

The chapters in Part III, Conditioning for Outdoor Activities, cover the conditioning demands of several specific activities. It is important that you read chapter 2, Aerobic Conditioning and Interval Training, and chapter 5, Strength and Balance Training, before reading an activity chapter. See chapter 9, Anatomy, Muscle Balance, and Musculoskeletal Injury, for illustrations of skeletal and muscular anatomy. See the relevant body region chapter(s) in Part II for information on the muscles or joint areas discussed in an activity chapter. Part III contains activity-specific exercises as well as cross-references to exercises found throughout the book that are applicable to that activity. At the end of Part III, there is a chapter on general conditioning and strength training (chapter 25) and a chapter on special issues for the conditioning woman (chapter 26).

If you are an outdoor enthusiast who engages in any of the activities covered in Part III, you will benefit from learning about common muscle imbalances and training activity errors. You will learn more about functional exercises and activity-specific training to help you achieve your goals. Some chapters contain conditioning plans that are examples of training programs, with time scales you can use or modify.

In this book, most distances are listed in inches, feet, yards, and miles, and most other units of measurement are also in standard American units. In some chapters, metric measurements are used for chemical and physiological data; in discussions of running, shorter distances and marathon distances are in meters or kilometers (abbreviated as K). The Appendix gives conversions for standard and metric units of measurement.

ABOUT THE EXERCISES

To assist you in keeping track of the many exercises described in this book, the following system has been devised. Each exercise, beginning with Exercise 1 in chapter 4, has been assigned a unique number, which is also used to identify any photographs or drawings used to illustrate it. If more than one part of an exercise is shown, each part is labeled, i.e., 1a, 1b, etc. Variations of a particular exercise are labeled 1.1, 1.2, and so on. Illustrations or photographs that are *not* exercise-specific are identified by captions that include the word "figure" (Figure 1, etc.).

The description of each exercise includes subheadings for *equipment*, *purpose*, and *technique*; some exercises also have *tips and precautions* as well as *variations*.

In each exercise's "purpose" summary, icons are used to indicate appropriateness of the exercise to specific outdoor activities (see Figure 1).

Each of us has only one body, but we all have a wide range of potential in our aerobic and musculoskeletal systems. The conditioning programs you choose can affect your motion and strength capabilities and your tendency to stay healthy or become injured. You can enhance your enjoyment of life and of your activities by choosing the most appropriate conditioning programs. Take charge of your health and maximize your potential by learning as much as possible about your body and how it functions. Become involved—choose the exercise and training that is right for you. We hope that this book will be an excellent resource for you as you move in that direction.

FIGURE 1. OUTDOOR ACTIVITY ICONS

 climbing, gym or rock

 mountaineering, rock or glacier or both

 scrambling, non-technical peak ascents

 hiking

 backpacking

 snowshoeing

 downhill skiing

 telemark skiing

 cross-country and skate skiing

 snowboarding

 cycling, road or mountain bike

 running or jogging

 canoeing

 kayaking

 crew

 windsurfing

 general conditioning

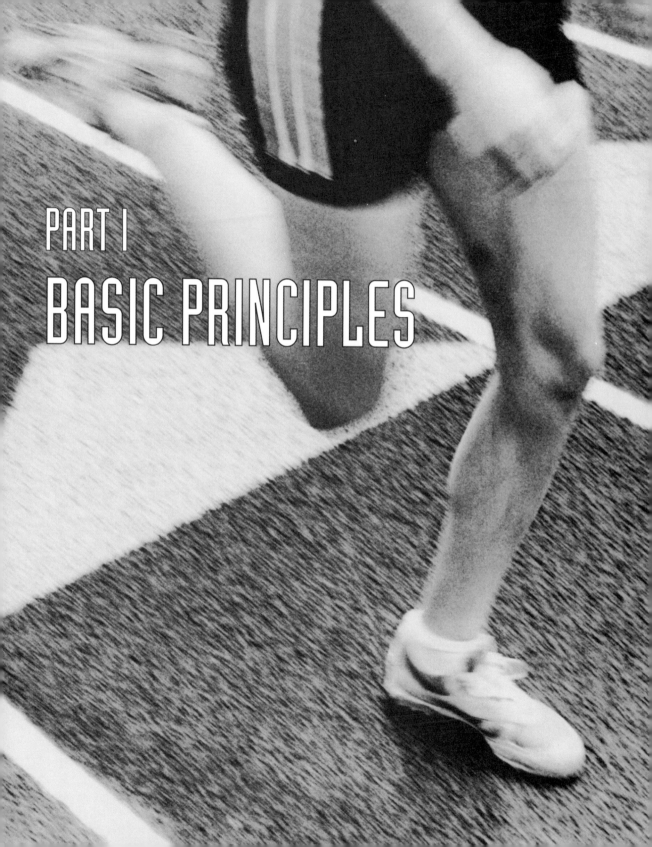

PART I
BASIC PRINCIPLES

Exercise Physiology
Energy Production; Cardiac, Respiratory, and Muscle System Function; and Training Adaptations

BY DAVID MUSNICK, M.D.

▶ **THIS CHAPTER WILL HELP YOU:**
- Understand your body's energy systems.
- Understand the difference between aerobic and anaerobic exercise.
- Understand how your respiratory and cardiovascular systems respond to exercise.
- Understand the physiological changes that occur when exercising at altitude.

In order to undertake any exercise, your body requires energy to power your muscles. To obtain this energy, your body must convert food into a substance known as adenosine triphosphate (ATP). The molecules of ATP are held together by high-energy bonds, and when these bonds are broken, energy becomes available to do biological work such as muscle contractions. The amount of ATP that can be stored in your cells is very limited. In fact, at any one time, your body contains only about 100 grams of ATP, which is enough to exercise at a maximum level for just a few seconds. Thus, a crucial function of your muscle cells is their ability to quickly recycle and synthesize ATP molecules—a task they do best in the presence of adequate oxygen supplies, that is, under "aerobic" conditions. (The terms *aerobic* and *anaerobic* refer to whether oxygen is being used in the chemical reactions—metabolic pathway—that your body uses to create energy.)

AEROBIC VS. ANAEROBIC EXERCISE
The amount of ATP manufactured by your muscle cells is directly proportional to the amount of oxygen available in relation to the intensity of the exercise. Activities that are performed at low to moderate intensity for prolonged periods (such as hiking, jogging, cross-country skiing, or kayaking) are aerobically fueled. Such activities involve the repetitive use of major muscle groups, which leads to an elevated heart rate. As the heart rate increases, the amount of blood flowing to the muscles also increases, as does the amount of oxygen in the blood. As the available oxygen increases, the production of

ATP becomes more efficient, allowing movement to be sustained over time.

Conversely, brief, intense activities (for example, sprinting or a few minutes of very difficult climbing) are usually anaerobically fueled. When you undertake such activities, there is inadequate oxygen available to meet the demand in the oxygen-utilizing pathways.

ANAEROBIC EXERCISE

In the absence of adequate oxygen, energy can be created in a variety of ways. These anaerobic reactions include: (1) the small amount of ATP stored in the muscle cells can be broken down; (2) ATP can be recycled from creatine phosphate (CP), a compound present in the muscles; (3) glucose (a sugar) can be broken down to a smaller molecule called pyruvate, a process called glycolysis; or (4) glycogen (a form of glucose that is stored in the muscles and liver) can be broken down into glucose.

Because the amounts of ATP and CP stored in our bodies are quite small, the first two reactions are only sufficient to sustain about 20 seconds of very high-intensity activity. High-intensity activity of any longer duration (up to 90 seconds) is fueled by the third reaction, glycolysis.

One by-product of anaerobic reactions is the accumulation of lactic acid. The enzymes necessary for muscle contraction work less effectively in acidic conditions, so as the amount of lactic acid increases, the efficiency of muscle contraction decreases. Also, in the absence of oxygen, the muscle cells cannot regenerate ATP quickly enough to meet the demands of high-intensity exercise, with the result that the muscles become fatigued and the intensity of the activity must be lessened or stopped altogether. These natural limits on energy production under anaerobic conditions explain why a runner can sprint for only a short

distance or why a climber can do very difficult moves for only a short period before needing a rest break.

Our bodies generate lactic acid whenever we exercise, but as the intensity of exercise increases, the level of lactic acid in the blood also increases. Each individual has a "lactate threshold," beyond which the level of lactic acid rises steeply with any further increase in exercise intensity. Less aerobically trained individuals reach their lactate threshold sooner than those who are physically fit.

Furthermore, individuals who train for endurance have a greater ability to metabolize (clear) lactic acid and may even produce less of it than untrained individuals. Endurance training may also increase the production of enzymes that support anaerobic energy production, making it more efficient (see chapter 2 for information on interval training for endurance).

AEROBIC EXERCISE

Aerobic exercise relies on energy produced via metabolic pathways in which oxygen is delivered from the lungs to the blood, and from the blood to mitochondria within the cells of muscle tissues, where the production and breakdown of ATP occurs. The chemical reactions that produce energy require the assistance of various enzymes (enzymes are catalysts that can speed up chemical reactions without themselves being altered in the process). Enzymes are critical to the transfer of electrons in the mitochondria of your cells, and they function best within a narrow range of acid (pH) and temperature balance. Enzymes become less efficient as acidity in the cell increases, and more efficient with slightly increased temperatures (one reason why warming up before exercise is a good idea).

Aerobic energy production involves a number of other biochemical reactions, including the

Krebs', or citric acid, cycle, which is approximately eighteen times more efficient at producing ATP than are anaerobic reactions. You can continue sustained low- to moderate-intensity aerobic activities primarily because of this ongoing production of energy.

FUEL SOURCES FOR ENERGY PRODUCTION

Energy production is fueled by food, which, once it is digested, can enter the series of metabolic reactions, described above, at a number of biochemical points. Each of the three types of food—proteins, carbohydrates (including glycogen), and fats (lipids)—functions a bit differently.

CARBOHYDRATES

Carbohydrates, which are composed of carbon, hydrogen, and oxygen, are the body's primary source of energy. When you consume carbohydrates, they are broken down into glucose (also called dextrose), which is transported directly to your muscle cells and used as fuel. The consumption of carbohydrates is especially important in the production of energy for activities lasting more than 60–90 minutes, such as a long run, hike, climb, bike ride, or kayak trip.

If they are not immediately used for energy production, carbohydrates are stored in the body, mostly in the form of glycogen, but they may also be stored as fat. Your daily intake of carbohydrates must be sufficient to supply the energy needs of your body as well as to maintain its stores of glycogen. Two hours of aerobic activity will almost fully deplete the glycogen stored in your liver and your muscles. If you use up your glycogen stores and do not consume additional carbohydrates, you will likely experience fatigue, decreased efficiency, and possibly even weakness, hunger, and light-

headedness, as glucose is pulled from your bloodstream (causing low blood sugar) for energy production.

FATS (LIPIDS)

Fats (lipids) are stored in both fat cells and muscle cells, usually in the form of triglycerides. Because a gram of fat has a caloric value of 9 kilocalories (kcals), compared with 4 kcals for a gram of carbohydrate, it has the potential to provide even more energy.

The body begins to use fat as fuel after about a half hour of light to moderate activity, and fat may contribute 50%–80% of energy needs during prolonged exercise. Regular aerobic conditioning increases the body's efficiency in extracting fat from your fat cells and increases the use of fatty acid for fuel in your muscles. It is for this reason that prolonged aerobic activity can result in weight loss. Your body's ability to break down fat for energy does not significantly decrease your need for carbohydrates during a lengthy activity.

PRACTICAL POINT

To burn more fat and lose weight, perform aerobic exercise of low to moderate intensity (50%–70% of maximum heart rate; see chapter 2, Aerobic Conditioning and Interval Training) for prolonged periods of time (greater than 30 minutes). This can be almost any type of activity, including walking and hiking, as long as the intensity does not increase to a high level.

PROTEINS

Proteins are made from amino acids, which are made from the basic building blocks of carbon, hydrogen, oxygen, and nitrogen. Proteins serve many purposes: They support the body's enzymatic functions and are in all its tissues—

muscles, ligaments, intracellular components, etc. Systematic resistance training increases the protein component of your skeletal muscle, which can lead to increased muscle size and strength. Protein normally plays only a minimal role in energy production. However, if the usual fuel sources (carbohydrates and fats) are lacking, the body can use protein as fuel.

PRACTICAL POINT

In summary, your body uses fuels for exercise in these ways:

At rest: free fatty acids and glucose.

For the first 20 seconds of exercise: reserves of ATP and CP.

As exercise progresses: glycogen, glucose, and fat.

After 2–4 hours of exercise: glycogen, glucose (if carbohydrates have been consumed during the activity), fatty acids, and protein; except during bursts of activity, when anaerobic use of ATP and CP resumes.

YOUR LUNGS AND RESPIRATORY SYSTEM

Aerobic conditioning increases the efficiency of the muscles you use to breathe, with the result that your breathing rate (i.e., number of breaths per minute) is lower than that of less trained individuals. Because aerobically conditioned individuals take fewer, but more efficient, breaths per minute, they are less likely to feel winded at higher exercise intensities. This response is fairly specific to the type of training and activities you regularly do.

YOUR HEART AND VASCULAR SYSTEM

Another benefit of aerobic training is that your cardiac output improves. Cardiac output is calculated by multiplying your heart rate (number of beats per minute) by your stroke volume (the amount of blood pumped per contraction). Regular aerobic training increases stroke volume. As your stroke volume increases, your resting heart rate decreases because your heart does not need to beat as many times per minute as it did in your untrained condition to output the same amount of blood. Your heart thus becomes a more efficient pump, both during exercise and at rest.

As the intensity of your exercise increases, so does your heart rate. Monitoring your heart rate is thus an excellent means of determining the intensity level of your exercise to keep it within the heart rate target zone (see chapter 2 for a discussion of target zones) that meets your fitness goals.

MAXIMAL OXYGEN UPTAKE (VO₂ MAX)

VO_2 *max* is a clinical measurement of the maximal oxygen consumption that a particular individual can achieve at the highest intensity of exercise. VO_2 max is related to the efficiency of numerous body systems, including the respiratory, cardiovascular (particularly hemoglobin concentration and blood volume), and aerobic systems within the muscles.

If you participate in regular aerobic training, you can increase your VO_2 max. Because you won't usually be performing at maximum intensity, you will be able to perform at various levels of exercise intensity with less effort. About half your endurance improvement will come from improved heart pumping ability and half from increased efficiency of the muscles at extracting oxygen and using it to supply energy.

YOUR MUSCULAR SYSTEM

Your muscular system is made up of a series of motor units. A motor unit is a set of motor nerves combined with the group of muscle fibers to which they supply motor impulses.

The amount of force you are able to exert in a contracting muscle is correlated to the percentage of motor units recruited (used), the intensity of the effort, and the percentage of faster or slower fiber types that you have in a muscle. Fibers are recruited from slower to faster. An increasing number of motor units are used as exercise intensity increases. For more powerful and rapid strength demands, the faster fibers are activated. You can train for increased recruitment to increase your speed and strength.

THE EFFECTS OF AEROBIC TRAINING ON MUSCLE

Aerobic conditioning can increase the size and volume of your muscle's mitochondria (where ATP is synthesized), the levels of certain enzymes related to energy production, the extent of your capillary plumbing system (very small blood vessels), and the efficiency of your muscles in using fat as fuel. It can also decrease lactic acid production. The muscles you use in aerobic exercise will become much more efficient metabolically, but this training is pretty specific to how you use the muscles, meaning that if you are a jogger you may not have much swimming or kayaking endurance.

MUSCULAR BENEFITS OF STRENGTH TRAINING

Strength training can enhance your performance in any outdoor activity, as well as in many work and home activities. It can improve body tone and shape, and slow the increase in the ratio of fat to lean body mass that typically occurs as you age. There is also evidence that strength training to the point of muscle fatigue can stimulate the release of growth hormone. Growth hormone facilitates protein synthesis and increases mobilization and utilization of fat as a fuel source, thereby increasing your muscle mass and decreasing fatty tissue. The release of growth hormone may occur with very high-intensity exercise, such as interval and anaerobic training, as well as strength training.

PRACTICAL POINT

There are a number of methods to acclimatize to increasing altitude, but in general all involve gradual increases in elevation gain (1,000 feet per day above 9,000 feet, or 2,000 feet every 2 days if base camps are being moved). It is a good idea to spend 2–4 extra days hiking at 7,000–8,000 feet, as well as at 12,000–13,000 feet, before going to higher altitudes. Rest days with lower-intensity activity are a good idea above 10,000 feet. Sleep at lower altitudes if symptoms start to arise. If symptoms of altitude illness are detected, descend at least 2,000–3,000 feet, accompanied by at least one other person.

ACTIVITY-SPECIFIC TRAINING

The effects of training on a particular muscle or group of muscles are specific to the fibers and motor units used, the range of motion of the joints, the length of the muscles used, and the speed of use. Activity-specific training means training to simulate the muscular demands of your activities using aerobic, strength, and balance training.

EXERCISE AT ALTITUDE

For the most part, altitude does not affect exercise performance until you reach an elevation of 6,000 feet. Then a number of physiological changes occur, all of which are primarily related to a decrease in total amount of oxygen delivered to the muscles, brain, and other organs. There are other changes, including a decrease in blood volume that can worsen with dehydration, an increase in the effort it takes to breathe, and a decrease in ability to do activities at submaximal and maximal levels.

Other changes can occur at higher elevations, including a decrease in arterial oxygen during sleep and a decrease in your ability to exercise to your maximum capacity. Sleep problems, including headaches, insomnia, and frequent awakening, can impede daytime performance.

At 10,000 feet, about half the amount of oxygen is available in the blood as at sea level. If you gradually move up in altitude, your body can adapt somewhat, but cannot fully compensate for altitude in regard to your ability to exercise and perform other activities.

2

Aerobic Conditioning and Interval Training

BY DOROTHY SAGER DOLAN, B.A., L.M.P.,
AND DAVID MUSNICK, M.D.

▶ **THIS CHAPTER WILL HELP YOU:**
- Understand what makes aerobic exercise aerobic.
- Understand the minimum aerobic program needed to achieve health benefits from exercise.
- Be able to modify the minimum aerobic program to meet the specific endurance demands of your planned outdoor activity.
- Be able to evaluate appropriate aerobic activities and equipment you can use to accomplish sport-specific goals.
- Understand the importance of the intensity at which you exercise and how to calculate intensity levels.
- Develop a complete program through goal setting and a heart-zone-intensity approach.

Aerobic exercise is the repetitive use of large muscle groups at submaximal effort for prolonged periods. This type of exercise utilizes oxygen at the cellular level to enable efficient production of energy storage molecules (see chapter 1) to supply energy for contracting muscles. With regular aerobic exercise, you can increase your stamina (endurance) and be able to exercise at your previous intensity, or a higher intensity, with more ease and less feeling of fatigue. The aerobic component of your conditioning program improves basic endurance and can lead to health benefits.

HEALTH BENEFITS OF AEROBIC EXERCISE

To achieve health benefits from exercise, you must do at least a regular aerobic program. One health benefit is a decreased risk of developing complications from coronary artery disease, including fatal heart attacks, by approximately two times compared with the risk for sedentary individuals of comparable age and risk factors. There is also a decreased risk of all-cause mortality.

There may be a slight lowering of blood pressure and total cholesterol, including low-density cholesterol (LDL), and a rise in beneficial high-density cholesterol (HDL). There is also a beneficial effect on blood clotting, which is a presumed factor in improved cardiovascular risk. There may be a decrease in the incidence of some types of cancer, especially colon cancer, and a decrease in the tendency to develop Type 2 diabetes. There is a slowing of a loss in bone density in peri- and post-menopausal women who do low- to moderate-impact weight-loading exercise.

Regular aerobic exercise can lead to improved sleep, stress reduction, and better weight control. There is often a decrease in anxiety and an improved mood. There may be a decreased risk of developing depression.

For some of the benefits, such as the reduction in risk of coronary artery disease, the risk-reduction level peaks when 3,500 kcals per week are used due to exercise. The risk starts to increase again beyond this level.

RISKS OF AEROBIC EXERCISE

There are possible risks to starting or increasing the intensity of aerobic exercise, predominantly related to complications of pre-existing coronary artery disease, or other heart or lung problems. Consult a doctor familiar with exercise evaluation and testing if:

- You have physical symptoms with exercise.
- You have a known disease condition.
- You are male and over 40 or female and over 50 and would like to begin or significantly increase the intensity of an aerobic exercise program or activity. This is especially important when starting interval training.

The other risks include overuse injuries such as strains and sprains, which are usually related to excessive exercise impact, quantity, or high-intensity interval training. Poor posture, excessive weight-loading (such as a backpack that's too heavy), and inadequate equipment can also play a significant role. See chapter 9, Anatomy, Muscle Balance, and Musculoskeletal Injury, for more information on injuries.

Free radicals and aerobic exercise. There is evidence that free radical oxygen molecules are generated during aerobic activity. These are molecules with one or more unpaired electrons that seek out other molecules to complete their unpaired electrons. They may contribute to damage in your tissues if there is an imbalance of free radicals with antioxidant reactions. (For more on this subject, see chapter 3, Nutritional Considerations for Conditioning.) The amount of free radical load is likely to increase with increasing aerobic exercise, especially with increased intensity. It is recommended that you have adequate antioxidants in your diet (see chapter 3) to help prevent such harmful side effects from your exercise.

THE FIVE VARIABLES OF AEROBIC CONDITIONING

Frequency, duration, intensity, specificity, and progression are the five variables of aerobic conditioning. Frequency: How often should you train? Duration: How long should you train? Intensity: How hard should you train? Specificity: What specific activity should you do? Progression: How should you progress your workout once you have obtained your desired initial level of fitness? Your aerobic conditioning goals and knowledge of the effects and risks of modifying the variables will influence your answers to these questions.

THE MINIMUM AEROBIC PROGRAM

The American College of Sports Medicine and the Surgeon General's Physical Activity and Health Report recommend a minimum aerobic program, so named because it is the lowest "dose" of exercise that can help you increase your likelihood of experiencing health benefits. It has been found that aerobic exercise of less intensity or duration will still improve stamina and decrease stress. If you are presently sedentary or exercising very irregularly, the minimum aerobic program, outlined below, can enable you to increase your stamina and increase your chances of improved health.

Frequency: 5–6 times per week.

Duration: 30 minutes within your intensity

range; may require an addition of 5–10 minutes of warm-up and cool-down time.

Intensity: Within your target zone, 60%–85% of your maximum heart rate (70% is ideal).

Calories: The activity should use a minimum of 200–300 kilocalories (kcals).

FREQUENCY

Frequency is the number of aerobic conditioning sessions per week. Six sessions a week causes the best physiological response. If you have been sedentary, begin with 2–3 sessions a week. For full cardiovascular risk reduction, increase your exercise frequency gradually.

DURATION

Duration is the amount of time for which you maintain the proper intensity in your exercise session. Gradually increase your intensity level until you reach your heart rate training zone, and do 30–50 minutes of continuous activity at this "plateau" intensity. If you are a beginner, start with 10–20 minutes. Optimum duration depends on the intensity you maintain and what your goals are. In order to achieve health and fitness benefits, exercise should be long enough to expend at least 200–300 kcals per session, but stress reduction can occur with exercise of any duration. Thirty minutes of moderate-intensity exercise can usually expend 200–300 kcals. In general, limit your aerobic training sessions on consecutive days to 50 minutes or less so that you do not overtrain.

If you are training for outdoor activities that last longer than a few hours, plan a lower-intensity, longer-duration (LILD) exercise session each week at an exercise intensity and difficulty level that are similar to your outdoor activity (usually 50%–65% of your maximum heart rate). You should feel comfortable at this intensity and be able to sustain it for 2–4 hours, so as to achieve approximately three-quarters of the expected duration of your first major outdoor activity. You can increase the duration 10%–15% per week; if it is a lower-impact activity such as cross-country skiing, hiking, or paddling, you can increase the duration 20% per week. These longer sessions should usually consist of the outdoor activity that you are training for, or one very similar to it, using similar muscle groups. It is good to start these longer training sessions within 6–8 weeks of your expected activity, or sooner if your goal is ascending a high mountain or running a long race. As the weeks go by, you may decide to add both distance and difficulty gradually so your body can adapt to the training stresses without injury.

INTENSITY

The intensity of aerobic activity is related to the level of oxygen consumption and the energy demands of your contracting muscles. Intensity is perhaps the most important variable that can affect your fitness, endurance, and aerobic power. Think of intensity as a percentage of your maximum aerobic ability that responds to increases in variables such as speed, slope, resistance, etc. As you increase any or all of these variables, and thus increase your exercise intensity, you will feel like you are working harder. Your exercise will stimulate a demand for increased oxygen and blood flow and a corresponding increase in your heart rate. The heart rate increases in direct correlation with increasing exercise intensity and oxygen consumption.

The intensity at which you exercise is measured in heart beats per minute (your pulse). The intensity range (target zone) that you choose (and within which you try to stay after you have warmed up) is related to many factors, including:

- present fitness level
- desire to burn fat and lose weight
- activity goals and the intensity demands of your desired activity
- health-related exercise goals
- health status, including your risks for heart

disease, presence of any heart rate–lowering drugs, and any musculoskeletal problems

All of these factors, except the last, are covered in the sections below. Any individual with health problems should seek an evaluation and advice as to safe exercise intensity zones from a physician trained in stress testing and familiar with exercise prescription.

A threshold of intensity to elicit a training stimulus seems to be an exercise pulse rate of about 50%–70% of your maximum heart rate, though this varies among individuals. The percentage and type of fuel used are also directly related to the exercise intensity, with a higher percentage of fat burned for fuel at lower intensity levels (less than 70% of maximum heart rate). Remember that working out at very high intensity levels (85% of maximum heart rate, or higher) might be associated with higher risks of injury or medical problems. Intensity can be expressed in many ways, including:

1. calories expended per unit time
2. percentage of maximum oxygen consumption (% VO$_2$ max)
3. rating of perceived exertion (RPE)
4. percentage of maximum heart rate (% max HR)
5. anaerobic threshold, a level related to the lactate threshold

Methods 3 and 4 are the most practical for the average exercising individual. These, along with Methods 1 and 5, are described below. Method 2 is the most accurate but is expensive and requires the most equipment. It is not practical for most people.

CALORIES

Calories expended per unit of time is an important factor if you are trying to accurately estimate your calorie needs to maintain your weight or to lose weight. This is especially true for long outdoor trips, to insure that you have enough food to meet your energy needs. Calorie expenditure in kilocalories (kcals) per minute is dependent on your body composition, intensity of the exercise, and the workload, such as whether you are carrying a pack. Although there is a great deal of individual variability, a fit person weighing about 150 pounds burns or metabolizes 7–10 kcals per minute for most moderate activities, including aerobic dance classes, cycling, rowing, backpacking, and mountaineering. Walking, swimming, and kayaking usually burn 5–6 kcals per minute unless they are very vigorous. Running, cross-country skiing, snowshoeing, and mountaineering with a heavy pack can use more than 10 kcals per minute, and up to 20. In general, the calorie values listed on exercise machines, especially stair-climbers, are overestimated.

RATE OF PERCEIVED EXERTION

Rating your perceived exertion (abbreviated as RPE) is a method that can help you evaluate your exercise intensity by how hard you feel the exercise is on a scale from 0 to 10, with 0 being nothing at all and 10 being very, very heavy. Your RPE can be correlated to your heart rate response to exercise by using a heart rate monitor or by taking your exercise pulse.

An adequate work intensity for achieving aerobic conditioning elicits a response of a value of 3–6. Interval high-intensity training leads to an RPE of 7–10. Most outdoor activities can be sustained at an RPE of 2–5.

FIGURE 2. RATE OF PERCEIVED EXERTION

RPE	EXERCISE INTENSITY	(% MAX. HR)
0	Resting	
2	Light work	50%–60%
4	Somewhat hard	60%–70%
5	Heavy (strong), moderately hard	70%–80%
7	Very heavy	80%–90%
10	Very, very heavy (almost maximum)	90%–100%

HEART RATE

Heart rate is a guiding factor for the intensity level of aerobic training. Most heart rate calculations of intensity use your maximum heart rate (max. HR), which is the highest heart rate you can attain during hard exercise. The safest way to determine your maximum heart rate is to take a graded exercise stress test on a treadmill. This should be done for people who fall into a higher risk category for coronary artery disease or other diseases due to age, symptoms, family history, and other factors. If you have questions about this, consult a physician trained in exercise testing.

As a rule, any man over 40 or woman over 50 who is thinking about exercising at moderate to high intensities should consider having a stress test. It will screen for electrical changes indicative of decreased heart blood supply and give you a maximal heart rate and a training zone prescription. You can also get an idea of your maximal heart rate from supervised short aerobic testing (2–4 minutes of running or cycling) while wearing a heart rate monitor (see Edwards, 1996, in Selected References). This is usually safe for people under 40 with no other medical problems or risks for heart disease.

Heart Rate Calculations

There can be a substantial error of up to plus or minus 25 beats per minute when using any formula to predict your maximum heart rate. You can estimate your maximum heart rate by subtracting your age from the number 220. Fit people over 40 may have a maximum heart rate that is underestimated by that formula. Maximum heart rate times a range of percentages, from 60% to 85% max. HR, will give you an estimate of your various training zones.

During times of higher-volume training, occasionally take your pulse before getting out of bed in the morning to determine if you are training too hard. If you are, you might find a morning resting pulse that is elevated past (8–10 beats per minute higher than) your normal. This, along with a feeling of fatigue, may be an indication that you are overtraining.

PRACTICAL POINT

To find your resting heart rate, take your pulse (turn your left forearm palm side up, and place two or three fingers from your right hand on your left wrist below the base of your left thumb) in a standing position for 15 seconds, and multiply it times 4 to get your per minute pulse rate (see Figure 3). You can also take your pulse right above your collarbone's midsection, if you have difficulty finding it at the base of your thumb. In general, it is not good to take your pulse right below your jaw, as putting pressure on this area can stimulate a response that may slow the pulse rate or make you lightheaded.

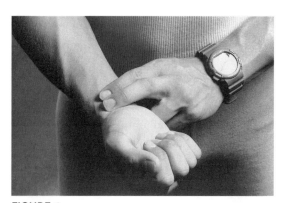

FIGURE 3

Calculate Your Heart Rate Training Zones

In outdoor recreation for fun, you are generally in a range of 50%–70% max. HR, which correlates to a feeling of light to moderate work. Vary your intensity depending on the activity, terrain, and your time constraints.

Calculate various heart-rate intensity zones

to be specific with your exercise planning. If you do not want to be this specific, calculate a 60% max. HR and start there. Gradually increase your intensity until you are at 70%–85% (closer to 70%) for the majority of your exercise. Try doing these calculations for yourself using an actual tested maximum, or estimate your maximum by subtracting your age from 220. Calculate your heart rate zones by using the formulas below.

Zone 5: 90%–100% max. HR

(my zone 5 =   ). Zone for intervals and training for speed and power, anaerobic/very, very hard exertion (sprints of less than 1 minute). Improved performance can occur from training in this zone, but there is a higher risk for musculoskeletal injuries and possible cardiovascular problems. Do most of your training below this zone.

Zone 4: 80%–90 % max. HR

(my zone 4 =   ). Zone for intervals and training for aerobic and anaerobic power at or beyond the lactate threshold. Fast HR and breathing rate. Very hard RPE (brief push in a kayak in rough water or tough, steep parts of a climb, hike, etc.).

Zone 3: 70%–80% max. HR

(my zone 3 =   ). Moderately hard RPE (your average workout after you have achieved a basic aerobic fitness level).

Zone 2: 60%–70% max. HR

(my zone 2 =   ). Somewhat hard RPE. An average level for longer-duration activities such as hiking, or for when you are gradually building aerobic fitness or working on weight loss.

Zone 1: 50%–60% max. HR

(my zone 1 =   ). Zone with high percentage of fat metabolized, and for lower-intensity, longer-duration (LILD) workouts. A light work RPE. A common zone for prolonged outdoor activities or when you are starting your fitness training.

Heart Rate Monitors

Using a heart rate monitor is one of the most effective ways to monitor your aerobic intensity. These generally consist of transmitter units mounted in chest straps that pick up electrical signals from your heart and transmit them to a receiver on your wrist or to a readout on your exercise machine. The continuous, accurate feedback allows you to be aware of your heart rate response and adjust the intensity of your exercise to stay within your desired intensity. Heart rate monitors are available at exercise equipment and sporting good stores.

LACTATE THRESHOLD

Your breathing response is also a good indicator of exercise intensity. If you are in aerobic training zones 1–3, you should feel relatively comfortable breathing and be able to talk while you exercise.

As you increase the intensity, you will notice a level of breathing that feels difficult and in which it is not easy to carry on a conversation. This will be associated with a feeling that it is very hard work and that you would not like to continue very long at this intensity level. There may also be a feeling of muscle discomfort. This is approximately the level at which you accumulate excessive lactic acid; this is called your lactate threshold. Your lactate threshold is usually some point between 80% and 90% of your maximum heart rate. Interval training helps increase your tolerance for lactic acid as it builds up in your system, and your body learns to use lactate as an alternate fuel source.

INTERVAL TRAINING

Interval training is the performance of an aerobic activity done at high intensities for brief periods of time. The energy systems used by your body may be aerobic or anaerobic, depending on how intense your exercise is. The goal of interval training is to increase your ability to do short spurts of high-intensity aerobic activity and to improve your aerobic fitness. In outdoor activities, very high-intensity aerobic activity may last less than 5 minutes. Moderately high-intensity activity may last for longer periods. Examples are going up a very steep, short trail, snow, or crevasse field; crossing a stream or boulder field; kayaking or paddling through a rough or dangerous area of water; or sprinting at the end of a race. Training for this short, high-intensity output can greatly improve your ability to accomplish these tasks well and without injury when the need arises.

You can use a variety of interval techniques, depending on the activities you are interested in. Try to simulate the conditions in which you do your bursts of activity, such as walking up slopes on trails or snowfields, bicycling up hills, or paddling through rough water. You can also add different types of interval training to more quickly improve your overall aerobic conditioning.

Interval training risks. Many people never do high-intensity activity spurts, and may prefer not to do interval training because of the injury risks or because they are content with their fitness level. Because interval training puts a higher demand on your cardiovascular and musculoskeletal systems, it is not recommended for anyone with any heart, lung, or musculoskeletal problems. A solid level of aerobic fitness (at least 6 weeks of training and an ability to exercise briefly at close to 80% max. HR) is necessary before beginning interval training. Precautions:

- Don't do intervals on consecutive days or when you are recovering from an injury that involves your back, hips, or legs.
- Don't do intervals if you have an infection or are anemic.
- Slow down or stop the interval if you have chest pain or excessive pain elsewhere.

Designing an interval workout. Consider adding intervals to your workout 2 times a week. The goal for each interval is to work out at an intensity of 80%–100% max. HR, depending on where your lactate threshold is (but usually in the 80%–90% range). Interval training can be done as a separate activity or within a regular aerobic workout or outdoor activity, such as Fartlek training (see below). You can do intervals while running, stair climbing, or doing any outdoor activity, as well as by using any indoor aerobic exercise machine (treadmill, stair-climber, etc.).

In interval training, the workout time segments are split into alternating periods of hard efforts, called the exercise interval, and recovery periods, called the recovery interval. The recovery periods usually consist of lower-intensity aerobic activity (50%–70% max. HR), and they are related to the length of the exercise interval by a ratio of work:rest. Recovery times are indicated in Figure 4, but you may need to have a longer rest period depending on how you are feeling. Based on the demands of your sport, you can choose the appropriate work interval that would be most applicable to your athletic goal. The intervals can be done as part of your general training or as a specific component of your activity-specific conditioning program.

Practical aspects of interval training. Warm up for 10–15 minutes at a heart rate of 60%–70% max. HR before you begin an interval effort. Increase your heart rate to 80%–95% max. HR, or work until you perceive your effort as very hard (6 + RPE). Hold the intensity there for the amount of time in your exercise interval, then reduce the workload to a recovery level by reducing speed, incline, or resistance until your heart rate has dropped to approximately 50%–70% max. HR. Hold your intensity at this level for the duration of your rest interval.

Based on how you feel, you can begin the next intense effort and try the sequence again.

FIGURE 4. SAMPLE INTERVAL WORKOUT

	INTERVAL DISTANCE TRAINING	*INTERVAL MID-DISTANCE TRAINING*	*INTERVAL SPRINT TRAINING*
Work:Rest Ratio	1:1	1:2	1:3+
Heart Rate Zone	Zone 2–3	Zone 4	Zone 4–5
Exercise Load Duration(s)	240 sec–15 min	30 sec–240 sec	10 sec–30 sec
Recovery time(s)	240 sec–15 min	60 sec–480 sec	30 sec–90 sec
Repetitions	2–5	5–15	5–20
Energy Supply	Aerobic	Anaerobic	Anaerobic

Initially try intervals of 30–60 seconds and do 2–4 of them. Gradually build up to 4–10 intervals per workout. You can decide on the duration of the intervals based on the demands of your activity. If your activity demands very short bursts of maximum intensity, then do intervals of 20–30 seconds. Your average intermediate intervals should be 30–120 seconds, the most common duration for interval training. Endurance anaerobic intervals are 120–240 seconds. Endurance aerobic intervals are 5–20 minutes.

Fartlek Interval Training

Fartlek interval training is interval training that is randomly dispersed throughout your workout in regard to when you start the interval, the interval duration, the rest period, etc. When you are training outside, you can use the distance between telephone poles, hill to hill, tree to tree, stone to stone, or any landmark to measure your interval. You can also use time periods.

Fartleks usually involve spurts of increased intensity that last 30 seconds–4 minutes. Try to exercise in a low- to moderate-intensity zone as a baseline (60%–75% max. HR), and then work out in higher-intensity intervals in various zones (zones 4 and 5), depending on the terrain and how you feel. This can be done on exercise equipment and can also be done outside by hiking, running, biking, or cross-country skiing. In a Fartlek interval, you usually continue some baseline aerobic activity between intervals. You can do the intervals at different intensities, speeds, and slopes. Below are some sample Fartlek programs.

Cycling: Do 2–4 repetitions (reps) of 30-60-90-120-90-60-30 seconds of Fartlek intervals, keeping your heart rate at 80%–85% max HR. Each rest interval should be twice as long as the exercise interval.

Hiking: Try this on a training day hike. After hiking for at least 30 minutes at a moderate pace, begin some random fast hiking. Pick a tree, stone, or bend in a switchback to head for, and use varying times of 20 seconds–2 minutes. Start with the 20-second interval and hike as fast as you can to your landmark, then slow down your pace until you feel only a light to moderate RPE. Try these short intervals on relatively level or gradual slopes, then try them on steeper trail sections. Within about a half hour from your major rest stop, try some longer intervals of 1–2 minutes at a slightly lower intensity than the first set of intervals. Rest at least 1–2 times the interval length until you are in your recovery heart rate, and try again 1–3 more times. Avoid doing these on downhill sections. Make sure you drink enough water, and avoid doing this on very hot days or on slippery or exposed terrain.

Aerobic machines: You can do Fartlek intervals on any piece of aerobic exercise equipment if there is a manual setting and you feel very comfortable and well balanced on the equipment. Increase the intensity by putting more effort into self-propelled equipment such as cycles or cross-country ski machines. For machines with intensity buttons, such as stair-climbers and treadmills, you can dial up the speed. Some equipment has programmed interval settings. Look at these beforehand to see if they are appropriate for you.

Slope Intervals

Slope intervals are intervals you could do on short hiking, snowshoe, or climbing trips in which you are on slopes rather than relatively flat terrain. Slope intervals are done like Fartlek intervals. The duration of slope intervals is usually less than that of intervals on level ground. It is best to try these with and without a pack.

SPECIFICITY

Your training should be specific to the demands of your outdoor activity, in regard to the muscles used, patterns of motion, loads (if any), and duration and intensity of your activity. If you usually do lower-body activities, there is not a great deal of transfer of aerobic capacity when you first try a predominantly upper-body activity such as crew, kayaking, or swimming. The optimal way to train for a specific activity is to do it, or something closely resembling it in regard to the muscles used. For suggestions on specificity of activities, refer to Figure 5, Aerobic Cross Training and Specificity.

CROSS TRAINING

While repeatedly using the same training machines or doing the same activities may enhance your performance in your chosen activity, over-reliance on the specificity principle can cause problems. Overuse injuries such as tendonitis and bursitis can result from training the same way all the time. If you never train the rest of your body, you may sustain injury from strength imbalances. Cross training is training with various activities or types of exercise equipment. You can choose standing vs. seated positions, for example, to change the stress on your hip, knee, and ankle joints.

Cross training can also mean choosing an alternate training mode that will train muscles not usually used in your primary activity. Many injuries can be avoided if you have a well-balanced body, with muscles and joints conditioned in as many ways as possible. To do this, train muscles you don't usually use in your primary sport. You can also use cross training to decrease your exercise boredom and provide an active "relative rest" period from your regular vigorous activities. Figure 5 suggests some ways you can train specifically for a sport, as well as some options for cross training.

PROGRESSION

As you plan your aerobic program, consider base development, intensity development, and maintenance. This is a way to plan how to use the total training time you have available. If you are training for a specific event, there will be a definite target date for your peak. If you are training for a seasonal activity, there will be a range of time in which you want to maintain high levels of aerobic conditioning. You can enter this sequence at any level, depending on your fitness level.

About 6 weeks after beginning a conditioning program, you can restructure your training cycle to include increases in intensity and interval training. Always keep in mind the demands of the actual sport you are pursuing. Use that specific activity to monitor the progress you are making. The closer you get to the event or season, the more sport-specific your training activities should be. For example, if your plan is to climb a mountain, spend more time on stair-climbers and hiking than on bicycles or kayaking.

FIGURE 5. AEROBIC CROSS TRAINING AND SPECIFICITY

ACTIVITY/EXERCISE	STAIR CLIMBING	STAIR-CLIMBER	CROSS-COUNTRY SKIING	CROSS-ROBICS	TREADMILL	CLIMBING WALL	EFX CROSS-TRAINER	CYCLING	ROWING	IN-LINE SKATING	STEP AEROBICS	SWIMMING	RUNNING	HIKING	SLIDEBOARD
Windsurfing	S	X	X	X	X	X	X	X	S	X	X	S	X	X	S
Walking	X	X	X	X	S	X	X	X	O	X	X	O	S	S	X
Hiking	S	S	X	X	S	X	S	X	O	X	S	O	S	S	X
Running	X/S	X/S	X	X	S	X	S	X	O	X	X	O	S	X	X
Rock Climbing	S	S	X	X	X	S	X	X	S	X	S	O	X	X	X
Scrambling	S	S	S	X	S	S	X	O	X	X	S	O	S	S	X
Mountaineering	S	S	S	X	S	S	X	O	X	X	S	O	S	S	X
Skiing, Downhill	X	X	X	X	X	X	X	X	X	X	X	O	X	X	X
Snowboarding	X	X	X	X	X	X	X	O	X	X	X	O	X	X	S
Skiing, Telemark	S	S	S	X	X	X	X	X	X	S	S	O	S	S	S
Skiing, Skate	X	X	S	X	X	X	X	X	X	S	X	O	S	X	S
Skiing, Cross-Country	X	X	S	X	X	X	X	X	X	S	X	O	S	X	S
Snowshoeing	S	S	S	X	S	X	S	X	X	X	S	O	S	S	S
Cycling	X	X	X	X	X	X	X	S	X	X	X	O	X	X	X
Rowing	X	X	X	X	O	X	O	X	S	X	X	O	X	X	O
Canoeing	O	O	X	O	O	X	O	O	S	O	O	X	O	O	O
Kayaking	O	O	X	O	O	O	O	O	X	O	O	X	O	O	O

S = Specific: Choose this option to train muscles and joints in ways similar to the demands of your sport.

X = Cross train: Choose this option to train muscles and joints with different demands from those used in your sport.

0 = Cross train other: Choose this option to train other muscles than those used in your sport in order to balance your body.

RATE OF PROGRESSION

Initial conditioning stage. If you have not been doing regular aerobic conditioning, start at this stage to build your aerobic base and achieve the physiological adaptations required for an event or season. This stage may last 4–6 weeks. Frequency should be 3–4 nonconsecutive days. Duration should be 12–15 minutes initially, and gradually increase to 30 minutes. Intensity as measured by heart rate should be 50%–70% max HR, starting at the low end. This stage should also include strength training at 2–3 sessions per week of light resistance with a higher number of repetitions (15–20 per set). Try to increase your exercise duration by 10%–15% per week, and gradually increase the intensity.

Improvement conditioning stage. This lasts 12–20 weeks. *Frequency* should be 5–6 days per week. Consider 1–2 aerobic sessions of 40–50 minutes, with your other sessions closer to 30 minutes. *Duration* is increased every 1–3 weeks by 10%–15% until 30–50 minutes are reached. *Intensity* as measured by heart rate should be 70–80% max. HR for fitness and health benefits. In addition, there might be a longer period of a lower-intensity, 50%–60% max. HR if you are conditioning for an aerobic outdoor activity requiring endurance or if you are trying to lose weight. Consider doing some cross training 1 day a week to avoid injuries, especially if you are exercising more than 30 minutes 3 times a week. You may add intervals after 4–8 weeks in this stage, if you have goals of doing high-intensity spurts of activity, or to more quickly increase your aerobic fitness. This stage should also include strength training with increased resistance and lower repetitions (8–12) per set. *Specificity* can be added if you are training for a specific activity; do activity-specific balance and skill exercises.

Maintenance conditioning stage. When you have reached your desired level of conditioning, your emphasis can be redirected to activity challenges. It is easier to maintain strength and endurance levels than it is to achieve them initially. Maintenance can be sustained with a *frequency* of 3 sessions per week, but the activities should be of the same *duration* and *intensity* used to achieve the improvements. Try to do aerobic conditioning 5–6 days a week if you wish to achieve maximum health benefits.

MAKING A ONE-WEEK PLAN

Begin by looking at a 1-week plan. Include 1 rest day and 1 day of active rest. Active rest is when you are physically active doing something other than your usual training. (Individuals 50 and older may do better with an additional rest day.) This leaves you with 5–6 days of specific training. Alternate between hard days and easy days. (Hard days are those on which you do interval training, or longer time or distances.) Try to use particular HR or RPE targets for every workout.

HEART-RATE-ZONE TRAINING

A heart-rate-zone training approach can be used to progress your aerobic conditioning and achieve an activity goal. Such an approach is based on periods of times in various training zones. See chapter 19 for an example of an aerobic program for a mountaineering-based heart-rate-zone training.

Building an endurance base: In this period, you are training primarily to improve your cardiovascular and muscular systems' adaptation to aerobic exercise, and to build your general endurance.

Spend 10% of your total training time at 50%–60% max. HR.

Spend 80% of your total training time at 60%–70% max. HR (zone 2).

Spend 10% of your total training time at 70%–80% max. HR (zone 3), after you have been working out in zone 2 for at least 3 weeks.

Increasing your endurance: In this period you are training primarily in your aerobic heart-rate zones.

Spend 20% of your total training time at 50%–70% max. HR (zones 1 and 2).

Spend 70% of your total training time at 70%–80% max. HR (zone 3).

Spend 10% of your total training time above 80% max. HR (zone 4); make sure you have spent 2 weeks at 70%–80% max. HR before you begin this interval training.

Increasing your speed: In this period, your focus shifts to adding more anaerobic interval training.

Spend 20% of your total training time at

50%–70% max. HR (zones 1 and 2).

Spend 60% of your total training time at 70%–80% max. HR (zone 3).

Spend 10% of your total training time above 80% max. HR (zone 4).

Spend 10% of your total training time above 90% max. HR (zone 5).

Reaching your peak: In this period you further increase your percentage of time in interval training. This is especially appropriate for racing or competition, for which a very high level of aerobic fitness is critical. This period likely would not be necessary for most recreational activities such as mountaineering, kayaking, noncompetitive cycling, and running, but is included for completeness.

Spend 10% of your total training time below 70% max. HR (zones 1 and 2).

Spend 60% of your total training time at 70%–80% max. HR (zone 3).

Spend 20% of your total training time above 80% max. HR (zone 4).

Spend 10% of your total training time above 90% max. HR (zone 5).

If you have 12 weeks to train for your target, spend the first 4 weeks building your endurance base, the second 4 weeks increasing aerobic endurance zones, and the third 4 weeks increasing your speed. Include time in the peak period if you are training for a race or competing. It is good to plan a reduced volume of training 1 week before your event so your body can rest and charge up its fuel stores.

These periods are similar to periods of progression discussed above and the periods discussed in chapter 7, but they are more specific to a zone type of training. Of important note is that some of the zones include a significant amount of high-intensity training (intervals), and you should be very healthy and medically cleared for this type of activity. It is possible to accomplish most goals with very little or no

interval training if you cannot do that part of the conditioning.

THE AEROBIC EXERCISE SESSION

Warm-up period. For a short period before you achieve your training zone, start at a low intensity of the aerobic activity you will be doing, and gradually increase the intensity until you are in your heart rate training zone. The warm-up period may last 5–10 minutes and can decrease the likelihood of overuse injuries.

Plateau period. Your target training heart rate zone is the range of heart beats per minute within which you can achieve conditioning benefits. The best method for an individual aerobic session is to warm up (see above) and then stay in a plateau period of intensity for the prescribed time, until the cool-down period.

Cool-down period. After you have completed your aerobic training, gradually decrease your level of intensity for 2–5 minutes (longer after very high-intensity or endurance events, or 10% of your workout time). This has been shown to decrease the likelihood of heart rhythm disturbances and may decrease muscle soreness. Abruptly stopping an aerobic exercise or activity is not a good idea.

Figure 6 shows a typical aerobic training session. This is an example of a 45-minute aerobic period for a 50-year-old training at a 70%–80%

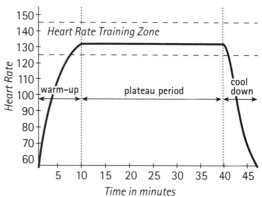

FIGURE 6

max. HR. Notice the gradual increase of intensity in the warm-up period and the gradual decrease in intensity in the cool-down period. Also notice the training zone and maintenance heart rate.

MODES OF AEROBIC CONDITIONING

The modality you select for developing cardiorespiratory fitness should use large muscle groups, be rhythmical, and be maintained continuously through the workout. Your choice of activity should be made with the following considerations:

- A high percentage of time (at least 60%) should be spent in activity-specific aerobic sessions if you are training for a specific activity. These are activities that use muscles and motion patterns similar to those used in your activities.
- Choose activities that are less likely to exacerbate existing injuries or restricted areas of motion, if you have any.
- Spend some time doing activities that you enjoy, to prevent becoming bored with your exercise program.
- Vary your activities to decrease the amount of impact if you are doing a high volume of aerobic conditioning. This might include lower-impact activities after a day of interval or long-distance training or after 3 consecutive days of conditioning.

The following evaluation covers joint and muscle demands, sports activities best trained for in each modality, potential concerns, and tips on form.

Using a stair-climber: Climbing accesses the large muscles of the hip and thigh that extend your leg and the calf muscles that lift your heel when you step. The movement challenges each leg individually from a standing position. A stair-climber is excellent for lower body workouts and provides functional training for activities that require you to carry your own body weight up an incline, including hiking and rock and mountain climbing. Stair-climbers that include a revolving step are particularly useful. For added benefit consider adding a pack when you are within 4 weeks of a significant mountaineering trip (see Figure 7a). It is important to step with your whole foot and keep off your toes to get the most out of your gluteal muscles and to reduce strain on your foot (Figure 7b illustrates good stair-climbing posture). Machines that have revolving full steps usually offer a more intense, full workout, but may be harder on your kneecaps. Try to take deeper steps with a definite force downward if you do not have knee problems. Place a minimum amount of weight on your hands, as this will decrease your energy expenditure (Figure 7c gives an example of poor stair-climbing posture). Maintain an upright posture, otherwise you will get less of a buttock workout. Also stay alert for kneecap pain, back pain, and foot tingling and numbness.

Climbing stairs: This is one of the best aerobic and anaerobic training modes for mountaineering, backpacking, snowshoeing, and telemark and cross-country skiing. It is best done outdoors if you can find an area with at least 5 flights of stairs. Bleachers or stairs inside tall buildings can also be used. Warm up with a fast walk or jog for 5–10 minutes before stair climbing. Stair climbing can be done as an aerobic or an interval workout. Options include:

1. Run single stairs.
2. Run double stairs.
3. Run stairs in a diagonal pattern (instead of running straight up, run at a diagonal until you get close to the side, then change direction of the diagonal).
4. Run stairs with a lateral hopping motion.
5. Fast-walk double or triple stairs.
6. Descend single stairs.
7. Descend double stairs.
8. Descend stairs in a diagonal pattern.

Using a cross-country skiing machine: The

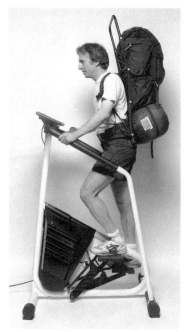

FIGURE 7a

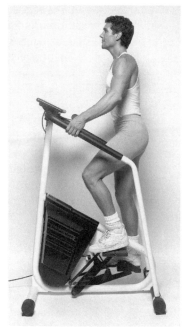

FIGURE 7b

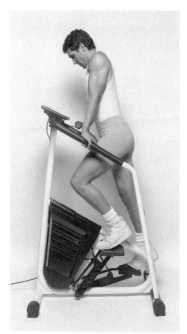

FIGURE 7c

motion on cross-country skiing machines is functional and bilateral. Muscles trained include hip flexors and extensors, quadriceps, hamstrings, shoulders, and upper back. The movement also trains coordination and balance. These machines vary in their design. Some have foot cars and poles connected so that more of your upper-body muscles can be trained. This training is suitable for general conditioning and any hiking or running activity, in-line skating, skiing, and snowshoeing. Some people report discomfort when they first train with this mode, and it should not be used if it aggravates an existing shoulder or low-back problem.

Using a treadmill: A treadmill is a lower-body training tool that is excellent for most people, because they can vary the impact while maintaining functional training. Running on a treadmill has a higher impact than walking on one, but has possibly a little less than outdoor running. Use a treadmill for running, especially in poor weather, just as you would incorporate regular running into your program.

Using an EFX elliptical cross trainer: This machine provides a unique combination of motions. It feels a bit like running, but with less impact. By adjusting resistance and incline, you can change which muscles are targeted. Muscles trained include hip flexors and extensors, quadriceps, and hamstrings. It is excellent for general conditioning and for hiking, climbing, snowshoeing, or cross-country skiing. Precautions include the possible strain of hip muscles due in part to a wide foot position, and an aggravation of back or knee problems.

Using a crossrobics machine: When using this machine, you sit with your body bent at a 45-degree angle from the waist, and put your feet on two independent foot plates. You pump your legs to move a stack of weights, and maintain the weights in a "floating" position. This trains for leg strength, power, speed, and endurance on one system, encouraging the use of a complete range of motion. This machine is useful for conditioning for walking, running, and activities requiring forceful or rapid movement of the leg backward (for example, cross-country and skate skiing, snowshoeing, mountaineering, and in-line skating). The crossrobics machine could bring on or exacerbate kneecap pain, back discomfort from the stabilizing position, and tendonitis in the hips.

Using a treadwall: This machine is actually a vertical treadmill/climbing wall with hand- and footholds attached. The rate of climb and the angle of the wall are adjustable to make it harder or easier. Climbing is intended to be predominantly a leg exercise. Instead of pulling up with your arms, push your weight up with your legs. As the wall angle becomes more of an overhang, your arms are used more in the workout. There is some technique required to use this machine well (see Figure 8). Possible

FIGURE 8

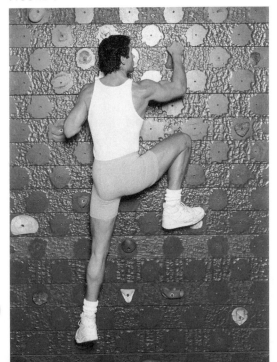

injuries include finger and forearm strains, and tendonitis in the upper body.

Using a stationary cycle: Several types of stationary bicycles are available in gyms. Muscles trained include hip flexors, quadriceps, and, with proper mechanics, hamstrings and gluteals. Upright bikes mimic the traditional cycle with a small saddle. Recumbent bikes offer a slightly reclined body position on a chair-like seat with back support. Stationary cycling offers several advantages, including reduced joint compression of your hips, lower impact, and a minimal need to balance your body on the cycle. Cycling can also be used when one ankle, knee, or hip is recovering from an injury. Stretch your hips and legs thoroughly after a bike session. Potential problems on a bicycle are aggravation of low-back pain and occasionally of kneecap disorders.

Using a rowing machine: Rowing is an excellent total body motion involving the legs, shoulders, arms, and back. Range of motion in the ankle, knee, hip, and back are challenged in this activity. Begin with a controlled range of motion and see how your body responds. On an indoor ergometer, use a lower flywheel resistance. The stroke power is in the pull. Keep your strokes per minute in the mid-20s. Use the return movement as a time to recover for your next pull. Good back positioning is important on this machine. The excessive use of low-back muscles may cause low-back pain or aggravate existing problems. Kneecap problems can also be aggravated.

Doing aerobics classes: Aerobics classes are excellent training tools and can train your lower and upper body. It is best to talk with an instructor to find out the duration of the target heart rate period, and whether there are sprinting intervals, upper-body exercise, or moves that might compromise an area of your body that you are concerned about.

Doing step aerobics: This class format uses a step at the height of your choice. It develops coordination and balance. Much of the effort comes from calf muscles, quadriceps, and hip muscles. It is good indoor training for hiking, climbing, mountaineering, snowshoeing, etc. This format is considered moderate- to high-impact. Possible problems include kneecap problems, low-back pain, and ankle sprains from stepping on or off the bench improperly.

Doing traditional aerobics: This mode is more like calisthenics or dancing, depending on the instructor, and should be classified as either a high- or low-impact class. It can be used as part of a cross-training program for most activities done in a standing position. Aerobics may cause a shoulder or back problem to flare up.

Doing Tae Bo aerobics: Tae Bo aerobics involves many different arm and leg motions, including kicking and punching. It is excellent for general conditioning as well as for hiking, climbing, running, skiing, or snowshoeing. Tae Bo can aggravate knee, hip, or shoulder problems.

Walking: Walking is the most natural movement pattern for the human body. Walking at a brisk pace is often enough to achieve and maintain a good functional level of aerobic fitness for people over the age of 55–60 and to reduce body fat. For fit individuals, walking on level ground is not usually intense enough to achieve a training effect. Walk with a good heel strike and roll through your foot, keeping your hips level. Walk on alternate days until you can walk continuously for 30–50 minutes at a good pace. To increase intensity, walk uphill. Do not use hand or ankle weights, as this throws off your gait and balance. Walking downhill may cause a knee problem to flare up.

In-line skating: This aerobic activity requires a moderate level of balance and coordination to be accomplished safely. It helps develop your thigh, hip, and buttock regions. You can get an excellent aerobic workout with a variety of outdoor scenery. It is good for general aerobic conditioning as well as for cross-country skiing. Wear protective gear, and if you are a beginner, avoid hills and uneven surfaces. The risk of falling is very high, and is most likely to occur when you are trying to stop, going downhill, or on uneven terrain.

Circuit training: This mode employs stations of weight-lifting and aerobic equipment for approximately 30 minutes of exercise time to achieve both aerobic and strength training fitness. Although circuit training can improve aerobic fitness, it has appeared to bring about less improvement compared to other more standard aerobic options. Ideas for outdoor circuits are described in chapter 8.

THE IMPACT OF AEROBIC OPTIONS

The impact of an exercise is measured by the amount of force that is transferred to the joints, bones, ligaments, tendons, nerves, discs, and other important body structures. This is important, because low- to moderate-impact exercise has been shown to be a significant factor in slowing the loss of bone density in women at risk for osteoporosis. It is also important because overuse injuries, including stress fractures, can be related to excessive accumulated impact in which the bone or other structure is not able to rebuild, repair, or remodel in a positive way.

Impact from aerobic exercise is usually thought of in terms of its effect on your feet, knees, hips, and low back, but the repetitive motion of aerobics can also lead to injuries of the upper back, neck, shoulder, and arms, especially from activities such as crew or ergometer rowing. If you are starting to feel pain from your back down, minimize the impact by decreasing the duration, frequency, or intensity of the activity. You might be able to minimize the impact of an activity by varying how you do the activity, such as by avoiding downhill running or slowing down the pace of downhill hiking. If this is not effective, go to a lesser-impact activity or consult a physician if the pain persists or you are having difficulty walking.

Higher-impact options:

Running or jogging, especially with intervals of sprinting or downhill running

Stair climbing or stair running

Step, Tae Bo, or high-impact aerobic dance classes

Basketball, volleyball, or soccer

Racquet sports, including squash, racquetball, handball, and tennis

Hiking, backpacking, and glacier mountaineering (especially with a heavier pack and going downhill)

Downhill skiing, especially over moguls, and snowboarding

Lower- to moderate-impact options:

Skating and in-line skating

Cross-country and telemark skiing, and ski machines

Walking outside and on treadmills

Stair-climbing machines

Lower-impact aerobics classes

Circuit training

EFX elliptical cross trainer

Minimal-impact options:

Cycling

Kayaking and canoeing

Rowing machines and rowing (note that these activities can lead to a higher impact on the upper back and shoulder regions)

Swimming

Water aerobics classes

ESTABLISHING AEROBIC GOALS

Match yourself up with one of the following goals. After each goal, the action is given that initiates your aerobic conditioning program.

1. *Goal*: Achieve some increase in stamina and some health benefits (I am presently not exercising or rarely exercising). *Action*: Start any form of aerobic exercise at a mild exertion, and gradually work up to the minimum aerobic program described earlier in this chapter, if you are medically cleared.

2. *Goal*: Increase your likelihood of achieving the basic minimal health benefits. *Action*: Do the minimum aerobic program.

3. *Goal*: Achieve the full benefit of coronary artery risk reduction. *Action*: Gradually build up your program until you are burning 2,500–3,500 calories a week by doing longer and more frequent aerobic sessions, and/or add one longer-duration, lower-intensity (LILD) session per week.

4. *Goal*: Lose weight. *Action*: Work out at intensities of 55%–70% max. HR for 45–50 minutes per session, for 4–6 sessions per week.

5. *Goal*: Increase your stamina for endurance activities that last longer than 1 hour. *Action*: Start incorporating 1 longer day of continuous aerobic activity at or slightly higher than the intensity level required for the desired activity. For example, training for backpacking, hiking, scrambling, or mountaineering would involve longer workouts of 50%–65% max. HR for up to 1 hour of an exercise activity. This would lead into hikes of increasing length and elevation as the season begins, increasing distance by 10%–15% per week.

6. *Goal*: Achieve Goal 5, but also be able to do brief spurts of high-intensity activity such as a very difficult trail section or snowfield, or a kayak sprint in high waves.

Action: Do the actions for Goal 5 above, but add intervals to your training that simulate the intensity and difficulty of your desired short bursts. Add a pack if it will be a pack-carrying activity (see the interval training section earlier in this chapter).

7. *Goal*: Train for moderate-intensity distance races.

   Action: Increase the intensity of some of your aerobic workouts to an intensity that is similar to the intended races, and gradually increase the distance/duration of your training on 1 day a week. Consider adding interval training to your workouts to increase power and speed.

8. *Goal*: Maintain your aerobic fitness with decreased boredom.

   Action: Vary your activities and cross train, or work out with other people.

EVALUATING YOUR AEROBIC FITNESS DURING YOUR CONDITIONING PERIOD

There are many methods for evaluating the progress of the aerobic component of your conditioning program. Keep a record of your resting heart rate; as you improve, it should decrease gradually down to a certain level (usually between 45–60 beats per minute). Have a standard self-test aerobic activity that is relatively consistent in aerobic demands, one for in the city and one for out of the city. Do each periodically to see how you feel on a rating of perceived exertion (RPE) scale. In-city activities could be a 3- to 5-mile walk or run, a 15-mile bike ride, or a particular aerobic class or stair-climber routine. Outside the city activities could be a particular hike, ski, or kayak trip. If the standard self-test activity is getting easier and you can do it more quickly, then you are making progress. You can expect the gains to be gradual at first and related to your consistency, specificity, volume, and variety of training.

SETTING UP AN AEROBIC CONDITIONING PROGRAM BASED ON AN ACTIVITY GOAL

In order to effectively design an activity goal–oriented aerobic part of your conditioning program, do the tasks listed below:

Identify your activity goals.

Assess your target activity in regard to the aerobic continuous and interval requirements.

Evaluate your current fitness level, especially in regard to your ability to comfortably meet the aerobic duration and intensity requirements of your planned activity.

Determine the time you have for conditioning both in the city and for a longer outdoor aerobic day.

Divide your training into periods for building an aerobic and strength training base and for developing higher-intensity aerobic fitness according to the demands of your activity. (See Periodization of a Conditioning Program in chapter 7 for more information on training periods.)

Write out your training plan week by week for the first week of each period.

Evaluate your progress with how you are feeling in your mind and body at the end of each aerobic session, at the end of each week, and especially at the end of each training period.

Make adjustments to your plan as appropriate.

Consult a health or fitness professional for any special problems or health concerns.

To meet your goals, you can do a very basic program that consists of a gradual building of your aerobic and strength base with an increasing lower-intensity, longer-duration (LILD) activity. You can add interval training for improved performance and ability to do spurts of high-intensity activity, if your goal demands it or for improved aerobic fitness. You can also plan a program around a heart zone periodization approach (see chapter 7).

3

NUTRITIONAL CONSIDERATIONS FOR CONDITIONING

BY BOBBI LUTACK, N.D., LESLIE MOSKOWITZ, M.S., R.D.,
AND DAVID MUSNICK, M.D.

▶ **THIS CHAPTER WILL HELP YOU:**
- Understand your energy needs.
- Understand the importance of carbohydrates, including complex vs. simple carbohydrates and carbohydrate loading.
- Clarify your needs for protein.
- Understand the role of fat stores as fuel and how you can make good fat choices.
- Clarify the issue of vitamin and mineral needs as they relate to exercise and free radical risk.
- Understand your fluid needs.
- Understand energy and fluid needs for high-altitude activities.

What you eat supplies the energy you need and affects both your performance and your health. Good training habits and nutrition help you function optimally. Whether you are a competitive athlete, an outdoor enthusiast, or just trying to stay in shape, you need to know the latest information on nutritional considerations for conditioning.

ENERGY REQUIREMENTS

Understanding your energy requirements is important if you are trying to lose or gain weight or if you are trying to plan food amounts for a backpacking, kayaking, or climbing trip. Your approximate total daily energy expenditure consists of the kilocalories (kcals) needed for your resting metabolic rate (RMR), plus kcals needed for the light activities of daily living and those related to exercise.

A precise formula to calculate RMR is the Harris and Benedict formula. For men it is:

66.5 + (13.75 x weight in kilograms) + (5 x height in centimeters) – (6.78 x age in years) = kilocalories

Below is a sample calculation of this formula for a 40-year-old man who is 5 feet, 9 inches tall and weighs 160 pounds:

66.5 + (13.75 x 72.72 kg) + (5 x 175.26 cm) – (6.78 x 40) = 1,671 kcals

For women the Harris and Benedict formula is:

655 + (9.56 x weight in kilograms) + (1.85 x height in centimeters) – (4.68 x age in years) = kilocalories

Below is a sample calculation of this formula for a 36-year-old woman who is 5 feet, 4 inches tall and weighs 135 pounds:

655 + (9.56 x 61.36 kg) + (1.85 x 162.56 cm) – (4.68 x 36) = 1,373 kcals

The kcals needed for your RMR can be estimated in an abbreviated version of this formula (women should use 0.95 kcals/kg):

weight in kg x 1 kcal/kg x 24 hours = kcals

To calculate the amount of kcals needed for light activities of daily living, calculate the number of hours spent in nonexercise activity and multiply by the number of kcals required for that activity. (This can be obtained from the chart referred to below.)

Calculating exercise calories burned during the day depends on what type of activity is being performed, the intensity, the load carried, and the weight of the individual. Exercise and outdoor activities can vary from 5–20 kcals per minute (walking to all-out cross-country skiing), with the average being 7–11 kcals. Most typical 30- to 40-minute aerobic workouts burn 300 kcals, and most rigorous backpacking or mountaineering trips can burn 450–600 kcals per hour. (The lower number would be appropriate for a 120-pound individual with a light pack, and the higher number would be appropriate for a 160-pound person with a heavy pack.) You can calculate your expected kcal output for an activity by estimating the amount of time spent in the activity and using a chart to estimate kcals burned per minute or hour. (Excellent charts are available in the appendix of *Exercise Physiology* by Katch and McArdle and in the article "The Compendium of Physical Activities; Classification of Energy Costs of Human Physical Activities" in *Medicine and Science in Sports and Exercise*; see Selected References at the back of this book.)

For example, an average 40-year-old, 160-pound male uses 1,671 kcals RMR; if he carries a 44-pound pack while mountaineering for 8 hours (taking 2 hours in breaks), this adds 6 hours times 600 kcals per hour, or 3,600 kcals, for exercise, for a total of 5,271 kcals of energy needed for each day. You can see that the largest variable here is the exercise, especially in outdoor activities lasting many hours. It is important to plan for enough calories to meet your energy needs if you are on an outdoor trip.

If you are going to participate in competition or longer-duration outdoor activities, you must plan for and take in a significant amount of food to provide this energy. Hunger is not the best guide to food intake during vigorous outdoor activities, especially if you are at higher altitudes. Inadequate food intake can lead to a feeling of general fatigue and can be dangerous in activities such as mountaineering.

FOOD AS FUEL

Carbohydrate, fat, and protein all yield energy, and this energy is measured in kilocalories. Carbohydrates and protein supply 4 kcals per gram, and fat supplies 9 kcals per gram. Most foods contain a mixture of these three, but usually have a higher percentage of one nutrient.

CARBOHYDRATES

The main emphasis in nutrition for sports, especially endurance exercise, has been on the role of carbohydrates for energy. Carbohydrates can be classified as complex, which means they are composed of three or more glucose molecules, or as simple, composed of one or two sugar molecules. Examples of complex carbohydrates are breads, pasta, and certain vegetables. Examples of simple carbohydrates are sucrose (table sugar), honey, corn syrup (used in many foods as a sweetener), fruit, and fruit juices. In general, these simple carbohydrates should not be eaten immediately prior to exercise or a race because they can stimulate a rapid rise in insulin and subsequent drop in blood glucose levels. Certain fruits are more likely to cause this problem, including bananas, watermelon, and papaya. Also, the rise of insulin inhibits fat mobilization and increases the use of muscle glycogen (stored starch). The normal effect of insulin combined with the effects of exercise can cause a significant drop in blood glucose. Simple sugars are appropriate to eat during a race and are usually mixed in fluids to maintain adequate blood glucose levels during activities prolonged for more than 1½–2 hours.

Both complex and simple carbohydrates can fuel your muscles and brain, but foods containing complex carbohydrates supply you with additional nutrients such as B vitamins, minerals, and fiber. The degree to which these other nutrients are supplied varies with the amount of processing of the food, your choice of carbohydrates, and the health of the soil in which the product was grown. Although you can take a vitamin supplement, you need fiber. The average person should eat 20–35 grams of fiber per day. You can get your fiber intake from a variety of whole-grain products, as well as a minimum of five servings of vegetables and fruit per day.

FOOD TIP

On a trip you can increase your fiber and the diversity of your diet by slicing up bell peppers, carrots, or celery and storing them in a sealed bag with some water droplets. This is great to add to dinners or to eat for lunch with peanut butter or other nut butters.

Most of both simple and complex carbohydrates in the diet are converted into glucose during digestion, to be used for fuel or stored for future energy use as glycogen in the muscles and liver. The liver can store about 100 grams of glycogen and muscles can store 300–500 grams of glycogen. Any carbohydrates consumed in excess are stored as fat.

When we eat carbohydrates, the subsequent rise in blood glucose signals the hormone insulin to circulate in the blood. Insulin promotes utilization of carbohydrates for energy by transporting glucose into the body's cells. When glucose concentration is high, insulin secretion is stimulated and carbohydrates are used for energy. When glucose levels are low, insulin is suppressed and fat is used preferentially for energy.

Carbohydrates are important sources of energy for contracting muscles during prolonged and strenuous exercise. Fatigue is often associated with muscle glycogen depletion and/or hypoglycemia (low blood sugar). During active training periods, especially around competition times, or significant aerobic events like climbing a mountain, the usual carbohydrate recommendation is approximately 60%–70% of total energy intake for the day, with 12%–20% going to protein, leaving a total of about 20%–25% calories from fat. The amount of carbohydrates needed may decrease in long-duration backpacking or mountaineering, in which high-calorie, dense fat is often used to supply adequate energy. There is also some controversy regarding the percentage of carbohydrate that the population at large should eat. This is largely as a result of new information on Syndrome X (a medical syndrome in which a person is obese and has high blood levels of insulin as well as high blood pressure) and on other milder forms of insulin resistance. For additional information, refer to "Modified Carbohydrate-to-Protein-Ratio Diets" later in this chapter.

The carbohydrate calories you need depends on your calculated daily energy expenditure and the percent of carbohydrate in your diet. For example, if your total energy requirements are 2,500 kcals per day, 1,500 kcals should come from carbohydrate (60% x 2,500 = 1,500). Since there are 4 kcals per gram of carbohydrate, there are 375 grams carbohydrate in 1,500 kcals (1,500 / 4 = 375). Note that 15 grams equals 1 serving, so that you have to calculate the number of portions of a particular carbohydrate-containing food. (Refer to The Exchange Lists *for Meal Planning* for more information on servings; see Selected References.)

FOOD TIP

At mealtime, have two-thirds of your plate covered with carbohydrate to obtain about 60% carbohydrate calories.

Because the benefits of a high-carbohydrate diet for improving sport performance are so highly touted, many athletes and exercisers believe they can eat all they want of any type of carbohydrate, as long as it's a complex carbohydrate. Not so. Complex carbohydrates such as refined pasta and breads are milled and lose vitamins and minerals during the process. Individuals whose diets are high in these complex carbohydrates may suffer from vitamin and mineral deficiencies. Fatigue, poor recovery, staleness, and aching muscles may reflect a lack of critical nutrients. It's better to eat relatively unprocessed whole grains such as oats, barley, wheat, millet, amaranth, spelt, and rice, along with a variety of vegetables and fruits, for your carbohydrate sources. Organic foods are grown without pesticides and are better for the environment and their use decreases your exposure to pesticides.

Choosing carbohydrates with a low to moderate glycemic index (see below) is also a good idea for the majority of your carbohydrates. Become familiar with the nutrient and fiber composition and glycemic index of various complex carbohydrates, so you are able to choose a variety to meet your nutritional needs.

Glycemic Index

The glycemic index is an index of the glucose responses of numerous carbohydrates. It refers to the entry rate of glucose from the digested food into the bloodstream and is related to the rise of insulin. A lower glycemic index indicates a slower and more prolonged increase in blood glucose and less of an insulin increase. A higher glycemic index indicates a rapid rise in blood glucose and insulin and a shorter duration of blood sugar elevation. In general, it is desirable to have your blood sugar elevated for longer periods of time to prevent hunger and the need for more frequent eating. It is also very important to eat lower glycemic foods if you are diabetic or overweight.

Glycemic response is determined by the type of simple sugar present (glucose, fructose, galactose), type and amount of fiber content (soluble or insoluble), and percentage of fat and protein in the carbohydrate or present in the rest of the meal. The higher the fiber, fat, or protein content, the lower the glycemic index. The sugars found in grains, pastas, bread, cereal, and sweets are usually absorbed quickly. Dairy products contain galactose, which is next to be absorbed, and fruits contain fructose, which has the lowest glycemic index.

FOOD TIP

Dried fruit is an excellent carbohydrate source and has a moderate glycemic index. Mix it with nuts to create a source of long-lasting energy.

Health care providers who support eating lower glycemic foods suggest that a steady blood glucose level is maintained by preventing an overstimulation of insulin and a more prolonged release of glucose. Therefore, hypoglycemia is avoided and excessive storage of calories as fat may be reduced. To maintain a reasonable level of blood glucose, eat lower glycemic carbohydrates as well as meals that have some protein and fat. This is especially true for outdoor activities of low to moderate intensity. Figure 9 gives some examples of

FIGURE 9. GLYCEMIC INDEX OF SOME COMMON FOODS

HIGH	MODERATE	LOW	LOWEST
Breakfast cereals	Pastas	Barley	Soybeans
Rice cakes	Candy bars	Apples	Peanuts
Glucose	Whole-grain rye	Oranges/Orange juice	Other nuts
Carrots	Most breads	Milk	Lentils
Potatoes	Raisins	Yogurt	Fructose
Bananas	Brown rice	Protein bars	

various foods' glycemic index. Eat lower to moderate glycemic foods during the day and use higher glycemic foods (including sports drinks) for a more rapid supply of energy if you are in an endurance activity or a race and need a quick energy source, especially after 1½ hours of the activity. (A good reference for glycemic index is *The American Journal of Clinical Nutrition*; see Selected References at the back of this book.)

FOOD TIP

Consider increasing your intake of vegetables in the cruciferous family as a source of carbohydrate and lower glycemic index foods. They have fiber and many beneficial biochemicals that may help prevent cancer. Cruciferous vegetables include broccoli, cauliflower, kale, cabbage, and brussels sprouts.

Glycogen Reserves and Carbohydrate Loading

Your glycogen reserves may vary from 300 to 500 grams, depending on the duration and intensity of your exercise. This could provide you with 1,200–2,000 kcals from glycogen alone, and this is combined with energy released from fat, depending on the intensity of the exercise. Your glycogen reserves could be used up within 1½–6 hours of prolonged outdoor activities. People seem to feel less energetic and have less exercise capacity when their glycogen stores have been used up. You can increase the glycogen storage in your muscles to aid you in competing in long-duration activities and races by consuming higher-than-normal amounts of carbohydrates and tapering your activities prior to the activity.

An example of a carbohydrate (glycogen)-loading plan is to start 1 week before the long-distance event. Consume a high-carbohydrate diet, starting at about 60% of your total kcals in carbohydrate, or 350–400 grams, and working up to 70% carbohydrate by day 4 (500–550 grams per day). Stay with this level of intake until the night before your event or activity. Perform your current intensity level of aerobic exercise for the first 4 days, but gradually decrease the duration of your training from 60–90 minutes the first day to 20–30 minutes on the fourth day. Day 5 would be a very light training day, and day 6 would be a rest day. Only adults who are in excellent aerobic condition and have no health problems such as diabetes should attempt carbohydrate loading. Try to include adequate protein during carbohydrate loading.

Meal Timing Suggestions for Carbohydrates

Ingestion of a meal (with carbohydrate, protein, and fat) 3–4 hours prior to exercise ensures adequate carbohydrate availability and enhances exercise performance. Try not to eat any simple sugars within 1½ hours of your exercise or event to decrease the possibility of low blood sugar. Replacement of body glycogen stores can be achieved most rapidly if extra carbohydrates are consumed as soon as possible after exercise and at repeating 1-hour intervals for at least 5 hours after the event. Carbohydrate replacement should be done within 24 hours after a prolonged, high-intensity event lasting longer than 1½–2 hours.

PROTEIN

Protein is the major structural material of our bodies. Adequate amounts of protein are necessary for the active individual to repair and build muscle tissue. Protein-containing foods are a good source of B vitamins and iron. Protein (especially the amino acid *alanine*) is a secondary source of energy during prolonged aerobic activity. Protein is composed of amino acids, and 9 of the 22 amino acids in the human body are essential because they must come from the food we eat and cannot be made by the body. Meat, fish, poultry, eggs, milk, and soy products contain all the essential amino acids and are called complete proteins.

Vegetarian Diets

Vegetarians who do not consume meat can get complete protein from eggs, soy, or dairy products. If you do not eat those foods, you must eat a variety of incomplete proteins to supply the essential amino acids. You can do this by eating legumes with grains or seeds (peanut butter with wheat crackers or bread; beans with tortillas or rice) or legumes with seeds (chickpeas with crushed sesame seeds or tahini). Vegetarians may be at risk for vitamin B_{12} deficiency and should consider taking it as a supplement. This is especially important if you do not drink milk or eat eggs. Other areas of concern if there are no or minimal dairy products in your diet are vitamin D, calcium, and riboflavin. You can get some of these in fortified food products, but vitamin and mineral supplementation is advised.

Iron levels may be low, especially in exercising menstruating women, because iron from non-meat sources is less well absorbed than iron from meats. Iron-deficiency anemia can develop and lead to decreased exercise performance and fatigue. Obtaining enough protein in a vegetarian diet requires more planning but is not difficult, especially if you eat soy products and a variety of protein-containing foods.

FOOD TIP

Vitamin C–containing foods (citrus fruits or certain vegetables) or low-dose supplements (100–250 mg) can be eaten with meals to enhance iron absorption.

Protein Requirements

Your need for protein varies depending on your body weight and its percent of fat, and the type, intensity, and duration of activity. The usual recommendations are that all adults should have 0.8 gram of protein per kilogram (2.2 pounds) of body weight, equivalent to about 0.4 gram per pound. This is likely enough for most individuals. While it was once thought that protein deficiency was mostly the result of being poor (protein generally being more expensive than either grains or vegetables), it is noteworthy that today many people with reasonable incomes do not eat even the minimal amount of protein recommended.

There is some evidence indicating that regular exercise at high volumes does in fact increase protein needs. The range of 0.4–0.7 grams of protein per pound of body weight should be adequate for the majority of people doing a moderate amount of exercise. If you strength-train intensely, you may need as much as 0.6–0.8 gram of protein per pound of body weight. If your activities are primarily aerobic, you will need about 0.5–0.6 gram of protein per pound of body weight. These extra requirements usually can be met through a diet consisting of 12%–15% of total calories for the day from protein (unless total caloric intake is insufficient, or in the case of some vegetarian diets in which there is no soy, milk, or egg products and inadequate protein complements).

FOOD TIP

Try to have some protein at each meal, especially at breakfast and lunch. Doing so can improve your likelihood of getting enough protein and improve your body's ability to regulate blood-sugar levels.

Most protein supplementation can be done with protein-rich foods low in saturated fats, but occasionally you could use protein powders of soy, egg, milk, or rice origin. Excessive protein may be detrimental because (1) it causes frequent urination to eliminate urea, a waste product formed when protein is digested, thus making the kidneys work overtime and possibly lose important electrolytes in the urine; (2) it can be high in fat, particularly saturated fat, and thus is a contributing factor in heart disease and certain types of cancer; (3) a high-protein diet may cause more calcium to be excreted in the urine. This is partuicularly problematic for women because of their higher risk of osteoporosis. Remember, unused protein is stored as fat, like any other unused fuel source.

FOOD TIP

Excellent protein sources to take on long trips are peanuts, almonds, nut butters, soy nuts, and milk and soy protein powder. They can be eaten separately or added to other foods to enhance their taste.

There are many methods to calculate your protein requirements. The formula you use is related to whether you are following conventional recommendations or one of the protein-to-carbohydrate-ratio diets described below. For the conventional approaches, multiply your weight in pounds times 0.4 gram, or higher if you are doing a lot of strength or aerobic training. Another method is to estimate your total calorie needs per day and multiply times 15%.

For example, if you need 2,500 calories per day, 15% x 2,500 = 375 kcals of protein. Since protein has 4 kcals per gram, you would need 93 grams of protein a day from complete and incomplete sources. Examples of protein sources:

Meat, 1 ounce:	7 grams protein
Milk, 8 ounces:	8 grams protein
Beans, ½ cup:	4 grams protein
Starch, per serving:	2 grams protein
Peanuts, ¼ cup:	8 grams protein
Peanut butter,	
2 tablespoons:	10 grams protein
Almonds, ¼ cup:	6.5 grams protein
Tofu, 3 ounces:	10–12 grams protein

Most nutrition bars have 10–14 grams of protein, but varying ratios of carbohydrate and fat.

FOOD TIP

Try increasing your intake of soy. It is an excellent protein source, and certain compounds in soy have many health prevention benefits. There appear to be decreased risks of prostate and breast cancer, as well as decreasing prostate hypertrophy. There is evidence that soy can help decrease cholesterol levels. Soy-based foods include tofu, tempeh, soy powders and milk, soy nuts, and soybean sprouts.

Modified Carbohydrate-to-Protein-Ratio Diets

A number of popular diets have proposed lowering the carbohydrate-to-protein ratio for the purpose of regulating insulin and its subsequent effects. They are being advocated for weight loss as well as other health benefits. They are also interesting because they may have a favorable effect on fat burning and general health. There have been some reports of good endurance being possible on these diets. The science of nutrition is continually evolving, and our biochemical individuality may dictate different percentages of nutrients for different individuals. Although the optimal percentage of carbohydrate intake probably varies from person to person, it is likely that a reasonable range of intake is 40%–70%. More research is definitely needed to determine if and what carbohydrate-protein-fat ratios are the healthiest and offer the best effects on exercise for endurance.

Enzyme and metabolic changes that definitely occur can sometimes take weeks to adjust to, especially if you are doing high-volume aerobic exercise. Don't switch diets unless you have at least 3–4 weeks before an event or major activity to try out the diet and determine its effects on your endurance.

The lower carbohydrate-to-protein-ratio diets are not recommended for long mountaineering trips at higher altitudes because they have not been adequately studied and because rapid replenishment of glycogen stores each day is needed. The majority of health professionals and nutritionists still recommend the higher carbohydrate diet. Consult a health care provider trained in nutritional and functional medicine for more information.

FAT

Fat is a stored source of energy, serves as a carrier for the fat-soluble vitamins (A, D, E, and K), protects vital organs, helps make hormones, and is an essential part of all cell membranes. At 9 kcals per gram, it is the most concentrated source of energy you can take on long outdoor excursions. Unfortunately, fat has gotten a bad reputation because of the relationship of saturated fat to heart disease and cancer, and for contributing excess calories toward obesity.

Essential Fatty Acids

We need essential fatty acids (a form of fat) such as linoleic acid (omega-6) and alpha-linolenic acid (omega-3), which we cannot manufacture in our bodies. Eating the correct balance of fats is important to your nutrition and can influence the structure of your cell membranes and your general health. The diet of most people is very high in nonessential, saturated, and hydrogenated fat and can actually be low in beneficial fatty acids. Some people, because of their concern over fats in general, eat an extremely low-fat diet that is actually deficient in essential fatty acids as well as the beneficial omega-3 fatty acids. Follow the fat guidelines below to avoid that problem.

Certain fatty acids, namely, omega-3 fatty acids found in flaxseed products and certain fish (salmon, sardines, and mackerel) and omega-6 fatty acids found in plant sources (primrose, borage, pumpkin, and walnuts), have been found to be beneficial to your health. The omega-3 oils have been shown to decrease risks of coronary artery disease. They also can have a beneficial and regulatory effect on eicosanoid production in the body and may lead to decreases in inflammation when taken in certain amounts. It is recommended that we have about 1 part omega-3 oil:4 parts omega-6 oil in our diet. Most people have about a 1:20 to 1:10 ratio in their present diets, which is inadequate.

FOOD TIP
You can increase your intake of omega-3 oil by adding flaxseed oil (1–2 tablespoons per day) to salads or in other foods that are not heated, such as salsa or humus. You can also increase your intake of ocean fish such as salmon.

The current recommendation is to consume less than 30% of total calories from fat and to get most of it from mono- and polyunsaturated fats such as olive, sesame, and flaxseed oil. To calculate your fat needs, take your total food calorie requirement per day (e.g., 2,500 kcals) and multiply it by a fat percentage of 20%–30%. For example, 25% x 2,500 = 625 kcals from fat. Fat has 9 kcals per gram, so divide your fat calorie requirement by 9, which in this example comes to 69 grams of fat per day.

Fats are abundant in foods, but you should pay attention to the right type of fat. Try especially to stay away from the hydrogenated fats in processed nut butters, margarines, crackers, and the like. Examples of good sources of fat include avocados, artichokes, olives, fish, nuts and seeds, tofu, soy milk, and almonds.

- -

FOOD TIP

It is important to bring adequate and diverse sources of fat on long outdoor trips (especially mountaineering trips), because they are compact, high-energy food sources. Good choices are cheese, olive oil, almonds and peanuts and their butters, other nuts, and sesame seeds. These can also be added to other foods to improve their flavor.

- -

Fat Intake Guideline Summary

Eat 20%–30% of your caloric intake per day in fat.

Increase this amount when you are on a multi-day outdoor activity, especially a mountaineering expedition.

Try to limit the majority of your fat intake to poly- and monounsaturated fats, and decrease animal-related fat, except for fish. Don't worry about this when planning for food during outdoor activities.

Avoid or limit food products with hydrogenated fats.

Increase your intake of omega-3 fatty acids by eating cold-water fish and flaxseed oil.

Use antioxidant vitamin supplements such as vitamin E (400 International Units per day) and vitamin C (250–1,000 mg per day) for both general health benefits and for prevention of damage to essential fatty acids.

VITAMINS, MINERALS, AND FREE RADICALS

The recommended dietary allowance (RDA) is an estimate of a safe and adequate nutrient intake that will prevent deficiency diseases. It is based on estimates for the population at large and not for individual needs. Humans have some biochemical individuality, and so some RDAs are limited in their usefulness. Always try to get as many nutrients from your food as possible. However, supplementation may be required because of poor soil quality where some foods are grown, and because of personal eating habits.

FREE RADICALS AND ANTIOXIDANTS

Increasing scientific evidence suggests that exercise causes an increase of free radicals in the body, particularly if you exercise outdoors and live in a metropolitan area or other place where the air is polluted. Free radicals are extremely reactive molecules that have an unpaired electron, which may seek to pair up with electrons from other molecules, and can lead to cell damage. By stealing these electrons, new free radicals are created and chain reactions can occur. Free radicals can harm your body by damaging your cells, impairing enzyme production, and leading to damaged arteries and cardiovascular disease.

The body creates free radicals as a by-product of oxygen metabolism. When we exercise, we breathe faster and require more oxygen for exercising muscles. Your body has an inherent capacity to rid itself of free radicals with naturally occurring antioxidants, but free radicals can exceed your body's ability to neutralize them, and supplements may be helpful. Research shows the following antioxidants to be beneficial.

Vitamin E scavenges free radicals produced in the fat (lipid) component of cells. Endurance exercise generates lipid free radicals, and vitamin E supplements can protect against exercise-induced tissue damage. Supplement with 400–600 International Units of mixed natural-source vitamin E per day.

Vitamin C is a water-based antioxidant that cannot be synthesized in your body. Our recommendation is 250–1,000 mg per day of vitamin C, and you might wish to take it in divided doses 2–3 times per day. In foods, you can get about 30–60 mg of vitamin C per serving in the following foods: cantaloupe, kiwi fruit, broccoli, kale, cabbage, brussels sprouts, green peppers, and citrus fruits.

Selenium is a trace mineral that is required as a component of an important antioxidant enzyme. It may also, on its own, decrease harmful changes to fat and have some role in preventing cancer and premature aging. The typical American diet is marginal or deficient in selenium. (The RDA is 55–70 micrograms per day, but 200 mcg per day may be more protective.) Good food sources of selenium include seafood (especially tuna), whole grains, nuts, lean meats, and chicken.

Other trace minerals, including zinc, copper, and manganese, are essential for the function of superoxide dismutase, one of the body's natural antioxidants. A good multiple vitamin should contain sufficient amounts of these nutrients. Recommended daily intakes are: zinc (aspartate or citrate form), 15 mg per day; copper, 1–2 mg per day; and manganese, 5–10 mg per day. Good food sources of these trace minerals include poultry, meat, fish, dry beans, eggs, and nuts.

Iron, another trace mineral involved in antioxidant enzyme activation, is paradoxically both a promoter as well as a scavenger of free radicals. Studies have demonstrated an increased relative risk of coronary artery disease as serum iron levels rise. There is no increase in the amount of iron needed for exercising individuals. It is recommended that you avoid food supplemented with a high percentage of the RDA for iron and avoid vitamins with iron unless you have laboratory tests demonstrating an iron-deficiency anemia. Adolescents and premenopausal women need adequate iron because of increased needs. If you are not sure, have blood drawn by your physician to check for anemia and to see if iron supplementation is appropriate. Good food sources of iron include dark green vegetables, egg yolk, meat, fish, fortified cereals, and blackstrap molasses. If you are deficient in iron, take iron supplements or eat iron-rich foods along with vitamin C or vitamin C–rich foods to increase absorption.

ERGOGENIC AIDS

Ergogenic aids are substances that may enhance performance in aerobic, anaerobic, or weight-lifting activities. They may be appropriate for athletes involved in high-performance activities, races, or body building. Ergogenic aids include food, drugs, vitamins, herbs, hormones, nutritional supplements, and blood products. They range from accepted techniques such as carbohydrate loading to unsafe approaches such as anabolic-androgenic steroid use. High-performance athletes should look at the reference works available and keep up with the literature before trying an ergogenic aid. It is important to look at the proposed mechanism of action and safety of the approach as well as studies that document improved exercise performance. Remember that no ergogenic aid will replace good nutrition, proper rest, and good training habits.

There is evidence that creatine monohydrate can increase your ability to do anaerobic intervals and repeated brief spurts of strength moves. This might be helpful if you are racing or if you are climbing in a rock gym. There has not been adequate research using creatine at higher altitudes to know whether it is safe. The dosing schedule is 20–25 grams per day, in amounts of 5 grams 5 times per day, for 5 days for loading. Take 2 grams per day for maintenance during your training season. The main side effect is water weight gain, and it should not be taken if you have high blood pressure.

WATER AND FLUIDS

Water is essential to sustain the metabolic processes of your cells, your blood pressure, and all vital functions. It is also a key factor in your ability to regulate your temperature by sweating and getting rid of heat. You need to take in fluids to replace your body's losses.

Your body can lose water from waste excretion, moisture in the air you exhale (12 ounces per day and up to 0.07–0.17 ounce per minute with very strenuous exercise), and sweat (17 ounces per day and up to 35 ounces per hour of very strenuous exercise in hot weather). Your sweat losses are the most significant variable when you are physically active.

FOOD TIP

Even if you are not exercising, you need 8–10 glasses of good-quality fluid (filtered or bottled) per day. If possible, store your fluid in glass bottles rather than plastics, because of by-products in plastics. If you are exercising in hot weather, you need to replace your losses from sweating. Your kidneys have the ability to get rid of extra water if you drink more than you need. In this case, your urine will usually be lighter in color. Light or clear urine is desirable during an outdoor activity or after you have rehydrated following an exercise session or endurance event.

If you do not replace fluid losses, you can become dehydrated and lightheaded, have poor exercise performance and stamina, and risk more serious problems such as very low blood pressure or heat-related illnesses. The average daily fluid loss amounts to about 2,500–3,000 ml in the average person on an average temperature day without significant physical activity.

Your fluid input consists of the fluid you drink, the fluid in the food you eat, and the fluid generated by your metabolism.

FOOD TIP

Avoid alcohol and caffeinated beverages before long activities in the heat, because they can cause fluid loss. In warm weather, drink cold beverages. In cold weather, drink warm beverages.

REPLACING YOUR FLUID LOSSES FROM SWEATING

You can lose 32–64 ounces of fluid per hour of exercise. For every 16 ounces of fluid lost, you will lose a pound of body weight. The following are recommendations to prevent dehydration. Before regular and longer-duration exercise, drink 12–16 ounces of fluid 1½–2 hours prior to your event or workout. After a vigorous short workout, drink 16–24 ounces of fluid. If you are in a race or competition, drink 6–8 ounces every 15–20 minutes. Drink enough after the competition is over to get your weight back to what it was before the competition. Drink 16 ounces (2 cups) for every pound of weight lost. If you are on a hike or cross-country ski trip, have your water handy and drink at least every hour, so that you feel good and have relatively clear urine. Carry at least two 32-ounce containers with you, and purify your water. You may need to drink 16–32 ounces per hour, depending on how vigorously you exercise and how hot it is. Your fluid requirements will increase in warmer weather, at higher altitudes, and with higher-intensity exercise.

SPORT DRINKS

Sport drinks contain a quick-acting carbohydrate as well as some sodium and potassium (*electrolytes*). They can provide calories and replace electrolytes, especially during a competitive event lasting more than 1 hour. The carbohydrate percentage should be about 6%–10%. There is some evidence that drinks containing maltodextrin as the sugar may have the best benefit. Drink carbohydrate beverages during an event at a rate of 30–70 grams per hour. Read the label on a sport drink to determine how much carbohydrate it contains, and drink accordingly; usually 16–32 ounces per hour is equal to 30–70 grams per hour. If you are participating in an outdoor activity away from civilization, or if you are on a more leisurely bicycling event and can eat foods with some salt and potassium in them (such as salted foods and dried fruit), you do not need to carry a sport drink.

ALTITUDE, COLD WEATHER, AND MOUNTAINEERING TRIPS

Mountaineering and trekking at altitudes above 8,000 feet presents numerous challenges, including getting enough calories and fluids. Fluid losses can increase because of increased breathing rates and fluid lost from expired air. Because everything seems more difficult at high altitude, extra effort and awareness must be given to maintaining adequate fluid balance. Every hour, drink approximately 8–32 ounces, depending on the temperature and how much sweating and rapid breathing you are doing. If your urine is dark yellow, you need to drink more. Your water should be conveniently situated so you do not have to remove your pack to get at it. All water should be filtered or treated. Consider bringing different flavored powders to flavor water if you cannot drink enough plain

water. Bring a few packets of oral rehydration powder if you are going to less-developed countries where traveler's diarrhea is a possibility. If you develop diarrhea, make sure you increase your fluid intake to keep up with the water loss.

A large quantity of calories needs to be consumed because of the amount of energy used to hike or climb for long duration on slopes, snow, and rugged terrain. Every 1–2 hours, consume snacks with a combination of fats and carbohydrate. Try to have a variety of nuts and nut butters to provide protein and fat. Pack many different crackers, dried fruits, and cereals, and don't worry about the fat content. Remember, you often need to eat more than you feel like eating, especially at higher altitudes or when you are feeling weak or tired. Try saving some diverse, tasty, easy-to-eat food for high altitudes when you will need maximum calories and may have little appetite. Don't worry about gaining weight on a multiday trip or expedition. The problem is usually one of weight loss, not weight gain.

FOOD TIP

You can usually pack enough food to meet your energy needs on an outdoor excursion if you plan for three meals and at least four snacks per day. Use bars or handfuls of energy-dense snack foods with protein and fat to add extra calories during the day. Eat during at least every other water or rest break. A bar or a handful of gorp usually has 150–200 kcals.

There is no consensus for diets with exercise in the cold. The evidence is strong that increased amounts of carbohydrates, and high calorie and fluid intake, are necessary. Foods with a high fat content are reasonable. Remember to drink frequently even though it is cold.

4

WARM-UP AND STRETCHING

BY MARIA ZANONI, P.T., AND DAVID MUSNICK, M.D.

▶ **THIS CHAPTER WILL HELP YOU:**
- Understand the principles of warming up.
- Learn how to safely stretch and maintain flexibility.
- Learn how to do active as well as passive stretches.
- Develop a warm-up and stretching program.

Stretching, although commonly regarded as a warm-up, does not in itself increase muscle temperature or enhance coordination. Stretching is important, but stretching alone is not an adequate warm-up. This chapter introduces the components of a more dynamic warm-up, as well as techniques to improve and maintain your flexibility.

THE WARM-UP

Increasing muscle temperature can improve flexibility as well as muscle contractile force and speed of movement. Warm-ups also stimulate balance pathways. You can warm up in several ways, but most warm-ups should include an aerobic activity (using large muscle groups: legs, arms, or both) done at low intensity for 5–10 minutes.

After the brief aerobic session you can add functional or conventional strength-training exercises at low resistance and high repetitions, or you can combine the above and add some agility or balance drills to prepare yourself for an activity.

It's best to do a warm-up that matches the demands of your activity. Think about the movement patterns and joint ranges of motion required in your shoulders, hips, and knees, and use some active stretches as well as functional exercises (see chapter 5) in your warm-up.

An activity that requires more strength, balance, and coordination requires a longer warm-up period. For example, a hike starting off on level ground without any immediate river crossings or boulder fields would require only a gradual increase in hiking speed as a warm-up. A hike or mountaineering day on scree, snow, or boulder fields with high requirements for shoulder-leg integration, balance, and full joint range of motion would benefit from some active stretches and agility drills.

THE AEROBIC WARM-UP

The aerobic warm-up is a good beginning for any activity. It is adequate for health club workouts as well as for most hiking, bicycling, running, cross-country skiing, and water sports. Exercise aerobically 5–10 minutes at a low intensity (50%–65% max. HR). Start slowly, and gradually increase your intensity. You can do this with any aerobic activity, but it is best to use an activity that uses the same muscles as your workout. When preparing for an outdoor workout, it could be a brisk walk, jog, or cycle.

Your aerobic warm-up could also be the same as the activity you will be doing, but at a lower intensity level. An easy kayak before engaging rough water, gently jogging before running, or hiking at an easy to moderate pace before hiking quickly or steeply are all good aerobic warm-ups.

PRACTICAL POINT

You can make a warm-up walk more effective by doing it at a quick pace and with variations in arm motions. Your fast walk could include exaggerated arm swings, forward and rotational punches, rowing motions, or virtually any functional arm motion.

THE WEIGHT-LIFTING WARM-UP

You can do an aerobic warm-up to prepare for weight lifting. A rowing machine or an arm/leg cycle are ideal because they use the arms and legs. In addition, you could also do a few lower-weight, high-repetition sets of some of your intended strength training exercises. Try to do a few that use larger muscle groups and go through a full range of motion. Consider a few functional shoulder-hip-leg combination exercises (see Exercises 20–22).

THE FUNCTIONAL EXERCISE WARM-UP

In a functional exercise warm-up, pick a number of functional exercises (3–5) that best simulate the motion patterns and balance demands of the activity you are preparing for. You can choose these exercises from chapter 5, Strength and Balance Training, or use the dynamic warm-up suggestions in the outdoor activity chapters in Part III. It makes sense to precede this with a 5-minute aerobic period. You can keep the warm-up aerobic by doing the functional

exercises quickly in 30- to 45-second sets, but without any added resistance except your body weight. Such a warm-up more adequately prepares your muscles and joints in different planes of motion.

THE AGILITY AND BALANCE WARM-UP

If your activity requires balance challenges and quick responses to changes in terrain, it can help to do balance or agility drills as part of your warm-up. Such activities include skiing (all types), snowboarding, climbing (including scrambling and mountaineering), and whitewater kayaking. Start with a 5- to 10-minute aerobic activity, then add a few balance and agility drills. For standing balance, do Exercises 38 and 39. For an agility component, do Exercises 38–40 and/or follow the agility circuit guidelines in chapter 8 or chapter 20. You can make a simple agility drill by walking quickly or jogging for 1–3 minutes while making quick changes in direction.

THE OUTDOOR ACTIVITY WARM-UP

It is a good idea to do a warm-up before you begin your outdoor activity. If that activity requires strength, balance, and agility, it is good to integrate these components after a brief aerobic period. The outdoor activity chapters in Part III have specific warm-up programs for the different activities covered. The dynamic warm-up discussed at the end of the next section is a good generic warm-up for many activities.

DYNAMIC WARM-UP DRILLS

Dynamic warm-up drills work on coordination and can be done prior to sports or outdoor activities. You can do these after a brief aerobic period or as part of your aerobic warm-up. Each one can be done for 30–90 seconds. They can be linked together or done individually.

Carioca: Run sideways to your right, with the left foot crossing in front of the right foot on the first step, and behind the right foot on the next step. Reverse direction, moving to the left, with the right foot crossing first in front of and then behind the left foot.

Crazy Legs: Run forward along an imaginary line, with the left foot crossing to the right side of the line, and then the right foot crossing to the left side of the line.

Shuffle Run: Stand with the front of your shoes about 6–8 inches apart. Using quick motions, take a 2- to 3-foot step forward with your right foot, making initial contact with your heel. Then bring the toes of your left foot forward to meet the heel of your right foot, making sure not to make heel contact with your left foot. Repeat this movement pattern quickly for 3–5 strides, then change your forward leg.

Horse Gallop Side Shuffle: Stand sideways to your direction of travel, with your feet shoulder-width apart and knees slightly bent. When moving to your right, push off your left leg and land on the ball of your right foot. Quickly bring your left foot next to your right foot, lightly tapping your feet together so that it sounds like a horse galloping. Move sideways rapidly for several strides, and then switch direction.

DYNAMIC WARM-UP

For a generic dynamic warm-up, start with brisk walking for 2 minutes, then either continue walking for 5 more minutes, or jog. This leads into a walking lunge exercise with alternate shoulder/arm raises, such as Exercise 25. Next do the warm-up drills above (Carioca, Crazy Legs, Shuffle Run, and Horse Gallop Side Shuffle). Next do a few functional combination exercises such as Exercises 20 and 21. Then do a balance exercise such as Exercise 38, and finish up with stretching Exercises 1, 3, 7, 8, 9, 13, and 19. A dynamic warm-up should generally last 5–15 minutes. Try experimenting with dynamic warm-up routines to see which works the best for you.

STRETCHING AND FLEXIBILITY

Flexibility is related to the range of motion in a joint or a series of joints, as well as the length of muscle and tendons. It is related to age, gender, activity level, and genetic factors. Stretching can improve flexibility. If your joints are very tight, stretching alone may not be adequate; you may need manual treatment to improve flexibility. The degree of flexibility in your body can almost always be improved by stretching.

The goal of stretching is to lengthen a muscle and move the corresponding joints through the full range of motion, thereby allowing both the *contractile* (muscle and tendon) and the *non-contractile* (ligament and joint capsule) *structures* to lengthen. Contractile tissue is more elastic; therefore, muscles and tendons respond better to stretching than do ligaments and joint capsules. Even so, stretching does increase the elasticity of both the contractile and non-contractile tissues. A tight and stiff joint capsule may be loosened through stretching.

The most effective stretching techniques involve postures that stabilize one end of the muscle in order to stretch the other end. Stretching can be done at any time, but in order to improve flexibility it is best done when your body is well warmed up. When stretching a cold muscle, use caution because it is much easier to injure a cold muscle. Stretching is often done too quickly and/or with poor positioning. This will not improve flexibility.

If your goal is to increase flexibility, for indoor workouts do the majority of your stretching after an aerobic exercise period. For outdoor activities, a few stretches at the end of your warm-up are advised. It is important to note that a stretching program needs to be accompanied by a balanced strengthening program for the best flexibility.

For a definition of anatomy terms related to stretching, see Basic Anatomy in chapter 9.

FLEXIBILITY IMPROVES PERFORMANCE

Limited flexibility has been shown to decrease the efficiency of an activity; that is, the body must expend more energy to complete a task. Increased flexibility can improve performance. For example, full hip flexibility along with adequate strength allows a climber to make moves that require full rotation of the hip, and the mountaineer to take long, high steps.

STRETCHING WHILE INJURIES ARE HEALING

It is possible to overstretch, particularly if you have an injury. One of the most common mistakes is stretching too hard too soon. Wait several days before stretching an injury, because you don't want to tear the healing tissue. An injured muscle or tendon needs to be stretched very gently, and definitely not pushed into pain. Any stretching program after a muscle-strain injury should usually be accompanied by low-resistance, high-repetition (20–30 reps per set) range-of-motion exercises for the first few weeks to help heal the injured muscle. This type of exercise involves contracting muscles and moving joints through a range of motion that is pain-free.

CORRECTING MUSCLE IMBALANCES

Occasionally, stretching will not improve flexibility or alignment in a particular muscle or body region because there is too much imbalance of muscle strength. For example, stretching the *pectorals* (pecs) may not be enough to decrease the chances of injury. If the back muscles are significantly weaker than the chest muscles, you can stretch all day long, but the stronger muscles will take over. In this example, it is more important to strengthen the weaker muscle group (in this case, the back) than only to stretch the tight pecs.

It is important to try to keep muscles in balance. That means that major muscle groups around a joint should be strengthened. Do not strive to make every muscle equally strong, but learn what is a reasonable strength for all the muscles in a particular body region.

TIGHT MUSCLES CAN ALTER JOINT POSITION

Muscles have an optimum length that allows for optimum strength and function. It has been shown that muscle strength and function change with a change in length. Muscles that are excessively shortened or excessively lengthened may change joint position and predispose you to injury. A common example of this is the weight trainer who likes to train the large muscles of the chest and the deltoids more than the back. The pecs become shortened and the shoulder bone (*humerus*) actually begins migrating forward in the shoulder joint. This is a very common muscle imbalance and a real culprit in shoulder injuries. The shoulder joint does not function normally when the humerus is too far forward.

Another example of altered joint position actually involves more than one joint. Tight hamstrings that attach to the pelvis pull the pelvis down and can change the position of the back. The back is then in a more flexed position and loses its optimal alignment. This can increase forces to the low back and raise the chances of injury.

COMMON TIGHT MUSCLES

There are common patterns of tight muscles and weak muscles in the human body. This is due to the way our body is designed. Muscles prone to tightness are usually those that span more than one joint.

Tight pectorals are usually the result of poor sitting posture and the tendency to overtrain pecs as compared to the back. The hamstrings (back of the thigh), iliotibial band (side of the thigh), quadriceps (front of the thigh), and hip flexors (front of the hip) are all large muscle groups that are commonly tight. General inactivity can lead to muscle tightness, but so can a lot of training with heavy weights. This shortens muscles and decreases flexibility.

The calf and Achilles tendon are also commonly tight, especially if you are involved in running or jumping sports. These activities demand power from the calf muscle group, and increased use of this muscle group creates an environment in which the muscles tend to stay shortened. People with high arches in their feet also tend to have tight heel cords. Stretching can maximize the length of the muscle, but stretching cannot change a skeletal alignment condition.

Reasons for Tight Muscles

Chronic bad posture. Probably the most common reason for tight muscles is poor posture. For example, sitting for extended periods of time with a slumped, forward head posture and a forward shoulder posture leads to tight pectoral muscles. Furthermore, sitting for extended hours can lead to shortened hip flexors, as well as shortened hamstrings.

Spine problems. Back and neck problems can lead to tight muscles due to an area of irritation in the spine joints or nerve roots. Muscles can stay tight for a prolonged period of time. An example is persistently tight hamstrings; frequently, there is an associated low-back problem.

Joint injury. In the event of an injury, a muscle reflexively tightens around the injury to guard the joint from further injury. A common example is a low-back strain. In an injury of the disc or ligaments, the low-back muscles tighten to protect the area.

Joint dysfunction. A muscle might be tight if a joint cannot move through a full range of motion for a prolonged period of time. The muscle attached to the joint may then shorten. An example of this is tight quadriceps after a knee sprain.

Imbalances in training. Imbalances in strength training can lead to muscle tightness in some regions. An example is a very tight, strong chest area with a weaker upper-back area. In this case, the commonly tight area is reinforced by overtraining the pecs and neglecting to strengthen the back.

METHODS OF STRETCHING

There are many ways to promote flexibility, including passive and active stretching as well as hands-on techniques by health professionals to loosen muscles and joints. Methods used by professionals, such as massage therapy and joint mobilization/manipulation techniques, are most appropriate for chronically tight muscles and joints. Of the several methods of stretching, this chapter focuses on passive and active stretching.

Passive Stretching

Passive stretching is the common technique in which your body is positioned appropriately to increase the distance between the *origin* (beginning) of a muscle and its *insertion* (end), and the position is held for a specific amount of time (usually 15–20 seconds). The stretch can be repeated 2–5 times. It is usually safe if proper positioning is used.

Some muscles cover one joint, like the *soleus* (deeper calf area), while other muscles cover two joints, like the *gastroc* (surface of the calf). The one-joint mover lends itself to a more simplified stretch. If you are stretching two-joint muscles, you must consider the position of both joints in order to maintain an optimum stretch.

The key to passive stretching is to be certain that you feel a slight pull in the muscle group. For example, if during a hamstring stretch you feel the pull in your back instead of your hamstrings, you should reposition yourself.

Use your breath to maximize your stretch in

the following manner: When in the stretch position, take a deep breath in, relax, then slowly breathe out and slightly increase your stretch.

Active Stretching

Active stretches work more on dynamic flexibility, which refers to the muscle and joint tissue forces that resist motion throughout the range. The benefit of an active stretch is that it teaches the body to lengthen muscles and improve joint motion. Actively working on range of motion may be helpful in improving your performance.

One type of active stretch, the paired muscle active stretch, takes a body region through a full range of motion with a muscle contraction while stabilizing surrounding joints. This type of stretch takes advantage of *muscle agonist/ antagonist relationships* to get a relaxation and stretch of one muscle during contraction of another muscle. An example is the active hamstring stretch done by straightening your knee while sitting. This type of stretch can be held briefly at the end of the contraction and then repeated 5–10 times.

Another type of active stretch (or active flexibility exercise) uses more than one muscle in a body region to bring joints through a full range of motion and muscles into more lengthened positions. This type of stretch is usually repeated numerous times and may be finished with a hold of position. An example of this is the hip swing in which you stand on one leg and swing your knee in full circles.

Try a few active stretches to get used to them, and then use them with your passive stretches, depending on your activity goals. Note that many of the functional strength exercises in chapter 5 take your joints into a wide range of motion and may have active stretching benefits as well.

FLEXIBILITY EXERCISES

This section includes certain active stretches and some of the most popular passive stretches, because they are often done improperly. When stretches are described for one side of the body, remember to switch and repeat on the opposite side. Most passive stretches can be held for 20–30 seconds and repeated 2–3 times per stretching period, 2–3 times per week. Active stretches can be repeated 5–10 times.

In this section, the term *neutral spine* is used (see chapters 6 and 14). In the low back, the neutral spine position is a slight arch. The degree of the arch is unique to each individual. In a neutral spine, the low back is not too extended (arched) or too flexed (slouched). A wall mirror can be very useful in helping you become aware of the position of your spine during stretching.

LOWER BODY STRETCHES

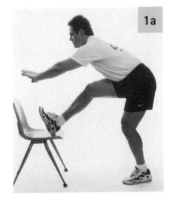

1a

1 Hamstring Stretch

Equipment: 12- to 18-inch-tall stool or chair.
Purpose: Stretch the large muscle group located on the back of your thigh. Tight hamstrings can contribute to back dysfunction because of the hamstring insertion on the pelvis.
Technique: While standing, position your heel on a stool or chair, with your toes pointing toward the ceiling, and bend forward at your hips (not your waist) with your arms extended straight in front of you, until you feel the stretch in the back of your knee and thigh. Keep your back neutral or slightly extended. Look straight ahead as you bend from the hips, not from the back. Think of yourself as projecting your chest forward. Try a stretch with your elevated knee slightly bent (1a) and one with it completely straight. To increase and improve the stretch, try modifying your foot or hip and leg position. For example, flex your elevated foot to move your toes toward your face. Or rotate your elevated leg and hip inward so your foot points inward, and hold that position, then rotate it outward and hold. You can also rotate your mid back and point to the left and then the right with one or both arms (1b). Do 2–3 reps.

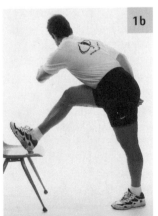

1b

Variation: 1.1. Sit on the floor with your right leg extended straight out in front of you, with your toes pointing up toward the ceiling. Bend your left leg and place the sole of your left foot against the inside of your right thigh. Keep your back in a neutral position. Flex at your hips, bringing your chest toward your right knee. If you can, grab the outside of your right foot with your left hand to include the left latissimus and upper back in this stretch.

Common errors: These exercises are usually done with excessive spine flexion; remember to maintain a neutral low-back position throughout the stretch.

2 | Sitting and Supine Active Hamstring Stretch

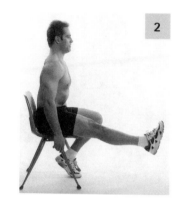

Equipment: Chair or other surface above ground level.

Purpose: Actively stretch the hamstring. Use this stretch if you have tight hamstring and back problems.

Technique: Sit on a surface that is high enough that your feet do not touch the ground when you have your low back slightly to fully arched. Slowly straighten one leg while keeping your low back in the arch position. The endpoint of this stretch is when you feel it in the back of your thigh. Hold the stretch for 5 seconds. Do 6–10 reps.

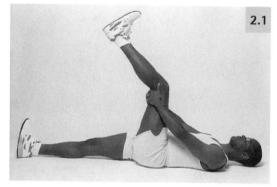

Variation: 2.1. A similar stretch can be done lying on your back. Hold the back of one thigh just behind the knee and slowly straighten your knee until you feel the stretch in your hamstrings.

Common errors: This active stretch is often done too quickly, so that people don't realize that their spine is moving into a rounded position. This exercise demands awareness of spine position, so do it slowly. Be sure your knee does not rotate in or out while doing this stretch.

3 | Quadriceps Stretch

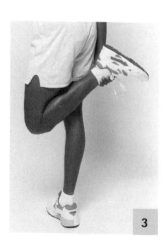

Equipment: None.

Purpose: Stretch the large muscle group in front of your thigh. Lack of flexibility may contribute to knee pain as well as back problems.

Technique: This is a two-joint muscle, so it requires attentiveness to both joints. The quadriceps both extend (straighten) the knee as well as flex (bend) the hip. The hip must be in extension, that is, slightly behind you, while the knee is bent. All the while, keep a neutral spine position. Stand on one leg with your knee slightly bent, and raise the heel of your other leg toward your back. Using your same-side hand as your raised leg, grab your ankle or something attached to your ankle, such as your pant leg or a towel, and pull it

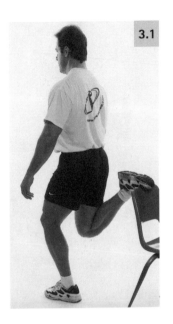

3.1

toward the same-side buttock until you feel a stretch on the front of your thigh. The stretch will be better if you bring your pelvis in a posterior direction (flex your low back). Do 2–3 reps. Also try using the opposite hand to bring your heel toward the opposite buttock (see Exercise Figure 3). This stretch also stretches your hip flexors.

Variation: 3.1. To stretch your quad and hip flexors at the same time, stand about 2½–3 feet in front of a chair, high bench, or other surface that is at the same height or up to 1½ feet higher than the height of your knee. Place the top of one foot on the surface and have your other foot far forward enough of the chair so that when you bend your forward knee, you can feel a stretch in the front of both your thigh and your hip. Make sure your back is in a slightly flexed position.

Tips and Precautions: Optimal range of motion is heel to buttock without compensating by hyperextending your back, bending your hip, or allowing your knee to go out to the side. Make sure you do not hyperextend your low back (do not arch your back). Your knee should not migrate out to the side; keep it close to the other knee.

4 | Active Quadriceps Stretch

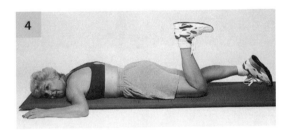

4

Equipment: None.

Purpose: Stretch your quadriceps if you have difficulty with balance or have problems extending your hips.

Technique: Lie on your stomach. Tighten your abdominal muscles so your pelvis won't move during this exercise. Bend one knee and move your heel toward your buttock, but do not let your spine arch. Do 6–10 reps.

5 | Iliotibial Band (ITB) Stretch

Equipment: Wall, tree, boulder, or other vertical support.

Purpose: Stretch the muscle and fascia tissue on the side of your hip and thigh.

Technique: Stand with your left side facing a wall, tree, or boulder, and touch it with your left hand. Have your left knee in front of you and slightly bent. Position your right leg behind your left leg and closer to the surface you are touching. The outside edge of your right foot should be touching the ground. Sidebend your spine to the left while you move your right hip slightly to the right. The right side of your body should be in a C-shaped curve. Do 2–3 reps.

Variations: 5.1. You can also do this with your right hand extended over your head, elbow bent, and pointing to the wall. 5.2. Stand with your right side facing a wall or vertical surface, and balance on your right leg with your knee slightly bent. Place the toes of your left foot behind your right heel, and your right hand above your head on the vertical surface for balance. Move your right hip toward the wall until you feel a stretch along your right hip and lateral thigh. For additional stretch, move farther away from the wall and reach your hand farther above your head.

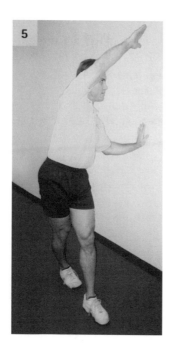
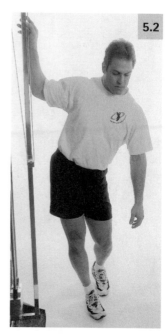

6 Hip Flexor Stretch

Equipment: Chair or bench.

Purpose: Stretch the muscles that bring your knee toward your chest. These are tight in almost everyone, because most people spend a significant amount of time sitting. These muscles extend from the low back to the front of the hip.

Technique: Kneel on the floor on one knee, with your other foot in front of you. Your hip on your kneeling side should be slightly extended, with that knee in back of your buttock. Hold onto a chair or bench while you shift weight onto your forward leg, allowing that forward knee to bend more. This will move your kneeling-side hip into a more extended position. Do 2–3 reps.

Precautions: Be careful that in the process your back is not hyperextended, because this is difficult for the back. Also be careful that you achieve a neutral spine position, or the stretch will not be very effective.

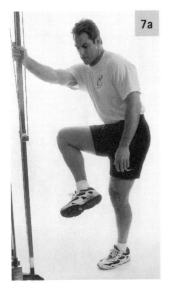

7a

7 Active Hip Stretch

Equipment: Vertical surface.

Purpose: Actively stretch your hip joint capsule and surrounding musculature.

Technique: Stand on your left leg and bend it slightly; with your right hand, touch a vertical support surface. Move your right knee into a flexed position (bend it 90 degrees) and bring it toward your abdomen. Imagine you have a pen on the front of your right knee and move it around clockwise to draw the largest circle that you are comfortably able to. Your right knee should rotate outward (with your right foot pointing inward) when it is on the outer half of the circle (7a), and rotate inward (with your right foot pointing outward) when it is on the inner half of the circle (7b). Tighten your abdominal muscles to stabilize your back. Do 5–10 circles and then switch to the other leg. You can also move your knee counterclockwise.

Precautions: People often allow for too much movement in the leg on which they are standing. Keep that leg stable so most of the motion goes into the leg that is raised.

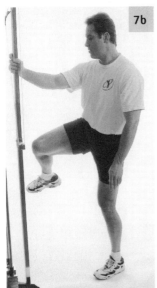

7b

8 Adductor Stretch

Equipment: None.

Purpose: Stretch the muscles of your inner thigh.

Technique: Sit on the floor with your legs spread apart and knees slightly bent. Lean forward at the waist, keeping your back straight, until you feel a pull in your inner thigh.

Variation: 8.1. Stand with your feet spaced very widely apart. Bend your left knee and sidebend your back to the right while you slide your right hand down the outside of your right leg. Bend your left knee and move your pelvis to the left to feel a stretch on the inner side of the right groin. Extend your left arm over your head toward the right to get a stretch in your left side at the same time.

Precautions: Don't round your back when you do this exercise while sitting.

9 | Heel Cord (Achilles) Stretch

Equipment: Vertical surface.

Purpose: Stretch your heel cords and calf muscles.

Technique: Stand in front of a vertical surface such as a wall, tree, or side of a car; position your feet shoulder-width apart and touch the surface to stabilize yourself. Then place one foot ½–1½ feet behind the heel of your front foot. Slightly bend your front knee while keeping your back knee straight. Transfer weight to your forward knee until you feel a stretch in the back of your leg (9a). Hold this for 20 seconds, then bend your back knee slightly and repeat the weight transfer (9b).

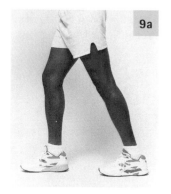 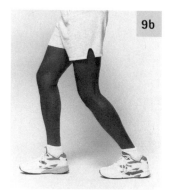

Tips and Precautions: This stretch is even more effective if you put your weight onto the outside of your foot. Be sure your toes are pointed straight ahead or even a little bit inward. The tendency is to allow the foot to turn outward, and this is not an effective stretch. Furthermore, try to maintain an arch in your foot. Make sure you bend at the ankle and keep your heel on the floor.

10 | Active Squat Stretch to the Heel Cord

Equipment: Pole or door handle.

Purpose: Stretch the heel cord and ankle joint into the functional squat position. Normal range of motion of the ankle joint is the ability to perform a full squat with your heels on the ground. Most people lose this range of motion and don't realize it.

Technique: Hold onto something like a pole or a door handle for balance, and go into a squat while keeping your heels on the ground. Do 10–15 squats. You also can do this stretch without holding onto anything, positioning your feet parallel to or one in front of the other.

Precautions: Avoid jamming your ankles by not doing this too quickly.

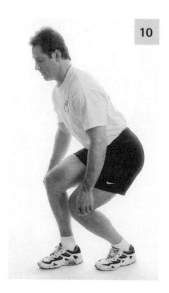

UPPER BODY STRETCHES

11   Chest Stretch

Equipment: Doorway or pole.
Purpose: Stretch the pectoralis and the anterior shoulder.
Technique: Stand in a doorway or by a pole. Extend your right arm straight out to your right side at 45 degrees above horizontal, and grasp the doorframe or pole. Rotate your body to the left to feel the stretch in your chest. Do 2–3 reps.
Precautions: Don't do this stretch if you have pain down your arm.

12   Rhomboid and Posterior Shoulder Stretch

Equipment: Doorframe.
Purpose: Stretch the muscles between and on the back surface of the shoulder blades.
Technique: Stand in a doorway with your toes at the front of the doorframe. Grasp the left outside edge of the doorframe. Rotate your torso to the right until you feel a stretch on your right shoulder blade. Hold for 20 seconds and reverse sides. Do 2–3 reps.

13   Active Shoulder Stretch

Equipment: None.
Purpose: Actively stretch the shoulder capsule and surrounding musculature. This is a good stretch for climbers, skiers, and boaters.
Technique: Standing with your feet shoulder-width apart, bend your right elbow to 90 degrees and point in front of you. This is the starting position. Move your arm and shoulder in a clockwise circle. You can do this for 4–6 circles on one side, gradually moving into larger circles, before you switch to the other side. After you complete this motion, move your right hand (with a straight elbow and your palm facing toward the midline of your body) in a forward arc motion, until you are pointing toward the ceiling or sky. Then move your arm in a reverse arc so that your fingers point behind you. Do 6–10 reps.
Precautions: Don't do this exercise if you have tendonitis of your biceps or rotator cuff, or if it is painful in your shoulder, neck, or arm.

14 | Rotator Cuff and Shoulder Capsule Active Stretch

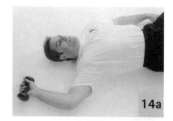

14a

Equipment: 1- to 2-pound weight or can of food; rolled towel; pillow.

Purpose: Stretch the rotator cuff muscles and ligaments that surround your shoulder joint. A tight rotator cuff can lead to shoulder joint problems. This is an important stretch if you can't achieve full shoulder motion.

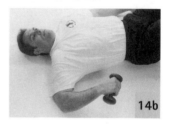

14b

Technique: Lie on your back. Support your shoulder with a small towel roll under your shoulder blade. You also may need a towel or a pillow to support your hand if it will not lie flat on the ground. Use a can of food or a weight for slight resistance; the weight should not be too heavy. Place your right arm extended out to your side at shoulder level and elbow bent to 90 degrees, so that your hand faces the ceiling. Allow your shoulder to rotate externally so that your forearm points straight up parallel to your head (like a holdup position in an old western movie) (14a). Hold this position for 30–45 seconds. Keeping your elbow on the floor, raise your forearm by rotating at your shoulder, moving your hand toward your feet until it is a few inches off of the floor near your waist. Your goal is a 20-degree angle measured from your hand to the floor (14b). If you feel the front of your shoulder moving forward, you have gone too far. Hold it for about 30–45 seconds. Next, straighten your elbow and raise your arm to 90 degrees so that your fingers are pointing toward the ceiling. Bring your straight arm back toward the floor until you feel a stretch in your shoulder and latissimus. Your shoulder is loose enough if the back of your hand touches the ground. Do 2–4 reps.

Precautions: Don't allow your arm to migrate toward your body. Don't let your shoulder lift off of the ground.

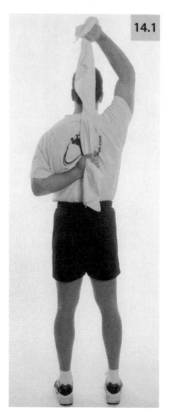

14.1

Variation: 14.1. Stand with your feet shoulder-width apart. Hold a towel with your right hand and place it over your shoulder, above waist height. Put your left hand behind your back, above waist height, and grab the towel; gradually pull up with your right hand. Hold when you feel a stretch. Repeat this stretch on the other side.

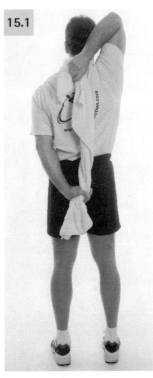

15.1

15 | Triceps Stretch

Equipment: Towel.
Purpose: Stretch the back of the arm.
Technique: Standing with your feet shoulder-width apart, lift your right arm over your head; bend your elbow so that your right hand is behind your neck. Hold your right elbow with your left hand and pull gently toward the back of your neck. You can also stretch your torso at the same time by sidebending your torso to the left. Do 2–3 reps.
Variation: 15.1. Set up as for the stretch described in Exercise 14.1, but pull down on the towel with your left arm.
Precaution: Don't let your right arm migrate out to the side.

16 | Forearm Stretch

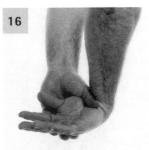

16

Equipment: None.
Purpose: Stretch the muscles of the forearm; this is particularly useful for those who do racquet sports, climbing, or kayaking.
Technique: Extend your left arm straight out in front of you, with your arm, wrist, and fingers parallel to the floor. Now move your wrist and fingers toward the floor. Rotate your hand so your fingers point out away from the left side of your body, and hold it. You can increase the stretch by grasping your left hand with your right hand and gently pulling on your hand. Then point the fingers of your left hand down with your right hand and gently pull them back toward the middle of your body. Do 2–3 reps.
Variation: 16.1. You can also stretch your forearm flexors by holding your arm straight out in front of you, parallel to the floor, with your elbow extended (straight). Bend your fingers back toward your body so that they are directed toward the ceiling.
Precaution: Don't bend your elbow.

Torso/Spine Stretches

17 | Cat/Camel Stretch

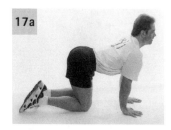

Equipment: None.

Purpose: Maintain and improve the flexibility of your back and neck to go into full flexing and extending.

Technique: Start on your hands and knees on the ground, with your hips and knees bent at about 90 degrees. Initiate an extending arch in your low back by moving your pelvis forward and bringing your belly button slightly closer to the ground in an arched back position. Gradually extend up your spine until your neck is extended and you are looking straight ahead (17a). Hold this position for a few seconds. Next, initiate a flexing action in your low back by moving your pelvis back and raising your belly button up toward the ceiling. Gradually move the flexing all the way up your spine to create a humped back and you are looking downward (17b). Hold this position for a few seconds. Repeat this sequence 5 times.

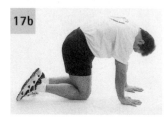

18 | Pelvic Circles

Equipment: None.

Purpose: Prepare the mid and low back for rotational motions.

Technique: Stand with your hands on your hips and your knees slightly bent (or sit on a chair). Move your pelvis from side to side, then forward (back arching) and back (back flexing).Then combine these movements to move your pelvis and hips in a smooth, circular motion (to the left, then forward, then to the right, then back). This will require you to shift your center of gravity while your pelvis circles underneath your unmoving upper body. Perform this motion for 4–6 revolutions to the left and then to the right.

Precaution: Be cautious if you have a lower back problem.

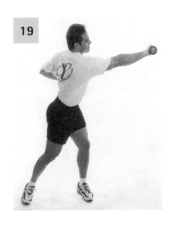

19 | Active Spine Rotations

Equipment: None.

Purpose: Maintain the rotation in your spine.

Technique: Start with your knees slightly bent in a mini-squat position, with your feet spaced wider than shoulder-width apart, and with your right elbow in a flexed position and your right arm drawn back so your hand is close to your shoulder. Initiate a punch across your body with your right shoulder and arm extending to the 10:00 o'clock position, and at the same time push off with your right buttock and foot, thus extending your right hip, straightening your right knee, and and weight-shifting to the left foot. Pivot on the ball of the right foot and end on the toes of your right foot with your heel up at the end of the punch. Then repeat the punch with the left hand, punching in the opposite direction to the 2:00 o'clock position. A rep is a punch to the right and and a punch to the left. Perform 2–3 sets of 15–30 repetitions.

Tips and Precautions: Punches can be performed in any direction, and either high or low, but are usually performed at shoulder height. You can punch as far as your spine can rotate after you have done it well to the 10:00 and 2:00 range. This exercise should initially be done in a slow and controlled manner so as to not injure your spine or shoulders. Increase the speed gradually and be cautious if you have a shoulder or back problem.

Variation: 19.1. Position your feet so that one foot is a running-stride-length in front of the other, with both heels on the ground and your knees slightly bent. Punch in a forward direction, 12 times with each arm, then add rotational punches as described above but keep the same stance position. After 12 rotational punches, switch your forward leg with the backward leg and repeat. 19.2. Try the exercise while sitting. This will take your knees and hips out of the motion and focus the rotational demands on your spine.

5

STRENGTH AND BALANCE TRAINING
Functional Exercises

BY MICHAEL HANSEN, P.T., AND DAVID MUSNICK, M.D.

▶ **THIS CHAPTER WILL HELP YOU:**
- Understand the benefits of strength and balance training.
- Understand the various strength training methods and equipment options.
- Understand the difference between traditional and functional strength training.
- Identify and learn how to use the various types of equipment used in resistance exercise.
- Learn specific functional strength and balance exercises.

STRENGTH TRAINING

The basic strength training concepts in this chapter will help you choose and evaluate strength training options. Functional exercises use your muscles and body regions in patterns that are closest to how your body functions in real life, and can improve your strength and balance significantly.

The term *strength* implies the maximum tension or force generated by a muscle or muscle group.

The term *one repetition maximum* (1 RM) is often used to define the ability of a muscle to produce a single repetition (rep) of a movement with maximal resistance. In strength training and outdoor activities, we are usually using a percentage of 1 RM.

Strength training can be defined as any form of active exercise in which a muscular contrac-

tion is resisted by an outside force. Outside forces include gravity, free weights, balls, pulleys, resistance tubing, and exercise machines. Such machines have made exercise easier, but their carryover to sport-specific function is sometimes questionable, and they should not be the sole basis of a strength-training program.

Strength endurance refers to the time limit of a muscle's ability to perform a strength exercise repeatedly. Exercise programs designed to increase muscular endurance emphasize doing sets with higher reps (15–35) and thus lower amounts of resistance.

Power refers to the product of force exerted and the velocity (speed) of the exercise, and thus the rate of performing the work of the exercise. When exercising, the force is a given resistance, that of a weight or the weight of your body against gravity. Your power can increase in one of two ways. (1) You can increase the number of reps in a given time. (2) You can do the same number of reps in a shorter time. This is important for a number of reasons. We usually are instructed that it is important to lift heavier loads with fewer repetitions. In fact, we function in most of our activities with lower loads and higher reps (for example, the kayaker's stroke). In certain outdoor situations, you may need to perform a movement with high resistance at quick speeds (a quick high step on snow or rock, a jump off of a boulder or river, a quick climbing move, or a kayak roll). To be prepared for these challenges, you should train at both ends of the power spectrum.

If your activity requires brief periods of moving your body rapidly, incorporate some higher-speed training into your routine.

BENEFITS OF STRENGTH TRAINING

The benefits of strength training are numerous. Resistive exercise creates adaptive changes in the muscle as it is progressively overloaded. These changes include *hypertrophy* (increase in size) of the muscle fibers, as well as an increase in the recruitment of muscle fibers, creating an improvement in muscle tone. Bone, ligament, and tendon density also improve, helping to stabilize your joints. Strength training improves your physical capacity to do more work, reduces your risk of injuries, and can improve your physical appearance. It can also enhance your body composition by increasing the ratio of muscle mass to fat, which improves calorie-burning metabolic function. As the strength of muscle continues to increase, the cardiovascular response to the muscle also improves, which results in an increase in muscular endurance and power. Strength training can also stimulate growth hormone release, which is helpful in maintaining muscle. In addition, there is an improvement in your mental outlook and sense of physical well-being.

DETERMINANTS OF STRENGTH

People of all ages can increase their muscle size and strength as a result of progressive strength training. Strength gains decline 7% per decade after age 30. Studies show that we lose a half pound of muscle every year of life after age 25 unless we perform regular exercise. The rate at which skeletal muscle can adapt to vigorous exercise is reduced as we age, but adaptations still take place and improvements in performance can occur. A person's strength is related to many factors, including gender, distribution of muscle fiber type, muscle and bone anatomy, genetics, body frame, nutrition, hormone levels, injuries, and training.

The *length tension* relationship of the muscle is another important factor in determining strength. When a muscle is at its resting length, a maximal number of sites are available for muscle fiber contraction. However, when the muscle is shorter (contracted) or longer (stretched) than its resting length, there are fewer available sites. Thus, the muscle can generate the most force around its resting length in a mid-range position and less force when it is in a stretched or shortened state. Training programs should include both exercise of a muscle at mid range for maximal force generation and through all ranges for functional full-range strength and balance.

Neural control (nerve control) of the muscles also affects strength by influencing the maximal force of a muscle. Neural control is determined by how many and how fast muscle fibers are involved in a contraction. An increase in muscle size takes 6–8 weeks to occur, yet people improve strength performance in 2–3 weeks of training. Much of the improvement in strength evidenced in the first few weeks of resistance training is attributable to neural firing adaptations.

STRENGTH TRAINING METHODS

There are many strength training methods.

One classification of strength training is by the type of muscle contraction, being either isotonic (moving) or isometric (not moving).

Isometrics are static muscle contractions, in which there is no change in the length of the muscle fiber. Functionally, it is a stabilizing contraction. Strength gains are specific for the joint angle held, but may have benefits within a range of approximately plus or minus 20 degrees. The exercise should be done in a few different joint positions as close as possible to the positions that you will be using in your outdoor activity. This type of training is most applicable to climbers, and the climbing athlete should incorporate some of these exercises into his or her routine. Maintaining a climbing hold on rock or ice could be trained by an isometric hold on a climbing wall, boulder, or fingerboard, or by a pull-up. You could start off with holds of 6 seconds and repeat each minute for 5–10 reps. You could increase the hold times of some of the reps to simulate your expected hold times in your climbs.

Isotonic resistance exercise is muscle action carried out against a constant load and variable speed as the muscle contracts. This includes free weights, pulleys, and most exercise machines.

Circuit weight training includes weight stations mixed with aerobic stations. The workout emphasizes muscle endurance and is not good for making significant strength gains. The aerobic workout in circuit training is not as good as aerobic workouts mentioned in chapter 2, Aerobic Conditioning and Interval Training.

Plyometric exercises are very fast motions that incorporate a rapid stretching phase prior to a whole-body explosive motion such as a jump. These may be done singly or in combination, and done on different sloped surfaces indoors or outdoors (see chapters 8, 11, and 20 for examples). Plyometrics can be helpful for downhill skiing, snowboarding, or any sport that requires jumping. Climbers can do modifi-cations of these on climbing walls by doing quick motions with legs and arms to reach for a particularly difficult hold. There is an increased risk of injury with these exercises, so be careful and consider doing a supervised session.

MUSCLE ACTIONS

In a *concentric* muscle action, the muscle shortens and joint motion occurs; for example, flexing your elbow while holding a 10-pound weight (an exercise called a curl) causes the biceps to shorten and brings your hand closer to your shoulder.

Eccentric muscle action occurs when the muscle lengthens while developing tension, because the contractile force is less than the resistive force (e.g., in the second half of the curl exercise, lowering the weight from a position close to your shoulder to a straight elbow position). In the biceps curl, the eccentric action of the biceps muscle prevents you from dropping the weight. Eccentric muscle action decelerates joint motion and is a very important function of muscles.

Many of your lower-extremity muscles (buttocks to feet) function eccentrically to control your legs from collapsing forward or inward. Your quadriceps have to work eccentrically to prevent your knees from flexing, and are subject to greater loads when you are going downhill. Many acute or gradual overuse injuries are due to inadequate eccentric strength. You can emphasize training eccentrically by having the eccentric part of the exercise take twice as long as the concentric. Eccentric muscle action in the lower extremities can be enhanced by performing exercises in standing positions that simulate the eccentric demands of standing activities. Such exercises can be made more challenging by performing them on one foot, by orienting the movement in various directions, or by adding weights.

Econcentric muscle action combines both

concentric (at one joint) and eccentric (at the other joint) contraction in a muscle that spans more than one joint. Examples of this include (1) a biceps curl performed while your shoulder moves into extension (backward movement of the elbow), and (2) when walking, prior to heel raise your calf muscle acts to both slow down the progression of forward ankle motion while assisting your upper leg muscles in extension (straightening) of your knee. Jumping exercises (see chapter 11) will work your muscle in this fashion.

STRENGTH TRAINING GUIDELINES
WARM-UP

Always warm up your muscles and joints with 5–10 minutes of aerobic exercise. Preferable methods are biking (especially bikes with moving handlebars), cross-country skiing, skipping rope, or rowing, because they use both the arms and the legs. Walking, running, or stair climbing are also acceptable for a warm-up.

PRACTICAL POINT
You may also warm up with high-rep, low-resistance sets, or functional exercises that incorporate the upper- and lower-body regions (Exercises 20 and 21 at the end of this chapter are good choices).

REPETITIONS AND SETS

How many repetitions (reps) you do is the number of times you repeat an exercise in a set before a rest period, or before you exercise different muscles. The number of reps in your sets should be based on your exercise goals. When you are working with machines or free weights in conventional exercises, consider beginning with 15 reps in a set for the first 2–3 weeks to avoid injuries, develop muscle capillary networks, and put your muscles and joints through a full range of motion. If your activity requires re-gional muscular endurance (many consecutive contractions of the same muscle group), then plan on performing 15–25 reps per set with lower resistance, and do 1–2 of these sets throughout your training program.

PRACTICAL POINT
Rest at least 1 minute between each set of the same exercise, or when exercising the same muscle in an exercise that uses it in a similar fashion. This will allow your muscle to regain the energy it needs for further contraction.

For maximum benefit, you should feel fatigue during the last 1–2 reps of a set. Increase the resistance of the exercise once you have mastered good form and the exercise feels easy. After you have been performing exercises to build your muscular endurance base (4–6 weeks), consider adding 1–2 sets of 8–12 reps, which will emphasize strength more than endurance. Gradually build up the resistance used with this number of reps. After 3–4 weeks you can add lower-rep sets (4–6) to build maximum strength and promote hypertrophy. As you progress through your training program, consider incorporating sets of different lengths to achieve a diversity of training effects: 1–2 sets of 15 reps, 1–2 sets of 8–12 reps, and 1 set of 4–6 reps.

For functional exercises that work on strength and coordination (see the exercises at the end of this chapter), start with 8–12 reps and do them slowly enough to establish your movement pattern. You can then continue with that number or do them on a timed basis for 30–60 seconds. As you feel stronger and more able to do a particular functional exercise, consider increasing the speed within the previous timed period. Do not increase speed unless you can maintain good form.

RANGE OF MOTION

Use as full a range of motion of the joint as possible to allow the muscle to strengthen at different lengths. Try to control the speed at the end ranges of a joint (especially the shoulder and knee) to avoid jamming it at its end range. Stay in a pain-free range of motion. This may mean limiting your range of movement. In some exercises, you may emphasize only part of a joint's range. This may be most applicable for the knee, especially if you have kneecap problems.

WEIGHT, RESISTANCE, AND GOOD FORM

Use as much weight (resistance) as is comfortable to complete a set pain-free and with good form. This means having good posture, safe spine positioning, and good movement patterns. Good form is a key to injury prevention. The last 1–2 reps should be difficult to perform, but good form should still be maintained. Add more resistance (5%–10% of what you are currently lifting) when the exercise feels easy. If you are doing consistent strength training, you can go to lower-rep sets and make higher-percent increases in the resistance. If you desire a good balance of endurance and maximum strength, progress your sets from 15 to 8–12 to 4–6 reps per set. High-performance professional athletes would progress somewhat differently. You are using too much resistance if (1) you are fatiguing before the last 2 reps in a set; (2) your movement patterns are poorly coordinated or done with poor balance; or (3) you have pain in the muscles you are exercising or in other muscles or joints in your body.

FREQUENCY

During the initial stages of your exercise progression, exercise each body region 3–4 times per week. The intensity of each workout and your current level of fitness will determine the amount of time needed for proper recovery. Allow at least 48 hours between strength training sessions that target particular body regions. Performing resistance exercise of a particular body region without adequate time for recovery can lead to injuries and excessive soreness.

WORK LARGER MUSCLES FIRST

In designing your strength training program, try to work large muscle groups first. If you fatigue your small muscles early in the workout, they will not be efficient at assisting with movements using larger muscle groups.

EXERCISE YOUR CORE (TORSO)

It is very important to exercise your abdominal muscles (all of them), along with your hip, buttock, and back muscles. These muscles are decelerators, initiators of movement, and stabilizers. A strong core can support strengthening of your extremities. Save specific abdominal exercises for last because their strength is needed in stabilizing your body during all other activities.

PRACTICE SAFE SPINE POSTURES AND MOVEMENTS

In general, try to lift with your buttocks and your legs as opposed to your back. Assume neutral spine positions (see chapters 6 and 14) when using seated equipment or in standing exercises, unless otherwise indicated. Avoid excessive spine flexion and extension.

AVOID MAXIMUM LIFTS

With a new exercise or when you have taken a break from your regular strength training program, initially use a weight or resistance (tubing size) lower than you think you can do. This will help you avoid injury. Be especially careful with new shoulder exercises when you are raising your arm to the front or side, as the rotator cuff muscles are prone to straining with heavier weights.

PRACTICAL POINT

If you are doing machine exercises or isolated muscle free-weight exercises, you can pair your exercises so you are exercising one muscle group, then its opposite (e.g., biceps then triceps, quads then hamstrings, push-ups then rows). You may then find that you do not need to take a 1-minute break between sets. You can also do an upper-extremity and then a lower extremity exercise. Take a full minute between each functional exercise that pairs exercises of the hips and legs with the shoulder. In general, rest approximately 48 hours between training sessions of a specific muscle area to allow the muscle to adapt and heal from the overload.

MUSCLE SYMMETRY

Workouts should be designed to maintain muscle symmetry. This can be thought of as exercising muscles that do opposing actions in a body region, that stabilize a region, or that are prone to weakness. (See the body region chapters in Part II for more specific information.)

Opposing muscles include quads/hamstrings; abdominal muscles and hip flexors/gluteus maximus and spine extensors; pectorals/rhomboids and trapezius; biceps/triceps; wrist and finger flexors/wrist and finger extensors. Think of giving attention to muscles on the front and back of your body. To provide stability, exercise muscles that stabilize a region along with the muscles that move it.

PRACTICAL POINT

It is important to maintain the strength of all of your major muscles. You may want to place more emphasis on some for strengthening and others for stretching. To maintain muscle balance, it's important to maintain flexibility of the overused muscles and maintain strength and endurance of the under-used muscles. Focus some of your strengthening on the muscles commonly prone to weakness, and make sure you include stretches for muscles commonly prone to tightness (Achilles, quads, iliotibial band, psoas, upper trapezius, levator scapulae).

In the majority of people, certain muscles are prone to weakness and are a good focus for strength training. These include the hamstrings, gluteus maximus and medius, abdominal obliques, spine extensors and rotators, middle and lower trapezius, rotator cuff of the shoulder, and wrist and finger extensors.

Repetitive activity can promote imbalances in muscle strength and length/tightness, and lead to musculoskeletal injuries and pain.

OVERLOADING AND STRENGTH TRAINING OPTIONS

As you do your exercises, you will reach a point at which you can easily do 10–12 reps without feeling much difficulty or fatigue at the last 2 reps. This is a time to increase the resistance. A 10% increase is usually a safe amount. If you are using tubing, you can go to the next size of tubing. Doing 2–3 sets of 8–12 reps and gradually increasing the resistance is adequate unless you are trying to build significant muscle size, power, or speed.

There are other methods of training a muscle, and in each the principle of overloading applies to building strength. *Overload*, simply stated, is applying stress to a muscle or group of muscles. If you overload a muscle in the way you want it to perform, the muscle will adapt and remodel in that fashion. As adaptation occurs, increased loading needs to occur. There are numerous methods of overloading muscle, each with its own advantages and disadvantages. Several include:

Light weight to heavier weight, same number of reps: If you are doing 3 sets of 12, in the first set you would use about 50% of the weight, in the second set 75%, and in the third set 100%, all for 12 reps.

Light weight to heavy weight, lower reps: With this overload method, you progressively increase the load with fewer repetitions as the sets increase. For example, if you can bench press 100 pounds 10 times, follow that with 8 repetitions of 120 pounds for the second set, and finish with 6 repetitions of 140 pounds for the third set. This method is used frequently for achieving increased strength, power, and mass, and could be used if you have already established your strength foundation or after 4–6 weeks of training.

Increased speed or rate of movement: This overload method is useful if you're trying to perform motions at faster speeds, such as fast paddling in whitewater kayaking, crew rowing, any racing activity, or climbing. After you have established a good strength workout with at least 4 weeks of 2 sets at 15 reps, you can try increasing the speed of your exercise. You may have to do this with the same resistance or slightly less resistance if using weights or machines. This method also increases coordination, especially with functional exercises, after you can perform the motion patterns well. There is some physiological carryover from one training speed to another, so it is beneficial to cross train at multiple speeds.

PERIODIZING YOUR PROGRAM

Periodization in strength training is the planning of time periods of strength training options in regard to resistance, reps, and speed. Periodized use of functional exercises, plyometrics, and sport-specific skill training will prepare you for activities or race goals.

We know that muscle adapts to the stresses it is exposed to and follows a predictable pattern of plateauing unless the stress is continually increased. With periodization, you change the training schedule so that when your goal activity begins, you will be maximally prepared. Periodization in strength training can include many plans, depending on your goals. For example:

The first stage of periodization might be a preparation stage in which you exercise with low resistance and higher reps (15–20) for 2–4 weeks while you are getting used to the equipment, movement patterns, and proper postures.

In the second phase you become more specific with your exercises, and increase resistance and decrease reps to 8–12. Add functional exercises during this stage. This phase could be 3–4 weeks. Start your activity-specific skill and balance work by the end of this phase.

In the third phase, add more speed and power to your program. Consider doing certain exercises in 1–2 sets with higher resistance at 4–6 reps if you have significant strength and power goals. Consider adding speed to some of the exercises, especially the functional exercises.

Add plyometrics at this stage if appropriate.

The final stage is your goal activity or competition, in which you are trying to maintain your strength while primarily performing your activity. Decrease the total volume of strength training and decrease frequency to 2 days a week. Also include a core of functional or free-weight exercises with 2 sets of 8–12 reps, and avoid strengthening sessions 1 day prior to goal activity sessions.

STRENGTH TRAINING EQUIPMENT

Selection of strengthening equipment can be confusing because of the diversity and variety of equipment available. The choice should be made on individual needs, but the best choice, based on function, economics, and space, is still free weights.

DYNAMIC VARIABLE-RESISTANCE EQUIPMENT (MACHINES)

Machines such as the Nautilus Hammer® and Cybex® are designed to provide variable resistance to load the muscle throughout range of motion. Their advantages include safety, isolated guided movements, and quick adjustment of loads. They also help build muscle tone and general muscle strength. Machines that allow independent, multiplanar arm motion are more challenging and are best used along with free weights once you have built up a base of strength. Disadvantages include limited training movements, and no balance or combination of body motions involved.

DYNAMIC CONSTANT-RESISTANCE EQUIPMENT (FREE WEIGHTS)

Dynamic constant resistance refers to fixed loads and variable speeds. Examples are free weights, weighted balls, or anything you can lift, such as a rock or log. Advantages include low cost of equipment, similarity to most functional work and exercise, and unlimited variety of training movements. Constant resistance is easily quantifiable, more functional, and often closed-chain (see p. 79) for the lower extremity. Disadvantages include inconsistent matching of resistive forces with muscle forces throughout the exercise, so the whole muscle does not get exercised with the same intensity. The weakest part of the muscle gets the greatest workout.

Ankle weights can help simulate the hip work needed in going uphill, in snow travel, or when wearing heavy footwear.

PULLEYS

Pulleys are excellent for shoulder, back, rotator cuff, and sitting or standing abdominal exercises. Many functional exercises can be done with pulleys in a gym or with tubing at home or outdoors. The best pulleys are adjustable so they can be pulled at different heights, depending on your activity. Most pulleys can only be pulled from the ground or from overhead, but some are fully adjustable on a vertical axis. The fully adjustable pulleys are best to use for rotator cuff and other shoulder and upper-back exercises.

ELASTIC RESISTANCE EQUIPMENT

Tubing comes in variable widths and resistance. Advantages are low cost, portability, and simulation of pulley motions. They are reasonable tools for the climbing, skiing, or paddling athlete. Disadvantages include a resistance increase as the tubing is stretched. This can lead to excessive force on some muscles at the end of the joint range and when the muscle is usually the weakest. *Note:* Attach elastic tubing to closed doors by tying a large knot in the tubing and closing the door, or tying it to a doorknob or other attachment. Outside, tie tubing to trees, bleachers, poles, etc. Be careful to anchor the tubing securely. You can buy tubing in different widths at most physical therapy clinics.

MEDICINE OR WEIGHT BALLS

Weighted balls of various sizes are excellent for the balance reach exercises discussed at the end of this chapter. They are also helpful for standing functional abdominal exercises.

LARGE INFLATABLE BALLS

"Physioballs" come in variable sizes and can be used for strengthening your abdominal muscles and for sitting balance training. They are available through most physical therapy clinics. The disadvantage is that you must be careful because they can be unstable.

STEPS

Steps are used to simulate a stepping motion and can be real steps, wooden boxes, or step platforms used in aerobics classes. Try to avoid such things as telephone books, as these are unsteady surfaces. Outdoors you can use steps, bleachers, rocks, and logs.

BALANCE TRAINING

Balance is your ability to react quickly to gravity or environmental challenges. Poor balance can lead to a fall or an injury. In order to improve your balance, you must improve not only the strength of your muscles, but your ability to utilize the strength and responsiveness of your muscles to specific balance challenges. *Agility* can be thought of as maintaining balance and good body positioning while responding quickly to changes in your environment while you are moving. Balance can be trained during an exercise in a number of ways:

* moving your arms or legs away from your torso (for example, Exercises 37 and 38 at the end of this chapter)
* moving your torso away from your center of gravity or your base of support (for example, Exercise 27 below)
* standing, walking, or sitting on an uneven or unstable surface such as logs, rocks, foam rolls, large physioballs, or specialized balance equipment

Climbing, windsurfing, skiing, snowboarding, snowshoeing, and mountaineering athletes can benefit the most from standing balance exercises. Walking on rocks or logs in parks or other outdoor environments will help train balance. Agility drills can also be helpful. There are specific exercises at the end of this chapter designed to challenge your balance (especially Exercises 37–40). Exercises 20.1, 22.4, 23, 24, 26, 27.2, 29.1, 30.1, and 36 are also excellent balance exercises. Other standing balance exercises are those in chapter 8 and 58.1, 59, 60.1, 62, 62.1, 63, and 64. Exercises 33–35 and 41 are good for sitting balance if done on a large ball with less weight on your feet. Other sitting balance exercises are Exercise 69 and those in chapter 21. Depending on your goals, your strength and conditioning program can be designed to work on muscle strength, endurance, power, and balance, or all four.

BALANCE EQUIPMENT
FOAM

Foam cylinders can be used cut in half or as cylinders. The balance challenge increases as you go from standing on the curved surface of a half roll to standing on the flat side of a half roll. Make sure the foam is firm. The larger the roll, the lesser the balance challenge. It is good to use 1- to 2-foot rolls. You can use these rolls to do Exercise 37 or to practice log crossings or walking on rocks. You can stand on the curved or the flat side of a half roll to challenge your balance with any functional exercise done while standing on one or both feet (see Figure 10).

BALANCE BOARDS

There are many types of ankle balance equipment; names include Baps boards, wobble

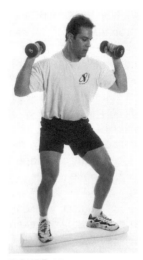

FIGURE 10

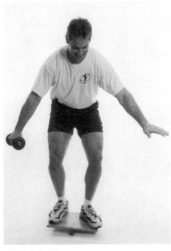

FIGURE 11

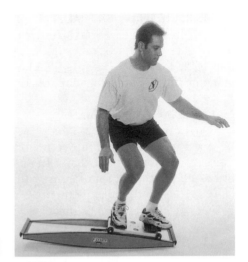

FIGURE 12

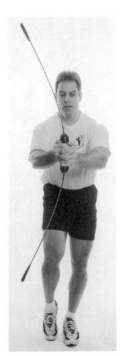

FIGURE 13

boards (see Figure 11), the "fitter" (see Figure 12), etc. They create balance challenges in different planes of motion. It is good to start with one that moves forward and back or side to side before you try the multidirectional equipment. You can do exercises on this equipment by simply trying to maintain your balance or by moving on them with or without hand weights. Use poles for additional support when you are starting to use this equipment. The most challenging equipment has a platform that moves on a roller surface. This should not be used until you are confident in your mastery of other balance equipment and can do many of the functional exercises with good stability. If you belong to a health club, it is a good idea to ask a trainer to help you use the balance equipment.

SLIDE BOARD

A slide board is available at most health facilities or fitness stores. It is an approximately 8-foot piece of plastic on which you slide back and forth in a motion similar to skating. It helps establish balance, provides you with a great exercise in decelerating the body to accelerating the body, as well as improves hip, buttock, and groin strength.

BODY BLADE

A body blade is a piece of graphite metal shaped like a bow, with small weights at each end. It can be oscillated while balancing on one leg or on various equipment (see Figure 13).

HOMEMADE BALANCE EQUIPMENT

You can make balance challenge equipment at home and shake it vigorously in multiple directions while standing on one or both feet, on a foam roll, on a rock, or on a log.

- Partially fill two canning jars with beans or rice, and hold one in each hand and shake them.
- Fill a beach ball with 16–64 ounces of water and shake it vigorously side to side and front to back.
- Half fill a 2-liter plastic bottle with water and shake it.

FUNCTIONAL VS. NON-FUNCTIONAL EXERCISE

Muscles do three basic things:

1. They decelerate or slow down the body (and its joints) against the pull of gravity.
2. They stabilize the body.
3. They accelerate the body (and its joints) against gravity.

The body has three basic planes of motion: the *sagittal plane* (forward-backward movements), *frontal plane* (sideways movements), and *transverse plane* (rotation movements). All joints and muscles have some component of movement in all three planes. Some joints and muscles are dominant in one plane versus another, but they all move three-dimensionally. This is called *triplanar motion*.

Function is a combination of motions in one or more joints at the same time. Performing an exercise within three planes of motion can make it more functional and true to real life.

FROM THE WEIGHT ROOM TO THE WORLD: WHAT MUSCLES REALLY DO

The functional demands of your outdoor activity relate to the following factors:

- the movement patterns and the planes of motion of your trunk, arms, and legs
- the postures you must maintain
- the load you are carrying
- balance and coordination requirements
- the endurance requirements of muscles used
- closed-chain vs. open-chain requirements of the muscles and joints
- the speed and power of the motion
- the combination of movements of your body regions

It is important to view the body as an interlocking chain, each link dependent upon the others. *Closed-chain* activity is when the end segment (i.e., foot or hand) of the chain is fixed to a relatively stable surface, i.e., the ground or a wall. *Open-chain* movement is when the end segment is not fixed to a stable surface. Lower-body muscles usually function with the foot fixed to the ground, a closed-chain movement, while the upper-extremity muscles function primarily with the limb free of the ground or other surface, an open-chain movement. The upper extremity is used in closed-chain movements during climbing, scrambling, cycling, windsurfing, skiing, and snowshoeing.

A weakness in a link may affect the rest of the chain. Muscle performance in the upper extremity and trunk depends on the muscle function of the lower extremity, and therefore are interrelated. For example, a traditional exercise to strengthen the shoulders might be a barbell overhead press in a sitting or standing position, or sitting in a machine with a controlled fixed load. Traditionally, we are taught to stabilize the trunk of the body and press the load straight overhead using only arms and shoulders. In real life, if you were loading a bicycle onto the top of the car, you would use your whole body, including your ankles, knees, hips, back, and shoulders, to push the load overhead. In function, the shoulder is usually dependent on the opposite leg and hip. If you do not train your hip extensors (gluteals) with overhead shoulder presses, and direct these presses in different planes, you are failing to train a very important part of your body for this functional movement. Some of your exercises should work combinations of body regions.

When looking at an outdoor activity, it is helpful to decide what is the most challenging or difficult movement you will have to do. A exercise can then be done or designed around that challenge.

FUNCTIONAL SELF-TESTS

You can test yourself on functional strength and balance with some very simple tests. Try Exercises 37.1–37.3 and 38. How far did you reach with your left foot as compared to your right foot? Was there any pain? Are there directions of motion with your leg or arm reach that feel unstable or less symmetrical? Do you feel wobbly or unsure? How strong do your abdominal muscles feel in their ability to control motion? How strong does your thigh and hip region feel in controlling motion after a set of 12? Try Exercises 23 and 24. Can you do multiple lunges, flexed enough to simulate your activity needs, with good spine position and without knee wobbling or pain? Try Exercise 31 without the overhead press (also see Exercise 73). How far can you confidently step up and down without knee pain or wobbling? How well can you control the motion, especially toward the end of the set?

These are good exercises for self-testing, but any of the functional exercises can be used. Most people find that they cannot initially transfer their strength on machines to functional exercises, and that they are sore in their buttocks and thighs for the first week after beginning a functional exercise program. Don't get discouraged by your initial performance on these self-tests. You will definitely improve quickly if you practice these exercises.

FUNCTIONAL EXERCISE GUIDELINES

- Always begin workouts with a proper aerobic warm-up to increase the core muscle temperature.
- Do functional exercises before your individual machine exercises.
- Practice each exercise slowly, to get the movement pattern and balance down, before increasing speed.
- Exercise in sets of 4–6 repetitions initially to get the form and movement pattern, then gradually increase to 12–15.
- Consider increasing the speed to see how many you can do within a 30- to 60-second period, especially if speed is important in your activity.
- Do them without resistance or with low resistance (weights, pulleys, or tubing) before you increase resistance.
- Do any standing exercises successfully with two feet on the ground and equal weight distribution before challenging your balance and working one side of your body more than the other.
- In some exercises, challenge your balance by placing more weight on one leg than the other, progressing to a toe touch and then only one foot on the ground. You may have to decrease the resistance you are using when doing an exercise on one leg. You will likely be able to do fewer reps in a particular time if you are doing an exercise on one leg only.
- Try the variations to see which exercise challenges you the most and works the best for you.
- For some of the exercises, you can vary the environment. After you have done them indoors and have the movements down, try them outdoors on hills, logs, or rocks. This is especially important within 2–4 weeks of your activity.

- Breathe properly.
- Exercise in strong, pain-free directions before exercising in weak planes.
- Don't do a particular exercise if you feel pain or significant weakness.
- Modify the exercises related to any injuries you have or based on your knowledge of the body region or your functional needs. You may initially want to try an exercise with much less range of motion to feel comfortable with it.
- Use good footwear with orthotic supports, if necessary.
- Train with a partner to improve the challenge and increase your motivation.

WORKOUT FREQUENCY AND INTEGRATION OF FUNCTIONAL EXERCISES

How often you train depends on the workout you choose and your goals. You can accomplish most functional strength goals with 2–3 periods of training per week of each muscle group. Two training sessions per muscle group per week is enough to maintain a level of strength, while 3–5 are needed to boost performance. You could decide to do all of your strength exercises on one day or split them up by body regions (lower extremity one day and upper extremity another day). You can do your functional exercises on the same day as you do other exercises, such as machine exercises (in which case, you should do them before your machine exercises). This is because most functional exercises use larger muscles and may incorporate challenges to balance. You don't want to be too fatigued before doing them, so you can maintain your form and avoid injury.

Whichever you choose, rest a minimum of 48 hours and not more than 96 hours between workouts of the same muscle groups.

FUNCTIONAL EXERCISES

There are many functional exercises in the body region chapters of Part II as well as in this chapter.

FUNCTIONAL EXERCISES WITH FREE WEIGHTS

These are shoulder, hip, and leg combination exercises. The terms *free weights* and *dumbbells* are different names for the same type of weight equipment that is held in one hand. Because there is a wide range of weight that people can manage, specific weights are given only for exercises of particular shoulder muscles in which excessive weight can lead to injury.

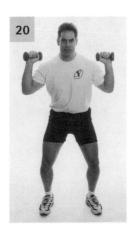

20 | **X-Combo**

Equipment: 2- to 5-pound free weights.
Purpose: Strengthen your leg, trunk, shoulder, and arm muscles in the same fashion you use them in activities that involve reaching overhead.

Technique: Start in a standing position with your knees bent slightly and your feet shoulder-width apart, with your elbows flexed to

about 90 degrees and your hands at about the height of your ears or top of your shoulders. Start with a light free weight in each hand, and reach for the ceiling with your left hand while pushing off from your left leg and left buttock. Elevate your left shoulder, extend your left elbow, and shift your weight over your right leg. With your right arm and hand, reach for the floor and side-bend your trunk to the right. Repeat this movement on the opposite side, bending your knees in transition. Do one set of 12–15 repetitions and progress to 2–3 sets.
Variation: 20.1. Balance on one leg with your knee slightly bent. Reach

one arm toward the ceiling and the opposite arm toward the floor, and alternate. You can do this with unequal weights to challenge your balance. After 30 seconds, switch legs and repeat for 30 seconds. This works your hips and challenges your balance.

Precautions: Inappropriate weight of free weights causes abnormal compensation patterns in the spine and shoulders. Start light and determine what your muscle endurance is for this movement.

21 Rotational Punches at Shoulder Height

Equipment: 3- to 5-pound free weights.
Purpose: Maintain the rotation in your spine.

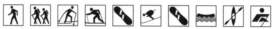
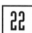

Technique: Do Exercise 19 with a free weight in each hand. Perform 2–3 sets of 15–30 repetitions.

Tips and Precautions: You can punch as far as your spine can rotate after you have done it well to the 10:00 o'clock and 2:00 o'clock range. This exercise should initially be done in a slow and controlled manner with light free weights so as not to injure your spine or shoulders. Increase the speed gradually and be cautious if you have a shoulder or back problem.

22 The Monkey

Equipment: 1- to 3-pound free weights.
Purpose: Strengthen the leg, trunk, shoulder, and arm muscles in combination with a mini-squat in the same fashion you would use them in activities that involve overhead reaching.

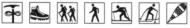

Technique: Stand with your feet shoulder-width apart, slightly bent knees, a free weight in each hand, arms resting in front of your thighs, palms down. As you extend your knees, elevate one arm overhead. Lower the arm as you return to the squat position, and repeat the movement with the opposite arm. Perform 2–3 sets of 12–15 repetitions.

Variations: 22.1. As your strength and coordination improve, try this exercise with a deeper squat. 22.2. Add lunges forward and from side to side. 22.3. For telemark skiing and snowshoeing, try a walking lunge (continuous) uphill or on a level surface with the alternate shoulder motions, and with ankle weights to simulate the resistance of skis or snowshoes. 22.4. For a balance challenge, do the basic exercise starting from a single-leg mini-squat; do 10–12 reps and switch legs.

Precautions: Inappropriate weight of free weights can cause compensations and pain in the low back, shoulders, and neck. Use low weight at first and gradually increase. Don't do this exercise if you have shoulder pain with the motion without a hand weight.

LUNGES WITH ARM AND SHOULDER CHALLENGES

You can do any lunge in place, or move around on a surface in a walking lunge. You can also do lunges on hills to increase the challenge. See Exercise 72 for the basic lunge technique.

23 | Forward Lunge with a Biceps Curl

Equipment: Free weights.

Purpose: Strengthen leg, trunk, and arm muscles that are involved with controlling lunging movements in the forward direction. Add challenges to your balance and strengthen your spine. Save time by combining biceps curls with lunges.

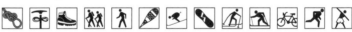

Technique: Grasp a pair of hand weights and position them at your sides. Lunge in a forward direction with one leg, while flexing the opposite elbow and curling the weight to the shoulder. Return to standing. Repeat the movement with the opposite leg and arm. Perform 2–3 sets of 12–15 repetitions.

Variations: 23.1. Curl the elbow on the same side as the lunging leg. 23.2. Vary the amount of flexing of the lunge knee. 23.3. Start with both elbows flexed and lower them simultaneously as you lunge on one leg, especially if you want to save time or to strengthen your back. Your forearm and hand position can vary at the bottom of the lunge. Initially try lunging with your fist and palms facing forward. Progress to ending with your palms facing inward (toward the midline of your body) and, eventually, ending with your palms facing to the rear. Changing the position and direction of your hands during the lunge will incorporate an important

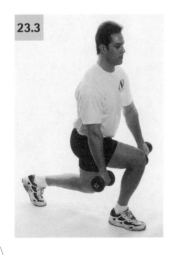

23.3

function of the biceps (supination). 23.4. Do a simultaneous curl with both hands starting at your side while you lunge, for less stress on your back as well as to save time.

24 | Anterior Lunge with Opposite Knee Reach

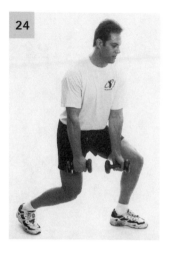

Equipment: Free weights.
Purpose: Strengthen leg, trunk, shoulder, and arm muscles involved with lunging leg movements, with a weight/gravity challenge toward the midline of the body. This is good for skiers, especially telemark and cross-country.

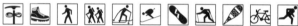

Technique: Stand with weights in each hand and your hands at waist height, with the weights pointing up in the air. Your knees should be just slightly bent and within 2–4 inches of each other. Lunge forward with the left leg while bringing the weights above your right knee. Your spine will rotate to the right slightly. Try to keep your left knee pointing forward, and use the muscles of your leg and hip to keep it from rotating inward. Go back to the starting position and repeat the lunge with the same knee, or do the lunge with the opposite knee. Increase the weight of the hand weights to increase the challenge of the exercise. Perform 2–3 sets of 12–15 repetitions.
Variation: 24.1. If you are a telemark skier, try holding the position long enough to simulate a turn.
Precautions: Do this slowly at first to develop control and decrease the stress on your knees.

25 | Anterior Lunge with Opposite Shoulder/Arm Elevation

Equipment: Free weights.
Purpose: Strengthen leg, trunk, arm, and neck muscles that enable you to lunge forward while elevating your arms, such as when lunging to place an ice ax or to secure a hold.

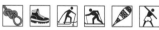

Technique: Stand with both feet pointing in the same direction. Start with your arms next to your side with your elbows extended. Lunge forward with your right leg. Elevate your left arm (raise it in front of you) to shoulder height. Then repeat on the opposite side. Perform 2 sets of 12–15 repetitions.

Variations: 25.1. Elevate your arm on the same side as your lunging leg. 25.2 Elevate both your arms and shoulders simultaneously.
Precautions: Do this slowly at first to develop control and decrease the stress on your knees.

26 | Lunge Matrix/Combos

Equipment: 3- to 15-pound free weights.
Purpose: Increase your entire body's strength, coordination, and endurance in multiple directions. Integrate every body region by incorporating lunging, reaching, bending, twisting, and lifting overhead in combination.

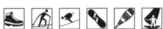

Technique: Stand inside a giant imaginary clock, with 12:00 located directly in front of you, 6:00 directly behind you, and 3:00 and 9:00 to your right and left, respectively. These are the directions for each sequence of the lunge matrix. After each lunge, return to the start position with your feet close to each other, standing in the center of the imaginary clock and facing the 12:00 position. Each time you perform a lunge, reach the hand weights toward the lunge foot. This will require you to bend your hips, knees, and mid back as you reach for the lunge foot.

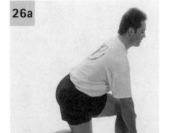

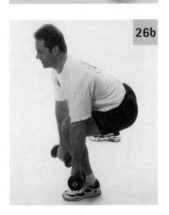

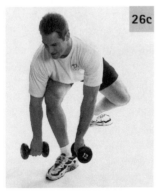

   Start the first sequence with your hand weights at hip height. Lunge with your right foot toward 12:00 while reaching the hand weights toward your right foot (26a). If this is too difficult, reach the weights to knee height (see Exercise 23.3, above). Once you have lunged and reached to a safe level, return to the start position, or center of the giant clock, with your hand weights returned to hip height. Repeat this lunge maneuver in the same direction with your left leg, again reaching your hand weights toward your left foot, then return to the start position in the center of the clock. Once you have completed three lunges and reaches, performed alternately on each leg, you are ready to change directions.

   The next sequence is performed with a side-to-side motion. Stand in the center of the clock with your hand weights at hip height, and lunge toward 3:00 with your right leg while reaching the hand weights toward your right foot (26b). Once you have lunged and reached to a safe level, return to the start position in the center of the clock. Repeat the same lunge maneuver with your left leg lunging toward 9:00 while reaching your hand weights toward your left foot. Perform three lunges to each direction, alternately. With each lunge, return to the upright position in the center of the clock.

For the third sequence, position yourself in the center of the giant clock and locate 5:00 (to your right and slightly behind you) and 7:00 (to your left and slightly behind you). Start by lunging toward 5:00 with your right foot while pointing the toes of your right foot at the 5:00 position. Remember to pivot on your left foot so that you don't hurt your knee (26c). Again, during your lunge, reach your hand weights toward your right foot, bending your knees, hips, and back. Once you have lunged and reached to a safe range, return to the start position in the center of the clock and face the 12:00 position. Repeat this lunge-and-reach maneuver toward 7:00 with your left foot while pointing your left toes toward the 7:00 position. Perform 3 alternate lunges and reaches in each direction for all 3 variations. This is considered 1 set. Start with 1 set and work up to 2–3 sets over 2–3 weeks.

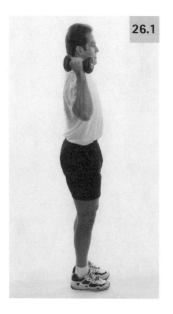

26.1

Variations: Progress to each variation in the order given here. Each variation is more difficult than the previous one. 26.1. Start with your hand weights at shoulder height. Do Exercise 26 as described above. Make sure that when you return to the start position in the center of the clock, the hand weights return to shoulder height. This variation incorporates your arm and shoulder flexors and adds additional loads to your legs and back. 26.2. Start as before, facing the 12:00 position. Extend your arms and hold the hand weights overhead. Perform the same sequence of lunge and reach. When reaching toward the lunge foot, allow the hand weights to pass close to your chest on the way toward the floor and upon your return to the start position. 26.3. Try an assortment of arm movements during your lunge and reach. For instance, when reaching toward the lunge foot with your hand weights, turn the hand weights so that your knuckles are facing each other at the bottom of the lunge. Then return to the start position, turning the hand weights so that your palms are facing each other. During the second-sequence side-to-side lunge and reach, raise the hand weights out to your sides so that they are at shoulder height when you are in the center of the clock, then reach the hand weights toward the lunge foot as usual.

Tips and Precautions: The start position for this exercise is always in the center of the clock while you face the 12:00 position. Make sure to use your knees during the lunge. Do not overtax your back by bending too far at your waist. If you have a history of low-back, knee, or shoulder problems, move in a pain-free range of motion in the direction you are lunging and reaching. Stick with the main exercise rather than the variations if you have any unresolved injuries. Lunge only in pain free-ranges. Do not lunge to low positions if your kneecap area is hurting. Use lighter weights, especially when first trying this and for variations 26.1 and 26.2.

27 | Lawnmower Pulls to a Row or an External Rotation

Equipment: Free weights.

Purpose: Exercise all the pulling muscles of the legs, trunk, upper extremity, and neck that help you pull or lift an object off the ground. Also help with balance and buttock strength, and with co-ordination of combined shoulder and hip movements.

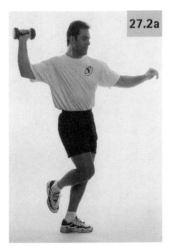

27.2a

Technique: Stand in a forward stride position with your left knee forward and slightly bent and your right knee back and almost extended; stand on the toes of the back leg. Hold a free weight in your right hand at about waist height. Lower the weight toward the left foot, to about midway between your left foot and left knee, while flexing your left knee, hips, and back slightly. Pull the weight back to your waist while extending your front knee and return to the starting position. Your trunk rotates slightly as you pinch the shoulder blade of the pulling arm back and extend the shoulder. The movement resembles that of someone starting a lawnmower. Perform 2–3 sets of 12–15 repetitions.

Variations: 27.1. Try this exercise with a shoulder external rotator motion instead of a row motion, to exercise your rotator cuff. End up with your arm horizontal to the ground, your elbow flexed to 90 degrees, and your hand gripping the weight, pointing straight up in the air. This is the starting position. If your shoulder will not easily move into a position with the weight pointing directly vertical, rotate it only as far as it will comfortably go. 27.2. To improve balance and strengthen your buttocks, try 27 or 27.1 while balancing on the front leg completely, or just placing minimal weight on your back foot for balance.

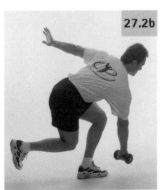

27.2b

Tips: Keep the majority of weight on the forward leg. Start this exercise by reaching with the weight to your knee before progressing to your shin or ankle. Start the exercise with 3–5 reps until you feel confident with the movement pattern.

STANDING ROW/LATISSIMUS EXERCISES

These exercises are done to strengthen the shoulder region in pulling, rowing, and rotational patterns. When doing these with tubing, make sure the tubing is securely attached. Start with lower resistance when using pulleys or smaller-diameter tubing.

28 Double-arm Combination Row Squat

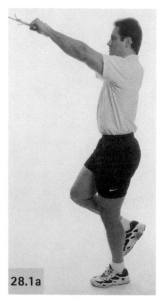

28.1a

Equipment: Resistance tubing, cord, or pulley.

Purpose: Strengthen muscles associated with pulling/rowing movements in the legs, trunk, shoulders, arms, and neck. This can be helpful for paddlers as a substitute for dynamic bentover rowing machines if a gym is unavailable.

       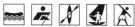

Technique: Tie a large knot in the center of resistance tubing or cord and attach it on top of a closed door. You can also use a pulley. Stand with your feet at slightly more than shoulder-width apart. Grab each end of the tubing or cord (or pulley handles) and move into a squat position so that your elbows are relatively straight (extended) and are at eye level at the start. Pull the tubing (or pulleys) to your chest with both hands simultaneously as you straighten both knees. Your hands should start in a palm-down position when your elbows are extended, and finish in a thumb-up position as your elbows flex, thus bringing your hands to your chest. Perform 2–3 sets of 12–15 repetitions.

Variation: 28.1. Grasp the tubing so that your arms are straight and elbows at eye level. Back away from the door until you feel tension in the resistance tubing or cord. Balance on your left leg (you may wish to assist your balance by toe touching with your right foot) (28.1a). Simultaneously pull the tubing toward your chest and perform a single-leg squat (28.1b). Return to the single-leg balanced position while straightening your arms.

Tips: The pulley or tubing can be attached in a low, middle, or high position. Securing the tubing or pulley at waist height is better for the crew athlete. Securing the tubing or pulley in a more overhead position is better for the climbing athlete. Both positions are beneficial for the windsurfer.

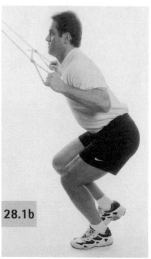

28.1b

29 | Single-arm Pulley Rows

Equipment: Resistance tubing, cord, or pulley.

Purpose: Improve flexibility of and strengthen muscles associated with rotational pulling movements in the legs, trunk, shoulders, arms, and neck, especially if you don't have access to a gym or have back problems.

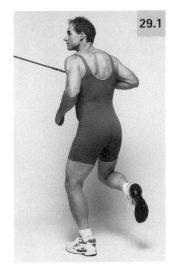

29.1

Technique: Start as in Exercise 28 but with only one hand on the tubing. Pull the tubing or pulley handle to your chest with one hand. The hand should start in a palm-down position with the elbow extended, and finish in a thumb-up position with the elbow flexed, thus bringing your hand to your chest. You can do this with very little or a lot of spine rotation. For water sports (especially kayaking, sweep rowing, and canoeing), do it with a moderate amount of spine rotation. Perform 2–3 sets of 12–15 repetitions.

Variations: 29.1. Start by standing on your left leg with your knee slightly bent. Pull down with your right arm as you extend your left knee. Do this 10–12 times, then switch your standing leg. 29.2. Pull down with the arm on the same side as the extending knee. 29.3. Change the angle of the tubing or pulley to simulate different angles of climbing holds. 29.4. Face 90 degrees away from the original start position, holding the tubing so it crosses your chest when performing the row motion.

Tips: The pulley can be attached in a low, middle, or high position. Your head can be pointed straight ahead or at your hand. The pulling motion can be performed with or without a squatting motion of the legs.

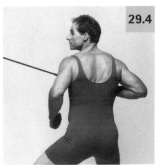

29.4

30 | Standing Latissimus (Lat) Pull-down

Equipment: Lat bar and lat machine.

Purpose: Train your lats, buttocks, and legs together and challenge your standing balance.

Technique: Stand in a squat position with your feet shoulder-width apart, in front of a lat pull-down machine. Hold the ends of the lat bar and pull the bar to your chest at the same time that you are straightening your knees and pushing off with your buttocks. Use a light amount of weight, definitely less than you would use in a sitting lat pull-down. Do 1–2 sets of 8–12 reps.

Variation: 30.1. When you can do this easily with both legs on the ground, do it with only one leg on the ground, for a balance challenge. (For starting position, see 30.1a; for ending position, see 30.1b.) Do a set of 10–12 reps on one leg, then alternate to the other leg.

Precaution: This advanced exercise should be avoided by anyone with neck, low back, or shoulder problems.

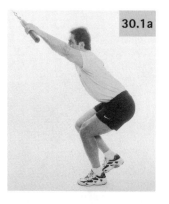

30.1a

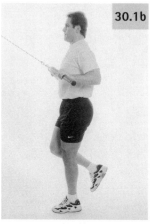

30.1b

STEP-UP ARM/LEG COMBO EXERCISES

These exercises strengthen and coordinate the step-up motion with arm/shoulder motions (including pushing and pulling). These are especially good for climbing, backcountry skiing, and snowshoeing.

31 | Anterior Step-up with Overhead Shoulder Press

Equipment: 6- to 12-inch step, free weights.
Purpose: Improve the strength of muscles in the knees and hips used to climb hills and rocks, and increase the strength of trunk, shoulder, and arm muscles used for pushing loads overhead. Also increase balance and coordination for hiking.

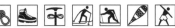

Technique: Standing 6 inches from a 6-inch-high step, with free weights held at your side, step forward up onto the step with one leg and straighten your knee while pressing the weights overhead, and then bring your opposite foot up. Then step down with the same leg that initiated the step up, lower the weights, and return the opposite leg to the initial starting position. Repeat the same sequence of steps so that the same leg always leads stepping up and down. Perform 2–3 sets of 12–15 repetitions, then switch to the opposite leg.

Variations: 31.1. Do this exercise with the nonstepping hip and knee rising in a flexing fashion in the air in front of you, with or without an ankle weight. The ankle weight is helpful to simulate the weight of backcountry skies, snowshoes, or heavy boots. 31.2. Do Exercise 31 with an arm elevation (raising a straight arm in front of your body to an overhead position), which is better for telemark skiers, instead of a press up. 31.3. Do Exercise 31 to either side as a sidestep instead of a forward step. This is good for cross-country skiers or climbers.

Tips: Step height can be varied depending on your strength and needs to do higher stepping in your activity. Climbers, scramblers, and glacier mountaineers should work with progressively increasing step heights. Start with a 6-inch step and work your way up to 12–14 inches (or higher).

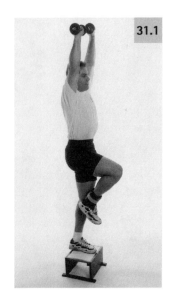

31.1

32 | Anterior Step-up with Resisted Shoulder Extension

Equipment: 6-inch step, resistance tubing or pulley.

Purpose: Improve the strength of muscles in the knees and hips used to climb hills and rocks, and increase the strength of trunk, shoulder, and arm muscles used for pulling down as in climbing. Also increase balance and coordination for hiking and climbing.

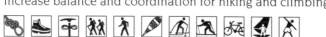

Technique: Standing 6 inches from a 6-inch-high step, and holding two ends of resistance tubing (or a pulley) in each hand overhead or at shoulder height, step forward up on to the step with one leg (32a) while pulling the resistance tubing backward behind the waist. Then step up with the opposite leg (32b). Then step down with the same leg that initiated the step up. Allow your arms to return to the original position, with hands over your shoulders, and return the opposite leg to the initial starting position. Repeat the same sequence of steps so that the same leg always leads stepping up and down. After a set, switch the leading leg. Perform 2–3 sets of 12–15 repetitions, then change the leading leg.

Tips and Precautions: This is a good simulation for scrambling and climbing. Step height can be varied depending on strength and your activity demands. The angle of the tubing or pulley can be varied to better simulate your activity. If you increase the step height or the resistance of the tubing, slow down the exercise and decrease the number of reps.

Variations: 32.1. Try this exercise with one leg and one arm, especially if you are a climber. Start by holding the tubing with your right shoulder and arm in an elevated or close to overhead position, to simulate a reach for a climbing hold. Step up on your left leg and straighten your left knee at the same time as you pull down with your right arm. Do this 12 times, then switch legs and arms. You can also do the same-side leg and arm. 32.2. For cyclists, have your handholds in cycling positions and the direction of the tubing at waist height.

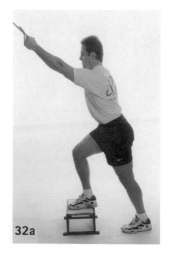

32a

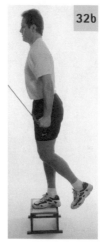

32b

SITTING BALANCE PULLING AND PUSHING EXERCISES

These exercises enhance sitting balance and strengthen muscles used in pulling and pushing for water sports. When preparing for canoeing, sit with your feet slightly ahead of your knees. When preparing for kayaking, sit with your knees slightly bent as if in a kayak. When preparing for crew, sit on the floor with your knees bent and, if possible, sit on a plastic bag or something that will allow you to slide as you extend your knees when you pull back.

33 | Make Your Own Erg

Equipment: Resistance tubing, cord, or pulleys, and/or 4-foot wooden dowel or kayak paddle; ball or chair.

Purpose: Strengthen muscles associated with pulling movements in the trunk, shoulders, arms, and neck. Do this for aerobic training if you are unable to get out on the water.

Technique: Attach the center of resistance tubing or cord to a door, or use a pulley. Grab each end of the tubing (or pulley handles), or attach the ends to a paddle or a dowel. While sitting on a ball, on a chair, or on the ground, pull the tubing to your chest in a rowing type of motion with both hands (for crew), or simulate a kayak or canoe stroke. Try doing it at first with both feet firmly on the ground, then try it with only your toes touching the ground. Do this with lower-resistance tubing for 20–30 minutes.

Tips and Precautions: The tubing or pulley should be attached below waist height, where you would expect the water level to be. Be careful to balance, and keep your feet on the ground.

34 │ Single-arm Pulley Pushes While Sitting

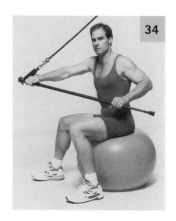

Equipment: Resistance tubing, cord, or pulley, and/or 4-foot wooden dowel or kayak paddle; ball or chair.
Purpose: Improve the strength of muscles associated with rotational pushing movements in the legs, trunk, shoulders, arms, and neck.

Technique: Attach the end of resistance tubing or cord to a door and the other end of the cord to a paddle. Sitting on a ball or chair facing away from the attachment of the resistive tubing, reproduce the same pushing motion you use in kayaking or canoeing. Perform 2 sets of 20–30 repetitions. Switch hand positions after each set.

35 │ Push-pull Double-arm Pulley Rows While Sitting

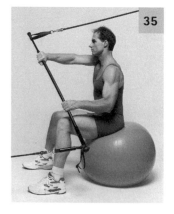

Equipment: Resistance tubing, cord, or pulleys, and/or 4-foot wooden dowel or kayak paddle; ball or chair.
Purpose: Strengthen muscles associated with rotational pushing and pulling movements in the legs, trunk, shoulders, arms, and neck associated with kayaking.

Technique: For canoeing training, attach one larger-gauge piece of resistance tubing or cord to a door in front of you and fix the other end to the neck of a paddle or dowel. Attach a smaller-gauge piece of resistance tubing or cord to a door or solid object behind you and fix the other end to the paddle grip. For kayaking training, use two pieces of equal-gauge cord and attach the free ends to the opposite ends of the paddle shaft or a dowel. Sit on a ball or chair with your knees only slightly bent. Emphasize the push-pull motion of kayaking on the tubing (photo 35 shows the mid-range position). Switch the resistance cord to the other ends of the paddle after you fatigue, and exercise the opposite side. Allow your torso to rotate during this exercise. Perform 2 sets of 20–30 repetitions in 30–60 seconds.

BODYWEIGHT PROLONGED-POSITION EXERCISE

This type of exercise is designed to improve your ability to hold knee and hip flexing positions for prolonged periods of time, as would be required in skiing or climbing activities.

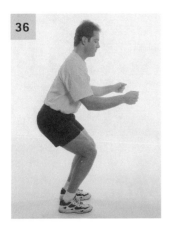

36 | Skier/Climber/Cyclist/Windsurfer Position Holds

Equipment: None.

Purpose: Strengthen the quads, hamstrings, and gluteal muscles in skiing, climbing, and windsurfing positions. Consider doing these within 1 month of starting your activity.

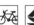

Technique: Ski position: Stand in a squat position and position your arms and hands as if you were holding poles. Keep your back from flexing excessively. Hold this position for 30 seconds at first and try to gradually work your way up to 2–3 minutes. If you can only hold it for 30 seconds before fatiguing, then try to return to this position 5 or more times for 30 seconds.

Variations: 36.1. When you get into the skiing position, try slightly dropping down into your knees (flexing), then slightly extending them in a rhythmical pattern (bouncing) as if skiing. Also try weight-shifting from your left to your right leg rhythmically. 36.2. Try this on a foam half roll (flat side up). 36.3. For cross-country skiing, try

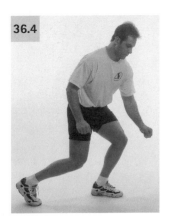

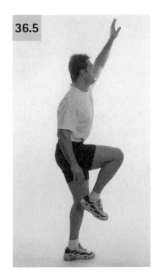

getting into a turning position and try weight-shifting from your right to your left leg. 36.4. For telemark skiing, try all of the above in a telemark position (a lunge). When in the telemark position with your right foot in front, move your hands and rotate your trunk toward your left knee for 10 seconds, then go back to the starting position. After 60 seconds, reverse your leg position. 36.5. For climbing, assume a position on a climbing wall or against a regular wall with legs farther than shoulder-width apart. Try your feet in various positions, including parallel or perpendicular to the wall. Put your hands at varying heights. From this position, try weight-shifting from foot to foot or slight bobbing motions in your knees. This could also be done in a gym while holding two overhead pulleys at different heights above your head and with different weight resistance. You can also do the climber's variation while standing on a foam roll. 36.6. For cycling, get into a lunge position as if you are on a bike going down a hill. Bounce slightly in this position for about 30–45 seconds. 36.7. For windsurfing, get into your board position. From there try weight-shifting from your left to right foot with a rhythmical side-to-side squat.

Precautions: This exercise can aggravate kneecap pain problems.

BALANCE EXERCISES

These exercises are designed to challenge your standing balance and to increase the strength of your trunk, buttock, and leg region. In addition, try outdoor balance exercises in chapter 8, and balance Exercises 62 and 63.

37 | Arm and Leg Balance and Reach

Equipment: None.

Purpose: Emphasize balance and strengthening of the gluteal and hamstring muscles, posterior trunk, abdominals, shoulders, arms, and neck.

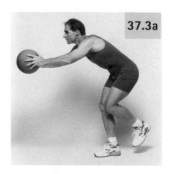

37.3a

Technique: Start with your feet shoulder-width apart and your knees slightly bent. Position your hands in front of your body and at waist height with your elbows straight. Start your forward reach by bending at your hips, keeping your back slightly arched. Reach forward approximately 6 inches, then return to your start position. Keep your reaches pain-free and move with good control. To monitor your progress, assume your starting position, with your fingertips touching a wall. While maintaining this position, back up 6 inches from the wall without changing your posture. Reach and touch your fingertips to the wall. As you become more successful at this distance, increase the speed of your reach before increasing the distance. You can also hold a ball while performing this exercise. Try 5–10 reps initially, then progress to 1–2 sets of 12–15 repetitions.

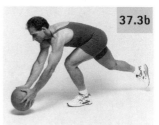

37.3b

Variations: 37.1. Reach not only forward but also at 45 degrees to the right and then to the left. 37.2. Stand on one leg with your knee slightly bent, approximately 1–1½ feet from a wall; reach overhead

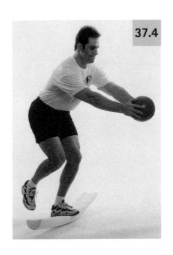

37.4

and touch the wall at imaginary 12:00, 10:00, and 2:00 o'clock positions. Do 12–15 touches and then switch the standing leg. 37.3. Try Exercise 37 while balancing on one leg with your knee slightly bent (37.3a). You can start with your other leg behind you for counterbalance, but then progress to placing your raised foot next to your standing foot. Try reaching down toward the floor with a ball or weight (37.3b). Switch to your other foot after 30–60 seconds. If you have had knee problems, do this with a bent knee. 37.4. Try doing Exercise 37 while standing on both feet or with one foot on a foam half roll.

Tips and Precautions: Start with no resistance and control your body weight first. Avoid this exercise if you have a back problem, unless you are supervised by a physical therapist or a physician.

38 | Clock Leg Reach

Equipment: None.
Purpose: Emphasize balance and strengthen the gluteal, hamstring, and trunk muscles. This is a good, basic balance drill.

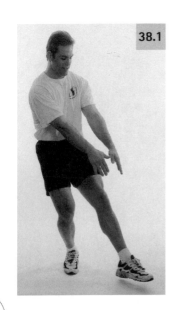

38.1

Technique: Make believe you are in the center of a large clock. Balance on your left leg and bend your knee slightly. Initiate a single leg squat with your standing leg, squatting enough to touch the toes of your other foot to the 10:00 position; do 2 mini-squats and toe touches. Then do the same at the 11:00 position, and then touch around the clock until your right foot gets to the 7:00 position. After you have mastered the basic exercise, try placing your toe touch randomly to do quick directional changes. For example, try this sequence: 12:00, 4:00, 11:00, 5:00, 1:00, 7:00. For an extra challenge, have a partner call positions out randomly. Switch to standing on your right leg and repeat the sequence in the opposite direction. Each time around the clock on a leg is 1 set. Perform 2–3 sets on each leg.

Variations: 38.1. To make this more challenging, add a reaching motion with both of your arms in the same direction as the motion of your toe-touching foot. 38.2. Reach with a free weight or medicine ball to increase the challenge. 38.3. Do this exercise while standing on a foam half roll.

Tips: Progress this exercise initially by increasing the speed and randomness of your toe touch before increasing the distance. Add the arm reach when you feel comfortable with the random toe touching.

39 | Single-leg Stance Upper-extremity Chopping Pattern

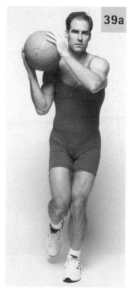

Equipment: Medicine ball or free weight.

Purpose: Emphasize balance and strengthening of your leg, trunk, shoulders, and neck.

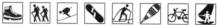

Technique: Balance on your left leg with your knee slightly bent. Hold a medicine ball or a free weight above your right shoulder (for starting position, see photo 39a), and move it toward your left hip (see photo 39b) and then back to an overhead position. Stabilize your spine with the movement by tightening your abdominals and minimize the amount of spinal movement. After doing a set of 12–15 reps, repeat the sequence but start with the weight over your left shoulder while standing on your right leg and bring it to your right hip. As you become familiar with this exercise, you can incorporate more spine and hip motion. After doing 12–15 reps on one leg, switch to standing on the other leg.

Variations: 39.1. Try bringing your right hip and knee toward your hands. Do this with an ankle weight to increase your hip flexion work, for climbing, telemark skiing, and snowshoeing. For water sports, do this sitting in an appropriate position without moving your hips.

Tips: This exercise is designed to improve your balance, so try to avoid contacting the ground with the opposite foot.

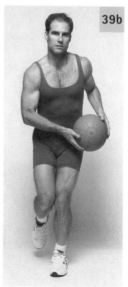

40 | Single-leg Ball Toss

Equipment: Small to medium-sized lightweight ball.
Purpose: Challenge your balance quickly and in multiple directions.

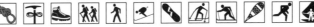

Technique: Stand on one foot with your knee slightly bent (40a.) If you have a partner, ask him or her to throw you the ball, initially directly to you at your chest level (40b). Catch the ball with both hands. When this is easy and you are not too wobbly, ask your partner to throw the ball to you anywhere in a half circle from 9:00 to 3:00 o'clock (40c). You can do this exercise by yourself by throwing the ball against a wall.

Variation: 40.1. For an increased challenge, stand on a half foam roll or ankle balance equipment as found in health clubs.

Precautions: Be careful with this exercise if you have had a knee injury. Don't rotate excessively on a fixed foot to catch the ball. Always feel free to put your other foot down if the ball is thrown poorly.

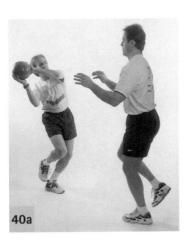

40a

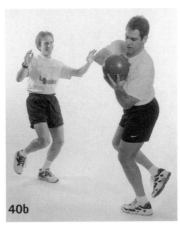

40b

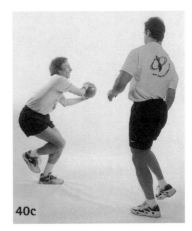

40c

41 Sitting Ball Toss

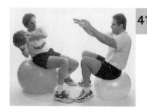

41a

Equipment: Physioball to sit on, small ball or medicine ball to throw.
Purpose: Improve sitting balance and strengthen your abdominals for boat and cycling activities.

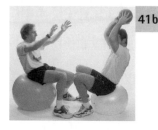

41b

Technique: Sit on a physioball with your toes just touching the ground. Face a partner or the wall (41a). Throw the ball in multiple directions to your partner so that he or she has to move forward, to the side, or overhead to catch it (41b and 41c). Try to keep a minimum amount of weight on your toes. To increase the challenge, catch the ball with both hands.

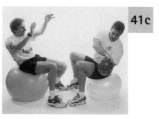

41c

DESIGNING YOUR OWN FUNCTIONAL EXERCISES

Believe it or not, all of the exercises that you could be doing have not already been designed or written about. Exercises can be individually designed for you, or for groups of people who do your activity, based on the demands of your activity. The number of exercise variations are endless if you follow a few basic rules:

- Analyze your most difficult activity movement challenges.
- Try a functional movement that simulates a part or all of the movement.
- Combine body regions that you will use together in your activity (think in terms of what your shoulders/hands and thighs/legs will be doing).
- Perform the motion slowly to learn the movement pattern before increasing the speed.
- Practice safe spine technique.
- Add resistance with weights and tubing or pulleys after you have done the exercise without resistance for a number of sets.

Functional exercises are practical, creative, and fun. The key is to look at the type of functional activity you are trying to train for, and the type of movements required to accomplish this task. Then you can break the task down into components of movement and test yourself to determine the thresholds of how far and well you can move in these components of movement, and then expand these thresholds with training. Many exercises are provided here, and they indicate which activities they are good for. In addition, the activity chapters in Part III combine functional exercises with conventional exercises in strength programs.

Body Posture and Movement Patterns
An Aston-Patterning® Approach

By Judith Aston, M.F.A., and
Joani Gelinas, P.T., certified Aston-Patterner

▶ **THIS CHAPTER WILL HELP YOU:**
- Increase your awareness of posture and your options in movement.
- Understand neutral spine posture in sitting and standing positions.
- Enhance your performance by using ground reaction forces and weight-shifting.
- Prevent injuries.

Finding our potential begins with the discovery that we all have posture and movement options. The choices we make affect the functioning of our muscles and joints, make us more or less efficient, and make us more or less prone to injury. This chapter presents basic principles that can help you move in a more balanced and efficient manner, along with movement exercises to let you discover how to use these principles and feel the benefits. You may find that by applying these principles to your activities, you decrease symptoms of musculoskeletal distress or improve efficiency.

There are many schools of movement. Some such as yoga or Tai Chi have definite exercise forms that each person practices. Others such as the Aston approach (as well as Feldenkrais, Alexander technique, etc.) are individually tailored to each person's body. To get the most out of a movement awareness technique, try some of the exercises in this chapter.

MOVEMENT PATTERNS

We all have unique movement patterns that we have developed throughout our lives. There's usually a good reason why they occur, and stay with us, without our even knowing it, long after they have served their initial purpose. They have become habitual and unconscious. Often they restrict the way we move, causing injuries or pain. Your usual movement patterns during the day are probably similar in everything you do.

A movement pattern requires many repetitions to change, which is why you need to do any movement exercise often. Gradually you will begin to sit, stand, and move differently as you choose movement options that are easier and more efficient. Here are four basic concepts and applications for various activities:

1. You can modify how gravity affects your body and how you use ground reaction force to move.
2. You can become aware of your neutral posture and how to find and maintain it.
3. You can change your base of support in standing or sitting positions to provide better central body stability for motion.
4. You can shift your center of gravity (weight-shifting) to move your whole body and extremities more efficiently.

GRAVITY AND GROUND REACTION FORCE

Gravity is the force we all live with, and it takes work to move against it. Its influence on a particular movement or exercise is variable, depending on the plane of the movement in relation to gravitational forces. Gravity has a counterforce that most people don't know about: ground reaction force (GRF). This is a force you can utilize as a result of your interaction with the ground to help support your body. Together, these two forces create a dynamic synergy that can work for you.

Ground reaction force is the force that you can create by pushing down onto any surface that you are contacting, such as the ground, the floor, a kayak, etc. It acts to support you against the downward force of gravity.

Neutral alignment, using gravity and GRF, and weight-shifting all contribute to continuous movement through the body. This creates a fluidity to movement that massages the tissue rather than creating tension. This fluidity brings motion to the body's soft tissue and enhances flexibility. Remember what it feels like to jump on a trampoline or off a diving board? There is a springing effect and you are elongated gently upward. As you come down again, you give in to gravity as you absorb the shock of impact, and then push up again.

Often, we forget to come down and let go into gravity, or "give." Think about hiking down a long, steep grade and putting a great amount of effort into controlling the impact abruptly rather than letting go slightly into the motion. The force is driven back up into a system that is rigid, creating jarring. Problems such as shin splints can result, or if the jarring moves up to a joint that is not well aligned (knees or hips), it may cause pain there. Think instead of receiving the impact, giving in to gravity slightly, and then distributing the motion throughout.

The secret is that the body is always in motion. Absorbing impact and distributing the different movements through the whole body make for movement with less effort and make it more powerful, with injury less likely. GRF is utilized alternately with gravity.

EXERCISES

42 | Ground Reaction Force

Equipment: None.

Purpose: Experience the effect of ground reaction force on your body.

Technique: While standing with your feet about shoulder-width apart, place your right foot a few inches in front of your left foot. Then raise your right arm in front of you parallel to the floor. Hold it there for a moment and feel how the weight of your arm seems to increase. You have now felt the effect of gravity. As you hold it there, your arm feels heavier and more difficult to hold up. Feel which muscles have to work and how hard they have to work. Can you also feel the muscles in your shoulder and neck tensing?

Now try it another way. First slightly shift most of your weight from your left onto your right foot. Next push off of your right foot and move more off of the ball of your left foot while elevating your arm in front of you. Progressively increase the length and tone up your right side, as you lift your right arm parallel to the floor. This utilizes GRF, lengthening your body and increasing support for your arm. Do you feel that your arm is lighter and easier to lift? Can you feel that the elevation of your arm is being assisted with the GRF and push-off from your feet, legs, and buttock?

Tips: In any standing activity, if you remember not only to concentrate on the action of the activity but also to support your activity and spine by initiating effortful moves with GRF first, you may feel that the movement is easier.

NEUTRAL POSTURES

A *neutral posture* is one in which your body, including your spinal joints and discs, are the least stressed and in the best possible position. Neutral is a position that the body can maintain with minimal effort or resistance to gravity. Neutral is your own unique position of a dynamically balanced alignment. Think of each of your body parts as being symbolized by a ball: your head, neck, chest, pelvis, knees, and feet all taking that round form. Think of neutral posture as the position of maximum balance, with each ball being balanced directly over the ball below it. These balls progressively lean just slightly forward, which centralizes the weight over the foot.

When any given part or segment of your body moves away from its balance point, increased effort or stress is required. This can take a variety of forms: a tensing, holding, tightening, or shortening in some areas, which causes excessive compression or stretching and compensatory motion in other areas. Injury can result. This puts stress and strain on the affected soft tissue and joints. Balanced posture has the effect of distributing support in all the dimensions of your body. This more evenly distributes your effort as well, so any activity occurs throughout your whole body. This may increase the efficiency of your muscles, because you are alleviating the stress and strain, and your muscles are able to contract better.

Many of us do not know how to sit or stand in an easy or efficient way. This is amplified when we walk, move, or perform recreational activities. The posture you have when you sit, stand, and walk makes a tremendous difference in the effort required, and the amount of discomfort you feel. The posture you have when you ride your bike, carry a backpack, in-line skate, or lift weights can make the activity enjoyable or tedious and injury-prone. The more time you spend in any activity, the more important it is to find an optimal neutral position. It is important to establish balanced posture before trying to increase repetitions or power in your activities.

Most people have learned to think of posture as something static and rigid. Remember that your neutral posture is dynamic, fluid, and flexible. There is a "zone" of neutral posture alignment.

Posture or alignment might be viewed as the way the body parts are balanced on one another. A body in better balance requires less energy to stay in one position or to move than a body out of balance.

Exercise 43 can assist you in finding your own neutral sitting posture, which will feel balanced, relaxed, and easy to maintain. Once you have practiced this, you can perform it on a bicycle, in a kayak, or while doing any sitting activity.

Note: The two bony prominences on the bottom of your pelvis (the *ischial tuberosities*) that you feel when you are sitting upright are called your *sit bones* in this chapter.

43 | Sitting Arcing Exercise: Finding a Neutral for Sitting

Equipment: Chair.
Purpose: Learn to find a neutral low-back position in sitting.
Technique: Sit on the edge of a chair that is tall enough that your hips are slightly higher than your knees. Place your knees a comfortable distance apart, with the front of your ankles under your knees. Let all your movements be smooth, without strain. Starting at the hip joint, roll your pelvis backward and down toward your

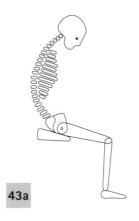

43a

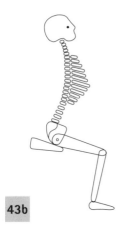

43b

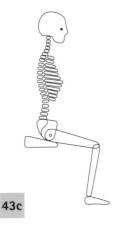

43c

tailbone. Your belly button will go in a posterior direction. Let the spine fall evenly into a C shape, your chest falling forward, letting all the segments of your spine bend about the same amount. Let your head nod slightly to match the bend through the rest of your spine. Exhale as you roll down. This is a "letting go" motion, called *flexion* (43a).

Next, start arching your back. Shift your weight slightly forward so you are rocking your pelvis through your chest forward, and feel your weight shift toward the front of your hips. Push down and back into the seat with your sit bones, which brings your tailbone up and away from the seat. Push down into the floor with your feet, creating a slight but even arch throughout your whole spine. Your spine will be pushed gently into *extension*, and the front of you will be lengthened. Your belly button should move in a forward direction. Inhale as you finish the movement. Allow your head and eyes to match the movement in the rest of your spine (43b).

Settle back into a midpoint between flexion and extension, where the length of your front approximately equals the length of your back. You will feel that you are sitting directly on your sit bones. Let your body find its place of rest. This will likely be closer to extension than flexion. This is *neutral* (43c).

Variations: 43.1. Once you find your neutral position, you can find *relaxed neutral* by letting go into gravity just a little, sliding down into a slightly flexed pattern. 43.2. *Toned neutral* is found by adding ground reaction force to your neutral position by pushing down into the seat with your sit bones and by pushing down into the floor with your feet. This toned position readies you for any movement action so you have the tone to support yourself in neutral while you move. This is important when you are lifting objects and during certain exercises.

Tips: Sitting arcing should be performed daily. You can use it whenever you first sit down or after a long duration of sitting. It can help you become more comfortable in sitting activities, from sitting in your car to lifting weights, kayaking, or bicycling. A small wedge may make neutral sitting easier.

Sitting Neutral and the Sitting Arcing Exercise

There are many variations to this exercise of flexing and extending the spine. Please note that Aston sitting arcing does not have you lift against gravity, but has you push and utilize GRF. Your inhalation will naturally lift your rib cage, which also assists in tractioning your spine. Once your spine is released from the locking mechanism of gravity, it is easy to find your balanced posture, in which the segments of your body rest one on top of the other without much effort.

The downward pull of gravity acts as a stabilizer. It can lock you into any posture you are holding, good or bad. That is why we want to find neutral. Often, people are locked into a slouched posture and think about getting into good posture by pulling themselves up from there (i.e., a military posture). This might look good, but it feels stiff because it requires that you continue to use your muscles to hold yourself up. If you find a neutral posture before you settle into gravity and get locked in, you can use gravity to your advantage. It will mechanically stabilize your spine into its place of balance, and your muscles can be at rest.

 ## 44 | Gravity's Effect on Sitting

Equipment: Chair.
Purpose: Feel a decrease in muscle tension during sitting posture.
Technique: Sit on a seat in a slouch and let yourself settle down into gravity, letting it lock your spine in this position. Then attempt to sit up tall by pulling up against gravity with your back muscles. Feel the tension in your back and shoulder blades; feel the rigidity in your muscles. Realize that if you don't continue to tighten your muscles, you will fall back down into a slouch.

Now try to do it differently. Practice Exercise 43 again, this time noticing that as you use ground reaction force and breathe in, you unlock your spine. Find your neutral, and then settle in, letting gravity stabilize your spine into neutral. Feel that your hips, pelvis, ribs, neck, and head are balanced on top of each other. Feel the absence of muscle tension and the overall stability and ease in your body. Because your muscles are not tensing to hold you up, there is more resilience and fluidity in your position. You should feel less tense and tired, since your muscles are not overworking just to sustain your posture.

Finding a Neutral for Standing

People often align themselves over only the posterior third of the foot. According to Aston-Patterning, the dynamic plumb line in relation to standing has a slightly forward inclination similar to the line used in relation to sitting. This takes into consideration the front part of the foot as part of the base of support. This helps distribute the body's weight over the whole foot rather than only the heel, which is a common base of support for a more perpendicular plumb line. Using the whole foot gives a broader base of support for the whole body, reducing unnecessary strain and tension and allowing easier movement.

45 | Standing Arcing Exercise

Equipment: None.
Purpose: Experience neutral spine position in standing.
Technique: Stand in a comfortable position with your feet directly under your hip joints (about shoulder-width apart). Let your toes turn out slightly. Rock forward through your ankle hinge (or joint), which allows you to shift your body weight toward the balls of your feet, and then rock backward, moving your weight slightly toward your heels. You have found the neutral position when you feel the whole length of your foot supporting you. Transfer your weight back slightly , rocking through your ankle hinge, so you feel your weight on the heels of your feet. Bend slightly forward at your hip hinge. Let your spine *flex* slightly and curve forward gently, remembering to distribute the shape of the curve evenly throughout your spine. Your back will be lengthened. Then let your knees bend. Exhale as you flex (45a).

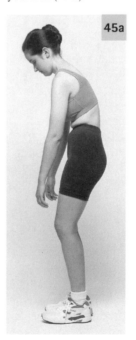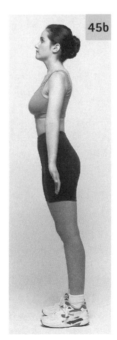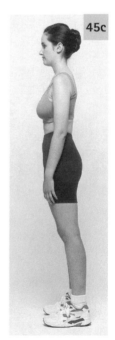

Rock forward by transferring the weight to the balls of your feet. Push into the ground, letting your whole body lengthen upward and arch slightly (*extend*) as you inhale. Gradually progress the movement along your spine toward your neck, and the front of you will be lengthened. Your whole body will be inclined slightly forward. Inhale as you go up. Let your arms respond with your palms facing forward (45b).

From your feet, move slightly back to a place that feels balanced, where the length of your front equals the length of your back (*neutral*). All of your body parts can balance over each other (45c). Move your whole body by rocking through your ankles to distribute your weight over your whole foot, front to back and side to side.

Benefits From the Standing Arcing Exercise

As in the sitting arcing exercise, the standing arcing exercise helps you find neutral, where the body parts are more easily balanced on each other. When this happens, activities in upright positions become easier, as the body is not spending as much energy on merely supporting structures that are out of alignment. This may result in an improved position; a body in neutral balance allows your muscles to work more evenly, which allows for greater efficiency.

Also, standing arcing helps you feel your upright base of support, which is your feet. We often perform standing activities using only the posterior third of the foot (the heel) for support. Or maybe we stand with more weight on the balls of the feet, or most of our weight on only one foot. Take a minute and stand in your natural stance and feel where the weight is distributed through your feet. Because our feet are supporting our whole body, it is extremely important to take advantage of the entire foot surface, feeling the ball, heel, and arch simultaneously supporting us when we are upright.

We may be unaware that we are using only a portion of the surface available to us for support (although this can definitely be important in activities such as rock or wall climbing).

BASE OF SUPPORT

Your body receives support in many ways: from your skeleton, from GRF, as well as from the tone and resiliency of your soft tissues. Another important way in which your body receives support has to do with its base of support (BOS). The base of support for any particular part of your body is the part directly underneath it, and the base of support for the whole body comes from whichever segment contacts the ground. In sitting, it is the pelvis and the feet. In standing, it is the feet. Base of support also takes into account the total effect of all of these parts supporting each other. If any part of your body does not have adequate support underneath it, it will have to tense or compensate to perform any action.

46 | Base of Support

Equipment: None.
Purpose: Become aware of your base of support.
Technique: Stand with your feet very close together and find how far you can reach with one arm—in front of you, beside you, or behind you—before you lose your balance or feel yourself tense up. Feel how the placement of your feet (BOS) is too narrow for your body to feel stable during your reaching action. Now move your feet to a wide stance so your feet are placed wider than your shoulders. Notice that this makes it very easy if you want to reach your arm to the right or left side of you, but how far does a wide stance's base of support support you for leaning forward? Not very far. You now have a base of support that supports side-to-side movements well, but lacks support for backward and forward movements. This makes it easy for you to face forward or for someone to push you over from behind. Finding the right base of support for your movements in hiking, climbing, weight training, and other activities can be helpful.

Whenever you perform an activity, it is important to understand in which direction you will be moving and try to make your foot placement match the body motion above it.

Without adequate base of support, any activity requiring reaching that you might perform standing or sitting may be more difficult. It might require more energy and probably have the potential to cause strains by the way that your body compensates due to the lack of support.

Base of support has to do with how the body parts rest one on the other, or line up underneath one another. Therefore, if you are standing, your feet have to be in a good position to support your knees, and your knees to support your hips. When you are reaching for a ball in tennis or racquetball, if you step and then reach for the ball, you have given your arm the BOS it needs for the reach. Because of the support gained for your arm when you step under the action, you are less likely to strain another part of your body. The same could be said for aerobics, climbing, etc. When you are lifting your arms, remember to modify your foot position to support the various arm and trunk positions you are performing.

WEIGHT-SHIFTING

And now it's time to move! Movement is most easily initiated by shifting your weight. This allows your center of gravity and spine to move to allow more stability for movements of your arms and legs. Weight-shifting involves maintaining a neutral but not rigid center.

Remember the importance of ground reaction force to assist with counteracting gravity. You now have a balanced neutral position, and a good base of support. Now you need to add movement, so first find neutral, and then find your BOS. Third, identify the joints bearing the greatest weight. If you are sitting, it's your pelvis and hips. If you are standing, it's your feet, ankles, knees, and hips. Rock and shift your weight across these joints to begin the movement with your aligned body.

The weight-shifting progression: First, find neutral. Next, identify the joint bearing the most weight (your BOS). In sitting, rock forward through your hip hinge and transfer the weight of the trunk across your hip. In standing, transfer the weight of your whole body across your ankle. Finally, shift your weight across your BOS to initiate the action, and notice any motion response in specific parts of your body.

47 | Weight-shifting in Standing

Equipment: None.
Purpose: Experience weight-shifting to improve your movement patterns.
Technique: Position your right foot about 18 inches to the side of your left foot, with your knees slightly bent. Now reach to the right side with your right hand as if you were reaching for an object, a rock, or a wall hold. Notice that it feels a bit off balance. Now initiate the movement from your BOS by transferring your weight over your right foot, knee, and hip before you reach or while you are reaching. Notice a feeling of more control and balance.
Variations: 47.1. Also try this exercise with your right foot in front of your left. Reach in front of you for an imaginary rock hold first without weight-shifting, and then with weight-shifting. You can do this in a diagonal pattern with your right foot at about a 2:00 o'clock position to your left. 47.2. Try this exercise while stepping onto a step, stool, rock, or log. Place your right foot onto a high step or other surface and feel the effort when you try to push off with your right foot. Now place your foot onto a high step and, before you

push off, shift your whole body more over the right foot until you feel yourself just moving forward. At this point, push off with your right and left foot.

Tips: If you step onto a higher surface without weight-shifting, you will likely use more effort and possibly tilt backward, especially if you have a pack on. Weight-shifting can make the step up more balanced and decrease your risk of injury.

Weight-shifting can assist you in many standing activities in which you reach with an arm or a leg or simply step. This shifting of your center of gravity can be very helpful in hiking or mountaineering when you are taking a long or high step up a steep section. It is also very important in rock and indoor gym climbing.

APPLICATIONS OF ASTON–PATTERNING TO ACTIVITIES

Below are applications to a few activities, but the basic principles can be applied to many outdoor activities.

CYCLING

Practice sitting arcing (Exercise 43) on a bicycle seat to find a comfortable neutral. This will also let you know how to adjust the seat, pedals, and handlebars to your body. It can also be helpful as a range-of-motion exercise during a long ride to keep from getting too stiff in your low back.

BACKPACKING AND MOUNTAINEERING

Always try to practice safe spine postures and movements when putting on your pack. (See chapter 17 for more details on lifting and positioning your pack.)

You can try doing a modified standing arcing (Exercise 45) with your pack on and during your hike to find the most comfortable low-back position. Most people end up in an excessively flexed position. Try unweighting your pack slightly by pushing up on the top tube of an external frame pack or on the straps of an internal frame pack. You can also have someone lift up on the bottom of the pack. Do the standing arcing with less flexing and extending to avoid a back injury. Try to arrive at a posture that is away from full flexion and closer to neutral.

KAYAKING

Many people find themselves sitting slouched in the seat of a kayak because of the design of the seat. This takes the support away from your shoulders and you lose good leverage for paddling. A slouch in flexion also compresses your low back because your spine is not in neutral and therefore your discs and spinal joints are at risk. If you find yourself slouched, with your arms doing all the work and your low back becoming sore, try pushing your hands down onto the kayak so you can lift and unweight yourself and elongate your trunk. Then move your sit bones back so they rest snugly against the back of the seat. Find neutral and then settle into this position. Next, weight-shift by leaning forward through your hip hinge for the initiation of the paddling—right hip hinge, left hip hinge, right, left—while using your feet to push on the footholds. This will increase your GRF and the feeling of power coming through your whole body. If you reach forward with only your arms and shoulders when you start to paddle, most of the effort is in your arms and your back, and you will move out of neutral and undo the good that has been achieved by finding your neutral.

WEIGHT TRAINING

Begin by lifting free weights in the usual way in a familiar exercise such as a biceps curl. Identify the effort, specifically in your arms and generally in your whole body. Now perform the standing arcing exercise (Exercise 45) so your weight is centered over your whole foot. From neutral, shift your weight slightly forward through your ankles and push slightly through your feet on the same side as you lift the weight.

If you do one arm at a time, you can put one foot slightly in front of the other with a weight-shift on the forward foot (the same side as the curling arm). Note that whichever foot is forward should be directly under your center of gravity.

STRETCHING

There is much that could be said about how to maximize the benefits of stretching, but here's one important point to remember so you do actually stretch rather than simultaneously compress other body areas. Many stretching techniques involve bending forward or sideways to stretch your spine, legs, or arms. Sometimes, in performing this bending, you actually shorten and compress the joints and deeper structures of your body while trying to stretch. Try lengthening your spine by pushing down through your feet while standing, or into your pelvis while sitting, to lengthen your spine before you lean and stretch. You can maintain the length of your deep and superficial muscles by using GRF and hinging at the great weight-bearing joint.

7

TRAINING CONCEPTS, CONDITIONING GOALS, AND PROGRAM PLANNING

BY CARL PETERSEN, P.T., AND DARCY NORMAN, A.T.C.

▶ **THIS CHAPTER WILL HELP YOU:**
- Set goals and evaluate your progress.
- Become familiar with smart training principles.
- Understand how to plan the progression of your conditioning program based on your time and scheduling (periodization of training).
- Understand principles of energy sequencing training.
- Learn principles and sequencing of strength training.
- Learn recovery techniques to facilitate training.
- Use a daily log and monthly calendar to plan and evaluate your progress.

If you have a particular physical or activity goal, you may wish to design a training program to aid you in achieving it. Physical training is very specific, producing physiological adaptations in the musculoskeletal and cardiorespiratory systems that progress if you are giving your body the proper gradual training stimulus. You will benefit the most from this chapter if you have read chapters 2 and 5. If you have any musculoskeletal or medical conditions that may limit your exercise, consult a physician before embarking on a training program.

GOALS

Goals for conditioning should be realistic and reasonable in light of the time you have available, your body frame, your age, and any medical conditions you have. Conditioning goals should also be a good fit with the goals you have for the other parts of your life. Try to set specific goals for your aerobic and strength training, as well as for flexibility, agility, balance, and skill development. Goals for conditioning may not be achieved for many reasons. The following are some tips to help you achieve your fitness goals:

- Give yourself adequate time to prepare for your activity.
- Assess equipment you have available before planning.
- Make a program based on equipment that is easily accessible.
- Be thorough in your planning.
- Keep track of evaluation numbers and objective numbers that will show you progress.

- Focus on good technique while exercising.
- Take any necessary precautions or time to facilitate any injury or conditions that may hinder your training activity.
- Plan out all your sets and reps so you know what you are doing before you do it.
- Be as specific as possible; it will make your program that much easier to follow.
- Give yourself adequate time to recover from exercise sessions.

When assessing your goals, make sure to have long- and short-term goals for every aspect of your training program. First, start with your activity goals. Identify the most difficult parts of your activity and when you would like to achieve them. Then plan to develop your flexibility, balance, agility, strength, and aerobic goals to meet the overall activity demands. Next, modify your program to meet the most difficult demands during a particular part of the season. If there is a particular challenge associated with the activity, use an exercise (or design your own) to prepare to meet that challenge using the periodization technique described later in this chapter.

This chapter and the activity chapters in Part III should give you a base of information to help you along the way. You need to set realistic objectives, allow enough time, and evaluate your progress.

ARE YOUR OBJECTIVES REASONABLE?

Your objectives are the action elements that help you achieve your goal. They need to be well defined. For aerobic training, you will know what, how much, at what intensity, and for how long you will be training. For strength training, you will know what number of reps, sets, and amount of resistance to use. Write them down ahead of time and be as specific as possible so that on the day of your activity, you do not have to do any significant planning or decision making. Of course, you can modify things depending

on how you feel when you are working out.

HOW MUCH TIME WILL IT TAKE?

The amount of time it takes to achieve your goals depends on your present level of fitness and skill, as well as your build, present health, age, equipment available, and quality of your program planning. If you already have a base of aerobic and strength fitness, you may be able to move into the second stage of a program quickly. If not, you will likely have to spend a minimum of 4–6 weeks building that base.

Most activities that have a long race or a high-endurance event, such as a marathon or a 2-day mountaineering climb, can require 3 or more months of preparation. In order to finish a race, you have to be quite close to doing the race distance in your workouts a few weeks prior to the race. Many activities take a minimum of 2 months of preparation, such as a difficult run of telemark skiing, downhill skiing, rock climbing, or glacial mountaineering.

Shorter-duration goals can take less time. The average person could be ready within a month for a full day of hiking. Evaluate your progress before undertaking difficult activities. If you try an activity before you are ready, you will be more susceptible to injury or to not completing the activity. As a rough estimate, figure that you will increase aerobic distances by 10%–15% per week and will need to achieve at least half to three-fourths of the distance of your goal. You should be able to simulate most of the moves requiring strength and balance numerous times and under various conditions.

EVALUATING YOUR PROGRESS

Evaluating your progress means many things. Are you doing what you had planned? Is it enough or too much? Modify your plans depending on your outcomes. How will you measure your progress? You can use measuring devices such as simply doing what you set out to do, or you can quantify the ease and time it takes you to accomplish an aerobic activity.

For your aerobic component, have a sport-specific activity that you do intermittently to judge your effort, time, and how you feel in general. This could be a 30-mile bike ride with hills, a 4- to 6-mile run, a 6- to 8-mile moderately steep hike, etc. This activity should be the same or directly related to your goal activity. If it is getting easier or it takes you less time to do it, you are making progress. You could also use an indoor aerobic activity to see if you can accomplish the same intensity and duration of activity with less effort.

In evaluating your strength, use your progress in increasing the weight or resistance on particular exercises. For functional exercises, see how many reps you can do in 45 seconds. You can also use a functional measurement; for example, how much effort it takes to lift something such as a full pack, your ease of performing a climbing move, or the effort required to maneuver your boat in rough conditions.

OVERTRAINING

Being smart about your training means recognizing non-adaptive responses to training such as prolonged fatigue, poor endurance, elevated resting heart rate, sleep disturbances, frequent infections, and pain. Establish a baseline for your resting heart rate by checking your pulse when you first wake up. If this increases by 5–10 beats per minute during your training, you may be overtraining. If you have an elevated resting heart rate or have a persistence of any of the above symptoms, you may be overtraining.

Occasionally exercise and outdoor or other sporting activities can be done to such an extent that your body cannot adapt well. In the early stages of excessive training, you might have some mild fatigue and decreased stamina

or performance. You may initially have more overuse injuries involving the musculoskeletal system such as tendonitis or stress fractures. If it continues, you might develop all of the symptoms and signs of overtraining syndrome, including increased muscle soreness, greater susceptibility to minor illnesses, decreased appetite, decreased motivation, poor performance, fatigue, and possibly a fast resting heart rate. Take your resting heart rate soon after you wake up in the morning, and keep a chart to make sure it is not elevating more than 7–10 beats per minute above your baseline.

Short-duration fatigue is common and can be associated with long exercise days, temporary illness, high altitude, etc. Prolonged fatigue, especially with the other symptoms, is something to be concerned about. If these symptoms occur, cut back on your training schedule by decreasing the duration and intensity of your exercise. Take a number of rest days. Try to decrease your regular aerobic session to 40 minutes or less. Eliminate interval training for at least a few weeks. As you get back to your regular exercise, try to schedule no-exercise or light-exercise days after heavy days such as interval training, long-day activities, or 3 consecutive aerobic days. Avoid exercising 7 days a week. Try to get adequate rest and adequate nutrition. Try to decrease stress from the rest of your life.

COMPONENTS OF A CONDITIONING PROGRAM
PROPER WARM-UP

A 5- to 10-minute warm-up should precede your workout. See chapter 4 and the activity chapters in Part III for more details.

FLEXIBILITY GOALS

Maintaining flexibility is an important goal, especially as we get older. Hips, knees, and ankles are key areas. Static and active stretching can be done with every workout, if only briefly. If you have had an injury or an arthritic condition, you may decide to devote more time to your flexibility program. Stretching is best done after a warm-up or at the end of your workout.

STRENGTH TRAINING GOALS

Strength training is now recommended for every individual as a part of a minimum conditioning program. In addition to a basic strength program, you can design exercises to build specific strength for your activities to allow you to do them with less effort and less likelihood of injuries.

AGILITY AND BALANCE

Establish agility and balance goals, especially if you are kayaking, boulder hopping, skiing, snowboarding, windsurfing, climbing, or over 65 and wish to prevent injuries. For this you can do short periods of balance and agility activities 2–3 times a week and gradually increase the challenges. (See chapters 5 and 8, as well as the activity chapters in Part III, for more details on exercises.)

AEROBIC STAMINA GOALS

Aerobic endurance should be developed before anaerobic high-intensity interval endurance. A solid base of aerobic endurance facilitates recovery and allows training at higher intensity levels. A solid aerobic base will help improve anaerobic and strength training because it promotes faster recovery.

If you do aerobic stamina training more than 4 days a week, alternate hard and easy days. This is necessary because hard days deplete muscle glycogen, which takes 48 hours to replenish. Hard days are those of interval training, races, or longer-duration aerobic activity.

The minimum aerobic program will help you achieve basic health benefits. You may increase your aerobic endurance by training at lower intensities for longer duration (LILD) at 50%–65% max. HR to be able to do longer-duration activities (see chapter 2).

Gradually increasing your duration by 10%–20% per week can get you to the endurance you will need. Add brief intervals of high-intensity training to improve your ability to do short bursts of difficult, high-intensity activity if you have first built your aerobic base with 4–6 weeks of basic low- to moderate-intensity training. See chapter 2 for interval training details.

PROPER COOL-DOWN

A cool-down is what you do at the end of your aerobic workout. See chapter 2 for details.

PERIODIZATION OF A CONDITIONING PROGRAM

Periodization is the process of structuring and planning training programs around blocks of time to provide optimum performance at a required time. Periodization is appropriate if you are conditioning to prepare for a season of moderate- to high-level activity or a particular event such as a race or a climb. You can also use these concepts to guide you in progressing your fitness program. This is done by dividing up the time available for training into smaller, more manageable periods of training with specific objectives in each segment.

One-month blocks of time work well when setting up the periodization plan, as this allows a gradual increase in training volume over the first 3 weeks of the cycle, followed by 1 week with decreased volume. The 3-week buildup positively stresses the body and the 1 week of decreased volume allows for recovery and adaptation to the imposed physiological demands. This improves overall conditioning.

Ideally, your training plan should be divided

into phases or periods. The length of each phase depends on the amount of time you can devote to training. The periods are:

Phase A: General preparation or aerobic base building

Phase B: Intensity building

Phase C: Sport- or activity-specific fitness

Phase D: Maintenance, competition, or time of maximum activity participation

Phase E: Recovery and active rest period

If you have a certain amount of time in which to reach your activity goal, then divide your time between the first three periods (phases A–C) in preparation for your activity. Periodization allows you to move from general activities to more sport-specific conditioning one phase at a time. Using this system optimizes your physical skills, leading to faster adaptations, improved performance, and decreased injury potential.

Following are general guidelines for periodizing your training according to the five phases noted above.

PHASE A: GENERAL PREPARATION PERIOD (AEROBIC BASE BUILDING)

Phase A is approximately the first one-third of a training program. It can last 4–12 weeks, depending on how many training activity goals you have. Generally, this period lasts 6–8 weeks. The objectives of this phase are to improve flexibility, stamina (general aerobic endurance conditioning), general strength endurance, and coordination.

In this phase, most of your aerobic training is of low to moderate intensity and you do not do any interval training until possibly the end of this period. Build up your aerobic sessions to a duration of 30–50 minutes at 60%–75% max. HR for 4–6 sessions a week. During this phase, 60%–70% of your time is devoted to aerobic endurance training.

Perform your strength training with higher reps (15) and lower weight (resistance). You can build up the resistance gradually at about 5%–10% per week, or as your strength improvements allow. During this phase, plan on strength training each body region approximately 3 times per week. A general whole-body strength workout is recommended, and it does not have to be very sport-specific. You could do a short period of balance exercises toward the end of this period if you do an activity requiring a moderate amount of balance.

PHASE B: INTENSITY PERIOD (INCREASING EXERCISE VOLUME)

This period lasts from 4–12 weeks, with an average of 4–6 weeks for most of the activities described in this book. The general objectives of this phase include improving specific stamina and increasing maximum strength. This stage involves a greater volume (number of hours and caloric output) of exercise and more aerobic, moderate- to high-intensity work.

To maintain your aerobic base, devote about 50%–60% of your time to low- to moderate-intensity aerobic endurance activities, including lower-intensity, longer-distance (LILD) activities. Gradually increase your 1-day-a-week LILD workout. Do five other aerobic sessions per week. These should be sport-specific activities with 2 sessions lasting 40–50 minutes. You may wish to include a cross training session 1 time each week. Two of your aerobic sessions could incorporate interval training if your activity requires brief high-intensity periods—such as for climbing, mountaineering, scrambling, snowshoeing, cross-country or telemark skiing, paddle sports, cycling, running, or windsurfing.

Initially start with 30- to 120-second intervals of 2–5 repetitions at moderate intensity. Gradually increase the number (progressing to 8 intervals), duration (some intervals to 3–4 minutes), and resistance (grade of hill, rough water, etc.) of your intervals. Remember to avoid excessive-speed workouts to avoid overtraining or injuries early in the season. You may try some short races if your activity goal involves racing.

Focus more on strengthening exercises pertinent and functional to your activity; do some sets with 12–15 reps and some with de-creased reps (4–8) and increased weight to im-prove maximum strength. Add appropriate functional strength training to the rest of your strength workout during this period.

PHASE C: SPORT-SPECIFIC FITNESS PERIOD

Phase C is approximately the final third of the training program and is 4–8 weeks long. The general objectives of this phase are to build stamina and strength particular to your activity and to improve skill and coordination.

About 40%–50% of the training time is in aerobic, lower-intensity, longer-duration (LILD) workouts if you will be doing an activity requir-ing long-duration aerobic stamina. Consider some cross training to avoid boredom and over-use. There is a decrease in total training volume. You can continue the interval training, but add higher-intensity and shorter intervals and some with more resistance (hills), if applicable.

Your strength training should include some functional exercises and focus on the body re-gions you will be using the most. Increase the speed of your functional exercises (see chapters 5, 8, 10, 11, and 15) prior to adding more resis-tance. An example would be to perform as many repetitions as possible safely in a 45-second period. For your regular resistance exercises, perform some sets of 4–6 reps for maximum strength along with sets of 12–15 reps for strength and endurance. You might add some plyometrics (such as jumping) and power work if your activity requires it (downhill or telemark skiing, snowboarding, windsurfing, rigorous

climbing, and mountaineering). Add balance training early in this phase for water, climbing, and snow-based activities.

PHASE D: MAINTENANCE, COMPETITION, OR MAXIMUM ACTIVITY PARTICIPATION PERIOD

The maintenance phase is the time during your competition or maximum activity period. The general objectives of this phase are to main-tain all the component aerobic and strength gains while allowing optimal performance and activity enjoyment.

During this time, there is less total volume of exercise. Continue your basic aerobic endur-ance, and use cross training intermittently. De-crease or eliminate interval training. Maintain strength training, but with little attempt to in-crease strength. Eliminate your low-rep (4–6 reps) sets. Include ample time for rest in this phase, especially after a race or a multiday activity.

PHASE E: RECOVERY AND ACTIVE REST PERIOD

The transition phase is the off time between the end of your activity season and the start of the next training cycle. The general objectives of this phase are recovery from the previous ac-tivity season, including injury rehabilitation, rest, and maintenance of general strength and endurance.

Recovery means giving your body the rest it needs to adapt to the stresses you have put it through during an intense training season. Note: This can also be a brief period lasting a few days to weeks to recover from overuse inju-ries or overtraining during a training period.

Use active rest activities to recover from high-intensity or long-duration activities or races. Recovery periods are days of lighter or no exercise. After big events, give yourself a few days of rest or minimal activity, then begin a period of 2–4 weeks of low- to moderate-intensity aerobic and strength workouts to maintain what you have gained. Try some cross training or other sports to prevent burnout and to use your muscles differently.

THE PERIODIZATION PLAN

Always start a training program with a clear idea of what it is you hope to accomplish. The periodization plan gives direction to training, and must be continually revised to ensure optimum benefits. Consider reviewing your plan each month throughout your training schedule.

To devise your plan, list your goals (as indicated earlier in this chapter) and the amount of time you have. Determine as well as you can what the demands of your activity are in the categories of aerobic (lower-intensity, longer-duration, and higher-intensity intervals), strength, flexibility, balance, and skill. Is it an activity such as hiking that requires stamina for long periods of time, or is it helicopter skiing, which requires anaerobic power and strength with long breaks in between? Write down in clear terms what you would like to be able to do in these categories. Remember, the plan you make is tailored to your needs based on your present fitness level, age, build, and the demands of your activity. The amount of time you spend doing LILD interval training and strength, speed, and power work can vary considerably depending on your needs and comfort level. Certainly, if you are conditioning for general hiking or backpacking, you do not have to do much except for regular aerobic and LILD sessions.

Break the time you have into the five phases of periodization and into month-long blocks. Use a special training log or a regular calendar with enough room to fill in your training schedule and your remarks on your progress and how you feel. Plan out the first 3–4 weeks of a period

and give yourself at least 1 rest day and 1 lighter day per week (after a long or intense workout). Evaluate your progress every 2 weeks and modify your program as needed. Approximately 1 month before your activity season or event, plan a test activity of shorter duration than your expected activity. This should give you feedback as to whether you have any major deficits in your fitness so you can modify your program in the remaining month.

RECORDING YOUR DAILY PROGRAM ON A CALENDAR OR DAILY LOG

Figures 14 and 15 are an aerobic conditioning log and a strengthening conditioning log, respectively, that you can use to record your daily and weekly plans and activities. Use them as thoroughly as you want. They can be used by themselves but are better used as a monthly calendar. Use them in a basic way and record the amount of time you spend in each activity. Or use them as a more detailed planning tool and plan out your predicted time in each activity from your monthly and year-long periodization plans. It is important to record details in the boxes.

When filling in your aerobic training schedule on a regular calendar (see Figure 14), record the activities, expected duration, and intensity as rate of perceived exertion (RPE) or percentage of maximum heart rate (% max. HR; see chapter 2). If you are planning intervals, record the duration, intensity, number, and rest-period duration. It is important to record details in the boxes, such as the intensity of your aerobic exercise, as either % max. HR or as a particular zone (1–5). The following abbreviations make it easy to record on your regular calendar: aerobic regular sessions (AR); lower-intensity, longer-duration (LILD); intervals (I).

For strength training, record your sets and reps for the exercises as well as the weight, in each box (see Figure 15).

The Periodization Plan

FIGURE 14. AEROBIC CONDITIONING LOG

NAME:_____ PERIODIZATION PHASE:_____ (WEEK:_____)

LONG-TERM GOAL: MAXIMUM HEART RATE   90% 80% 70% 60% 50%

SHORT-TERM GOALS: BEATS/MIN   BEATS/MIN

1)   2)   3)   BEATS/10 SEC

	MON.	TUES.	WED.	TH.	FRI.	SAT.	SUN.
WEEK 1 ACTIVITY							
Time/Distance							
Route/Program							
Intervals							
Resting Heart Rate							
Comments							
WEEK 2 ACTIVITY							
Time/Distance							
Route/Program							
Intervals							
Resting Heart Rate							
Comments							
WEEK 3 ACTIVITY							
Time/Distance							
Route/Program							
Rest Periods							
Intervals							
Comments							
WEEK 4 ACTIVITY							
Time/Distance							
Route/Program							
Intervals							
Resting Heart Rate							
Comments							

FIGURE 15. STRENGTH TRAINING LOG

NAME:_____   PERIODIZATION PHASE:_____   (WEEK:_____)

LONG-TERM GOAL: AGILITY   PLYOMETRICS   FUNCTIONAL STRENGTHENING EXERCISES

SHORT-TERM GOALS: REST PERIODS:

1)   SETS X REPS:

2)

3)

BODY PART OR EXERCISE TYPE	EXERCISES DATE	WEEK 1			WEEK 2			WEEK 3			WEEK 4		
		DAY 1	DAY 2	DAY 3	DAY 1	DAY 2	DAY 3	DAY 1	DAY 2	DAY 3	DAY 1	DAY 2	DAY 3
	Warm–Up/Stretch												
Agility (A)	1)												
	2)												
	3)												
Plyometrics (P)	1)												
	2)												
	3)												
Functional Strengthening Exercises	1)												
	2)												
	3)												
Upper Body													
Upper Body													
Lower Body													
Lower Body													
Abdominal Muscles	1)												
	2)												
	3)												
	Resting HR												
	Weight												

In both figures, each log covers 4 weeks. Your phase can consist of 1 week or all 4. If it is 6 weeks, just fill in another sheet for the remaining 2 weeks and leave the last 2 weeks blank. Recording your morning heart rate is one method to monitor for overtraining. Recording your resting heart rate at another time of day can assess your cardiovascular training response in regard to pumping efficiency. The more accurate record you keep, the easier it will be to stick to your program. If your program at any particular time does not include agility training, just cross out that portion. Figures 14 and 15 are provided as a guideline to help you plan your successful program. Evaluate your progress every 2 weeks, then modify and plan your schedule for the following 2 weeks.

PLANNING YOUR OWN PROGRAM

Programs can be planned from the top down or from the bottom up. The top-down planning process can seem complex and difficult and is most useful for competitive athletes. Top-down planning involves looking at a whole year or parts of a year, and planning phases and varying volumes of the different types of activities. Use guidelines based on sample templates from this book and other sources in regard to the number and amount of time per week or month devoted to a type of conditioning activity. It is possible for anyone to do if they have particular goals and don't mind the time involved. For further information on developing a periodization plan or a yearly plan, or to see more templates, see the activity chapters in Part III and Selected References (especially Sleamaker) at the back of this book.

The planning process can be modified for outdoor athletes, the bottom-up version. Simply assess your present level of fitness in regard to your expected activity demands or conditioning goals, and start planning for actions to meet them. You can go at a gradual pace as you improve your aerobic and strength base. After you have improved your base level fitness for 4–6 weeks, you can add aerobic interval training and speed and plyometric training if you have a need for bursts of higher intensity. Add balance, agility, and activity-specific functional exercises within 6 weeks of the desired activity.

8

CREATIVE USE OF THE OUTDOORS IN TRAINING

BY PETER SHMOCK

▶ **THIS CHAPTER WILL HELP YOU:**
• Understand the benefits of training in an outdoor setting.
• Become familiar with the most important outdoor training exercises, such as hill running, jumping, and agility drills.
• Develop balance skills using logs, rocks, and hills.
• Design training programs with simple equipment outdoors.
• Choose outdoor conditioning exercises for your upper body, lower body, and torso.

Outdoor environments offer unique advantages to help you train for balance, agility, and power, especially when utilizing hills, logs, etc. Training outdoors can also add variety and decrease boredom in your workout. Training under the open sky has additional benefits. In skiing, climbing, mountain biking, and any other outdoor sport, it is essential to be able to respond quickly to the unexpected that can be encountered outdoors.

When training outdoors there's a lot of room for creativity. It's best to scout around for locations that provide many different options, such as schools, parks, or a diverse area of land. Here are some things to look for:
• stadium steps, bleachers, stairs, park benches, and tables for step-up exercises
• trees on which to anchor tubing
• hills with varying degrees of incline to practice lunges, jumps, interval training, and agility drills for skiers, climbers, and mountain bikers

• snowfields for simulation of balance challenges
• sand (a beach or a long-jump sand pit) to practice jumps
• playgrounds with objects to balance on
• logs, low fences, and rocks for balance drills
• boulders for variable-level push-ups or dips with one or two hands while standing and for climbing practice

In addition, simple, transportable, and affordable training tools are easy to take outdoors. They include:
• weight balls for throwing; large physio-balls (approximately 3 feet in diameter, available from physical therapy departments) for sit-ups
• free weights for resistance exercises
• traffic cones, ski poles, garden poles, and other markers for agility drills
• rope placed on the ground or from tree to tree to step over and under

- tubing or webbing for resistance in row and balance exercises
- ankle weights to use in step-ups or hill lunges to simulate the weight of snowshoes or telemark skis and boots

DEVELOPING STRENGTH, BALANCE, AGILITY, AND ANAEROBIC CAPACITY IN OUTDOOR SETTINGS

STRENGTH

Strength can be increased in outdoor environments by adding weight or gravity as resistance. For example, you can improve strength in your lower body by doing gradually progressive step-ups on bleacher steps, park benches, logs, rocks, and boulders. You can improve your jumping and hopping ability by using hills and sand pits.

BALANCE

Standing balance, the ability to maintain your body core and extremities in a safe and well-functioning position despite challenges from the environment, is most important for climbers, backpackers, snowshoers, snowboarders, and skiers. Exercises to improve it are best done in outdoor areas with slopes and surfaces that challenge you in ways similar to your activity. Identify equipment that could be challenging to balance on—a fallen log, rocks, a low log fence, tires in a playground, a snowfield, etc. Plot out a course of walking on these surfaces. Try it initially without a backpack and then with a backpack. At first you may walk post to post, rock to rock, or straight along a log.

When doing any balance exercise, make sure your center of gravity is slightly forward so you are not leaning backward. When walking on logs, your steps should be a normal stride length, but you can increase your stride to challenge your balance more. When walking from rock to rock, land on the largest surface of the rock with a forward momentum. If there are a lot of rocks in an area, try varying which rocks you walk over, to change your direction and stride length.

- Walk a narrow log.
- Walk from rock to rock as if you were crossing a river.
- Walk from post to post or tire to tire in a playground.
- Place a 25- to 75-foot string on the ground and anchor it so it will not move much when you walk on it. Walk heel to toe initially. When this is easy with a backpack, increase the length of your stride. Try doing this on a hill traverse or on an up or down slope.
- Try Exercises 27, 37–41, 58–60, 62, 63–64 (using a tree to anchor the tubing), 66, and 68. You can try these while standing with one foot on a log or rock, or while standing uphill or downhill. Using hills for balance is particularly useful for climbers, backpackers, scramblers, and practioners of all snow sports.
- You may be able to make a balance circuit made up of segments of balance challenges that last 30–120 seconds each.
- Try linking any of the above balance challenges.

The important thing is to maintain a stable upright position without straining or hurting your knees or back. Try to simulate the balance and environmental demands of your activity.

Training for sitting balance and abdominal strength is most important for whitewater boating and for mountain bikers. For both sports you can do sitting ball exercises such as Exercises 33–35 and 41 or abdominal challenge exercises such as Exercises 66, 68, and 69. For water sports, train on the water with easy rapids or agility courses in calmer water. For mountain bikers, the up- and downhill agility cycling drills in chapter 22 are appropriate.

Remember that balance can deteriorate just like strength if you do nothing to exercise it.

AGILITY

Agility can be described as "moving balance." Training for agility involves setting up obstacle courses in which you have to make quick changes in direction while maintaining your balance. The outdoors is the best setting in which to train for agility. Choose woods, hills, snow slopes, or large open spaces that allow you to move unassisted while adding an element of the unexpected (see chapter 20 for snowboarding and ski agility drills; chapter 21 for water agility drills; and chapter 22 for mountain biking drills).

You can create your own outdoor agility course by using small traffic cones, ropes, ski poles, trees, garden poles, or whatever is handy to set up an obstacle course. The agility course should have at least 10 stations in which you make changes in direction. You could start with a course on level ground, then progress to hills.

Initially, start with fast walking between the stations. Then progress to running. You may progress to adding lunges, jumps, and hops between some stations, depending on the sport you are training for (lunges are most appropriate for cross-country and telemark skiing and for snowshoeing). For downhill skiing and snowboarding, set up your agility course on a hill with mostly jump turns, with an occasional walking lunge on a hill side slope to simulate a traverse. For telemark skiing, set up a combination of running, walking lunges, turn simulations, hops, and jumps. In a good agility circuit workout, you should feel like you are doing body movements similar to those of your activity and at similar speeds.

Precautions: Agility circuits require a high level of aerobic, balance, and strength fitness. You should be able to do basic lunges, hops, and jumps individually and with good form before you do them quickly in a circuit. You should also be able to comfortably do stationary balance exercises from chapter 5. Agility circuits can aggravate any existing lower-body or back problem. Caution should be taken if you are recovering from an injury or have a long-term condition.

ANAEROBIC CAPACITY

Some of the best methods of anaerobic training are interval running, cycling, rope skipping, and stair climbing. You can incorporate anaerobic interval training in your outside exercises to make a more complete workout. Do this by doing 1- to 3-minute high-intensity intervals of the above aerobic activities during an outside aerobic workout, or in between every 2–3 outdoor exercises to amount to 4–8 intervals per workout.

If you incorporate intervals into your outdoor circuit, you have a few options. You can do an interval training workout before or after your strength, balance, and agility exercises. This would be a 30- to 40-minute block of time that includes an aerobic warm-up. You could mix the interval in with the rest of the circuit, but you would have to warm up, at least for a few minutes, to enable you to safely reach your high-intensity target zone. (See chapter 2 for more details on interval training and precautions.)

TRAINING TIPS FOR THE MOST FUNDAMENTAL OUTDOOR EXERCISES
HILL RUNNING AND SPRINTING

Running and sprinting uphill are excellent exercises to increase both aerobic and anaerobic conditioning. Hill training interludes between circuit training exercises are excellent for outdoor conditioning. You can use hill running to incorporate an aerobic or anaerobic component into your outdoor program. Exercises on hills can be practiced upslope, downslope, and on the traverse. Slopes can help you to simulate the gravity demands of your activity. Keep these things in mind to gain the most benefit from your efforts:

- Lean into the incline of the hill.
- Emphasize the driving of your arms more than on a flat-surface run. Pump your arms more on steeper hills.
- Focus on the extension of each leg as you push off and the raising of your knee as it is brought forward.
- Look ahead to see where you are going.

A recommended hill-training distance for developing aerobic power is approximately 440–660 yards (400–600 meters). For anaerobic training, use a distance of 220–330 yards (200–3000 meters) or 1- to 3-minute interval times. The steeper the slope, the shorter the distance should be.

STAIR RUNNING

Stair running and walking are excellent aerobic training for general conditioning as well as for climbing, mountaineering, and backpacking. Try to find an outside set of connected stairways with at least five flights of stairs. You can walk with one-, two-, or three-stair strides. You can run one or two stairs at a time. You can mix interval sprints of 1–4 minutes during a stair running aerobic workout. It is better to walk fast or run the stairs in an uphill portion and to walk down the stairs or jog a path to get to the bottom of the stairs. Running down a flight of stairs can lead to knee or ankle problems. See chapter 2 for more information on stair running.

HOPS AND JUMPS

Hop and jump practice can help you to get ready for skiing, snowboarding, snowshoeing, climbing, and glacier mountaineering. It is especially good to do these on hills, because this can simulate the demands of your activity. Begin adding these to your program after you have established a good aerobic and strength base and within 4–6 weeks of beginning your activity.

For downhill skiing, a mix of more jumping than hopping is appropriate and should be practiced on a level surface before being done on a downhill slope. For glacier mountaineering, an emphasis on hopping with side-to-side and forward leaping motions is recommended. Try this both up and down a hill. When doing side-to-side hopping, do it on level ground first, then progress to a hill and vary the angle and distances of the hopping. Occasionally try a longer leap if you anticipate having to jump over a crevasse, etc. See exercises 75 and 76 for technique details.

DESIGNING OUTDOOR TRAINING PROGRAMS

When you design an outdoor training program or try one of the segment circuits at the end of this chapter, choose from exercises in this chapter as well as from chapter 5; the body region chapters in Part II; and the agility circuits in chapter 20, 21, or 22. Try to have a good mix of lower-body, upper-body, and abdominal exercises that are relevant to your activity. Some of the exercises are very conducive to outdoor training.

For the lower body try squats, lunges, step-ups, hops, and jumps (Exercises 70, 72, 73, 75, and 76, chapter 11). Doing them on hills (up, down, and traversing) is helpful for climbers, snowboarders, and skiers.

For the upper body try dips, pull-ups, and push-ups in outdoor settings. Exercises 86, 91.2, 91.3, 98–99, 101, 103, and 107 are all appropriate in outdoor settings.

For the abdominal region try Exercises 58–64, and 66–68.

You can do any of the balance exercises (see Balance earlier in this chapter) in an outdoor setting. Add additional challenges with logs and rocks.

OUTDOOR EXERCISES

The following exercises are divided into categories of lower body, torso, and upper body. However, these categories are intended primarily to aid in program design, because the exercises use more of the body than these categories imply. The best exercises for outdoor activities use multiple muscles and joints simultaneously, because we are interested in training the total motion, not simply one section of the body.

Each exercise is adapted to beginning, intermediate, and advanced levels. People with injuries might need to simplify movements to pre-beginning levels. Stop any exercise if you feel pain or discomfort.

Everyone, regardless of fitness level, should start at the beginning stage and progress when performance is easy and graceful. Only extremely fit athletes should attempt the advanced versions. Always warm up for at least 10 minutes before starting any exercise program.

LOWER BODY

48 | Outdoor Step-ups

Equipment: Raised platform 1–2 feet high.
Purpose: Develop your quadriceps, gluteals, and hip muscle groups for stepping motions.

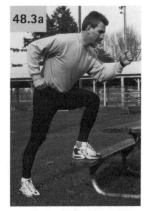

48.3a

Technique: See Exercise 73 for details on technique. Place one foot on a raised platform 1 to 2 feet high. Use a step, bleacher seat, park bench, log, or tree stump. Start with low steps and work your way up to higher steps to simulate the highest stepping demands of your activity. Glacier mountaineering will occasionally require step heights that place your knee and hip in a fully flexed position. Weight-shifting (see chapter 6) is quite important for step-up exercises that use the higher step heights found in outdoor settings. It is also important to push off from the back foot once you have weight-shifted onto the step. Once on the step, balance briefly on one leg and then slowly lower yourself down. You may raise your nonstepping knee up into the air and swing your opposite arm with it.
Variations: 48.1. *Beginning*: Use smaller steps. Consider assisting your step with ski poles. 48.2. *Intermediate*: Use larger steps such

as bleacher steps, rocks, or logs up to a foot high. 48.3. *Advanced*: Use very high steps that will bring your leg into a high step position with your hip almost fully flexed, such as a park bench seat or a foothold on a boulder (48.3a and 48.3b). Because most high stepping is done with some assistance from your arms, you may wish to use ski poles or wooden dowels to assist.

Precautions: Gradually work your way up to a high step, because there is a risk of muscle strains. Do shorter step-ups, lunges, and other exercises as preparation.

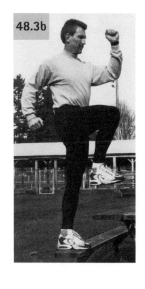

48.3b

49 | Squat Hops and Jumps

Equipment: None.
Purpose: Develop your quadriceps, hamstrings, gluteals, and torso for snow and climbing activities.

Technique: Warm up by doing 1–2 sets of regular squats, jumps, and hops. (See Exercises 70, 75, and 76 for technique).

Variations: 49.1. *Beginning*: In sand, do small continuous hops forward and backward. Do jumps with pauses in between and gentle landings (49.1a, 49.1b, and 49.1c). 49.2. *Intermediate*: Do jumps and

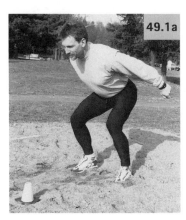

49.1a

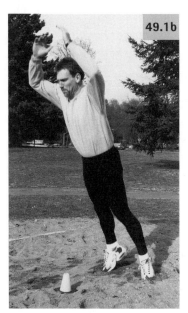

49.1b

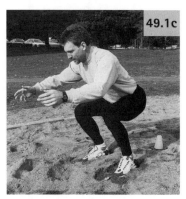

49.1c

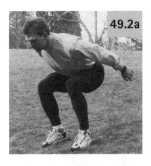

49.2a

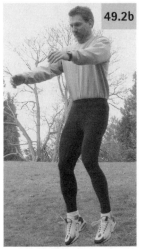

49.2b

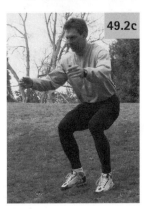

49.2c

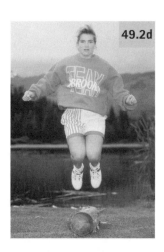

49.2d

hops on stadium steps or on a hill; do them uphill, downhill (49.2a, 49.2b, and 49.2c), forward, to the side, and diagonally. Try them over a stretched bungee cord, ball, or log, 6 inches off the ground (49.2d). To increase the difficulty, do them more quickly or raise the bungee cord. 49.3. *Advanced*: Add ankle weights and/or speed to the above exercises. Do lateral hops uphill, hopping with your downhill leg. Do quarter turns while jumping uphill. Avoid pauses between hops.

TORSO

These exercises are not intended for people with back injuries or low-back pain. No matter what your fitness level, always start with the easiest version to learn the movement and warm up before advancing. Perform torso exercises with great control. Your head should not be pulled forward or allowed to roll back. Find a head and neck position by imagining a string being pulled out the top of your head, not by extending your chin forward. For outdoor circuit training, add any of the functional abdominal exercises from chapter 10 for your torso exercises.

50 | Sitting Ball Rotation

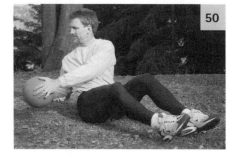
50

Equipment: Ball.
Purpose: Control rotation forces in a sitting position.

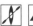

Technique: Hold a ball and sit on the ground with your knees slightly bent and your feet touching the ground. Lower yourself backward until you feel your abdominal muscles activating. Rotate your spine and touch the ground with the ball to the right and then the left.
Variations: 50.1. *Beginning*: Do the exercise slowly, then increase speed. 50.2. *Intermediate*: Hold a weighted ball. 50.3. *Advanced*: Perform movement on an incline, with your feet pointed uphill.

51 | Over and Back

Equipment: Ball.
Purpose: Increase the strength of the extensors of your back and gluteals.

  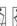

Technique: Lie face-down on the ground. Extend your arms overhead on the ground, keeping them close to your ears. Hold a ball (or imagine holding a basketball) in your hands. Extend your back and raise your shoulders and arms off the ground, moving from side to side as if you were raising the ball over an invisible 6- to 12-inch object (or use a cone or a natural object outdoors). Pause briefly on each side. Keep your legs straight and focus on your long, stable spine (51a and 51b).
Variations: 51.1. *Intermediate*: Hold the ball for 3 seconds without moving side to side. 51.2. *Advanced*: Lift a weight ball.

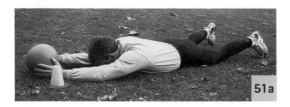
51a

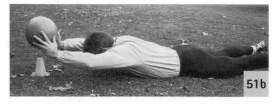
51b

Upper Body

For your outdoor circuit, include Exercises 20, 23, 24, 29–31, and any of the exercises in chapter 15 in addition to the following exercises.

52 | Dips

Equipment: Raised surface.

Purpose: Strengthen your chest, anterior shoulders, triceps, and upper back, and improve your ability to push yourself up or away from a surface.

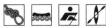

Technique: Dips can be done at different angles, depending on the surfaces you have available. Locate a raised surface that has a

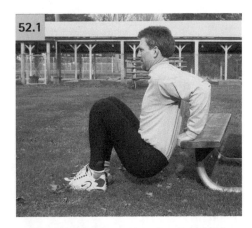

height that is between the level of your low back and knee when you are sitting on the ground with your knees in 60 degrees of flexion. You can use a park bench back's top or park bench seat, or a surface on a fallen log or a boulder. It's preferable to have two surfaces within shoulder-width apart. Back up to it until you are almost touching. Place the heel of your hands on the top edge of the surface, placing them just outside of hip-width apart, fingers pointing forward. Support your body weight, with your arms straight. Move your feet away from you about 3–4 feet, and keep your knees bent and feet flat. Lower your body by bending your elbows until your upper arms are almost parallel to the ground, then press down against the surface until your arms are straight again.

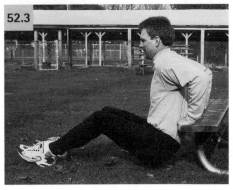

Variations: 52.1. *Beginning*: Bend your knees maximally under your body and use your legs to help push your body upward to assist your arms, as in a squat-type exercise. 52.2. *Intermediate*: Do the movement with your knees less extended. 52.3. *Advanced*: Extend your legs straight in front of your body, resting your weight on your heels. The farther your feet are extended, the more difficult the movement.

Precautions: Dips outdoors are potentially stressful to your elbows and shoulders.

53 | Pull-ups

Equipment: Overhead bar.
Purpose: Strengthen your upper back, shoulders, and biceps, and improve your ability to pull up your body weight.

Technique: Find a jungle gym or some other sturdy overhead bar. Grasp it, palms facing away from your body. Pull your body weight upward until you can see over the bar. Be careful not to reach up with your chin.

Variations: 53.1. *Beginning*: Do pull-ups on a low bar with part of your weight supported. 53.2. *Intermediate*: Do pull-ups with a partner. Have him or her stand behind you. Grasp the bar and bend your knees. Have your partner place his or her hands under the front of your ankles. When you pull up, press down against your partner's hands to relieve some of the effort on your upper body and to unload. 53.3. *Advanced*: Do the movements without a partner. When you can do at least 6 pull-ups unsupported, add weight to your body. You can do this with a backpack, ankle weights, etc.

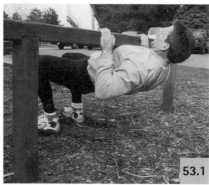

53.1

54 | Push-ups

Equipment: None.
Purpose: Strengthen your chest, shoulders, and back to aid in pushing.

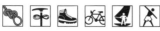

Technique: Identify different surfaces on which you can safely do a push-up in a standing and leaning position as well as on the level ground. Use tree trunks, stairs, boulder faces, etc. Do the push-up in a slow, controlled manner. See Exercise 86 for technique.

Variations: 54.1. *Beginning*: Do a push-up while standing and leaning against an inclined surface. Try 10–12 in a set. Next, vary the angle and increase the difficulty until you are doing some on the ground. Have your knees touching the ground. 54.2. *Intermediate*: Straighten your knees and have them off of the ground; do 8–12 in a set. 54.3. *Advanced*: Try plyometric push-ups (see Exercise 55, below), especially useful for climbers.

55 | Plyometric Push-ups

Equipment: None.

Purpose: Improve your ability to push quickly off of a surface, which is helpful for climbers.

Technique: Start a regular push-up as described in Exercise 86. After lowering your body to the ground, your hands should be placed to the outside of your shoulders and slightly below them. Your spine and body, from the top of your head to your knees, should remain straight, with no swaying or arching of your back. Plyometric (plyo) push-ups are done by quickly pushing your body off the ground explosively from the lowest position, instead of just pushing to the straight-arm position. Your hands will raise off of the ground. Start on an inclined hill, and gradually work toward doing these on flat ground. It is tempting to use your back muscles to throw yourself upward, but avoid this. Plyo push-ups are very difficult, so don't expect to do too many.

Variations: 55.1. *Beginning*: Try these against a wall or a sloped boulder. Try to do them at angles that will simulate the angles that you will need to push off of during your activity. Try push-ups on an incline (like a grassy hill) with your head uphill and knees downhill. Another way is to stand up, then lean into a park bench or picnic table with your arms straight. Your body will be at an angle to the ground instead of parallel to it, which makes pushing off much easier. 55.2. *Intermediate*: Add the plyo push-up on a more level surface. 55.3. *Advanced*: Increase speed and repetitions to increase difficulty.

Precautions: Plyo push-ups are a very high-level exercise and are potentially risky to your shoulders and back. Don't do them if you have any active injuries in these regions.

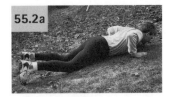

55.2a

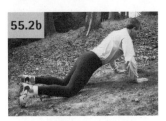

55.2b

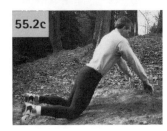

55.2c

OUTDOOR "SEGMENT CIRCUIT TRAINING"

This is a more sophisticated method of circuit training most suited for outdoor performance training that increases overall strength within an endurance format. There is greater emphasis on training the torso, and no machines are used.

Design an outdoor circuit of 10–15 stations using exercises from this and other chapters. In most cases, you will alternate between lower-body, upper-body, and torso exercises. Do 1–2 sets at each station, and rest only 30–60 seconds before moving on. You can walk quickly, run, skip, or cycle between stations. This keeps the heart rate at an aerobic level while still providing strength training. You can also incorporate aerobic or anaerobic intervals between stations.

APPLYING STRENGTH/ENDURANCE EMPHASIS TO A TRAINING PROGRAM

For those activities that require more endurance, follow these general guidelines:

- Do more repetitions (15–20) of each exercise.
- Do longer aerobic intervals between sets (e.g., jog or bike for 3- to 4-minute intervals or 10-minute lower-intensity aerobic sessions).

APPLYING SPEED/STRENGTH EMPHASIS TO A TRAINING PROGRAM

For those sports that are anaerobically-oriented, alter the segment circuit training this way:

- Do anaerobic interval training between sets (sprinting, short hill running, or cycling).
- As an alternative to counting repetitions, time some of your sets with a stopwatch or second hand and do as many reps as you can within 30–45 seconds.

SAMPLE OUTDOOR WORKOUTS

Below are two examples of how to pattern your outdoor workouts using segment circuit training. For both, do the following:

1. Fill in the exercise that you want, choosing from the upper-body, lower-body, and torso exercises in this chapter as well as with other exercises in this book (see Designing Outdoor Training Programs earlier in this chapter). Try to start with easier exercises that are safe for your spine before you add variations or advanced levels. If you wish to train for an activity, make your exercises as activity-specific as possible.

2. Try to incorporate some exercises to challenge your balance.

3. Consider adding an agility circuit somewhere in your outdoor circuit.

4. Make sure you do a short warm-up before beginning your outdoor circuit.

5. In the sample outdoor workouts below, numbers in square brackets indicate rest time between sets. You may decide to decrease or eliminate the rest periods as you get more experienced or if you want to make it a more aerobic workout.

6. Each segment of three to five exercises is followed by an aerobic or anaerobic interval. An effort level for each of these intervals is suggested, as a percentage based on resting is 1%, jogging is 50%, and maximum output is 100%. Pay attention to how you feel and learn how to assign an effort level percentage to that feeling. This takes practice. There is never a need to go beyond 90%. This would increase the chance of injury and require long recovery times.

Endurance Workout With Lower-Body Emphasis

Each segment is followed by a jog/run of 5 minutes. Use a stopwatch or second hand to time each set. Don't count repetitions. The timed sets are followed by short periods of rest. Do exercises at a rhythmic, non-explosive pace to increase aerobic capacity. See Figure 16.

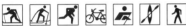

Explosive/Anaerobic Workout With Lower-Body Emphasis

Each segment is followed by a 60- to 90-second sprint, hill run, or hill cycle. Count repetitions instead of timing each set. Exercises are performed with increased speed and intensity (compared to those in the endurance workout in Figure 16), followed by longer rest periods of 60 seconds. This is excellent for sports requiring shorter, more intense workout periods followed by longer rest periods. See Figure 17.

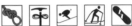

FIGURE 16. ENDURANCE WORKOUT

EXERCISE	TIME/INTENSITY	REST PERIOD (SECONDS)
Aerobic warm-up	10 minutes, 70%	
Lower body	30–45 seconds	[30]
Upper body	30–45 seconds	[30]
Lower body	30–45 seconds	[30]
Upper body	30–45 seconds	[30]
Run	5 minutes, 80%	
Lower body	30–45 seconds	[30]
Torso	30–45 seconds	[30]
Lower body	30–45 seconds	[30]
Torso	30–45 seconds	[30]
Run	5 minutes, 85%	
Upper body	30–45 seconds	[30]
Lower body	30–45 seconds	[30]
Upper body	30–45 seconds	[30]
Lower body	30–45 seconds	[30]
Aerobic	5 minutes, 75%	

ADVANCED LEVELS ADD ONE MORE SEGMENT:

Lower body	30–45 seconds	[30]
Torso	30–45 seconds	[30]
Lower body	30–45 seconds	[30]
Lower body	30–45 seconds	[30]
Aerobic	5 minutes, 70%	Cool down
Flexibility work	5–10 minutes	

FIGURE 17. EXPLOSIVE/ANAEROBIC WORKOUT

EXERCISE	REPS/INTENSITY	REST PERIOD (SECONDS)
Run, jog, or cycle	10 minutes	
Lower body	2 x 8–12 reps (fast)	[60]
Torso	2 x 20 reps	[60]
Lower body (hops and jumps)	3 x 10 reps	[60]
Sprint or hill run	60–90 seconds, 85%–90%	[60–90]
Lower body	3 x 8–12 reps (fast)	[60]
Upper body	2 x 8–12 reps (fast)	[60]
Lower body (hops and jumps)	2 x 8–12 reps (fast)	[60]
Sprint or hill run	60–90 seconds, 85%–90%	[60–90]
Torso	2 x 12–15	[60]
Upper body	2 x 8–12 (fast)	[60]
Torso	2 x 12–15 (fast)	[60]
Run variations: backward uphill	60–90 seconds	
Lower body	3 x 8–12 (fast)	[60]
Torso	3 x 12–15	[60]
Lower body	3 x 8–12 (fast)	[60]
Jog	5 minutes	Cool down
Flexibility work	10 minutes	

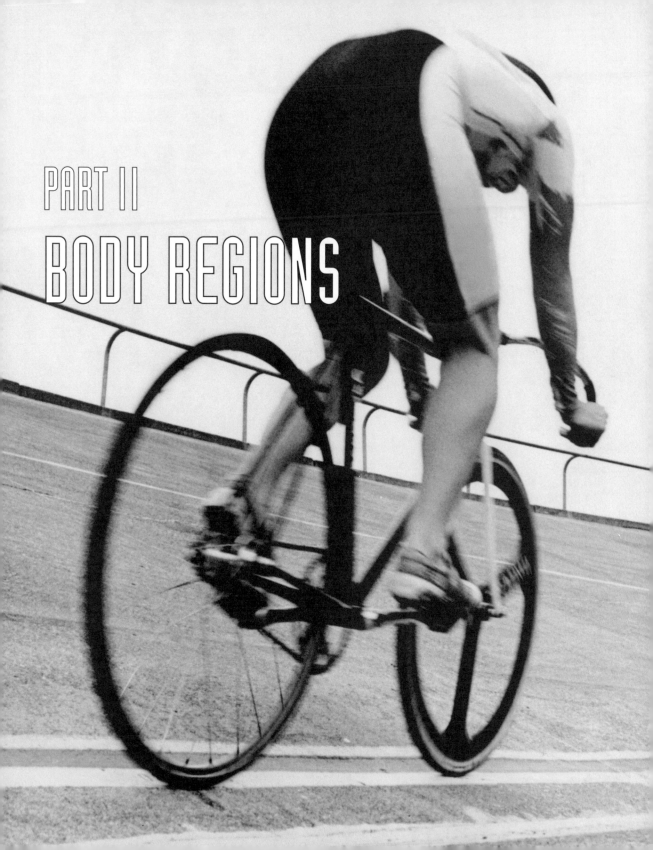

PART II
BODY REGIONS

Anatomy, Muscle Balance, and Musculoskeletal Injury

By David Musnick, M.D., Sandy Elliott, P.T., and Mark Pierce, A.T.C.

▶ **THIS CHAPTER WILL HELP YOU:**
- Understand movement, planes of motion, and anatomy terms used in other chapters in this book.
- Understand why muscles and ligaments get injured.
- Develop exercise and activity strategies while recovering from an injury.
- Orient yourself to the muscles described in chapters 10–24.

Your musculoskeletal system works as a whole, but can be analyzed and exercised in "regions." Learning about your system by using the regions approach can be very helpful in enabling you to analyze and plan a better exercise program. There are many important functional relationships between your regions. For example, strengthening your shoulder and upper back is critical for arm and hand functional strength. Strengthening your abdominal muscles and balance is important for lower- and upper-body function. Strengthening your shoulder along with your hip and leg is critical for many activities. More examples are discussed in chapters 5 and 10–16.

The body region chapters are organized similarly. Each begins with a brief description of the function of the body region, and describes functional relationships between the regions. The body region's anatomy, which is presented next, is not comprehensive, as you would find in an anatomy atlas or medical text, but is presented in enough detail to explain its functions without sacrificing accuracy. The anatomy review is followed by a discussion of common muscle imbalances and injury prevention. Exercises and self-tests are then presented.

BODY MOVEMENTS

Flexion or *flexing* means to shorten a muscle or set of muscles and bring one part of the body closer to another. *Spine flexion* means rounding your back. Hip and spine flexion will bring your chest closer to your thighs. *Sidebending* or *lateral flexion* means bending your back to the side so that your arm and elbow go closer to your buttock if you are sitting, or to your knee if you are standing.

Extension or *extending* means moving a joint from a flexed or neutral position (such as straightening your elbow or knee). In the spine it means the same thing but may also mean arching your back if you are starting upright or neutral.

Neutral is a term usually given to the spine. It indicates a position of spinal alignment in which the joints are positioned to give the spine its normal curves, and is usually near midrange alignment. Details are given in chapters 6 and 14.

Lateral movement (abduction) is away from the midline of your body. *Medial movement* (adduction) is toward the midline of your body. *External* (lateral) *rotation* is a rotation of your feet, knees, hips, and shoulders away from the midline of your body. *Internal* (medial) *rotation* brings these joints toward the midline of your body. *Circumduction* means moving a body area in a circular motion. It can be used in reference to pelvic motion that might occur in a canoe or kayak.

PLANES OF MOTION

Our body movements can be described in three planes of motion. *Sagittal plane motion* is movement in a front-to-back or flexion/extension direction. *Transverse plane motion* is in a rotational direction. *Frontal plane motion* is in a side-to-side direction.

In outdoor and sports activities, demands are placed on your muscles and joints to perform in these combined planes. Many exercises in this book have been chosen or designed to simulate multiplanar demands. This is a major component of functional conditioning.

PRONATION/SUPINATION

These terms are usually used to describe motion in the foot and lower extremity (foot, ankle, knee, and hip). When your foot *pronates*, it flattens and rolls inward and the arch gets slightly closer to the ground. The term *pronation* has been used in relation to the body and may mean rotating inward of the knee, hip, and shoulder as well as flexing of the spine. *Supination*

indicates an outward rolling of the foot and ankle and an increase in the height of the arch. In relation to the rest of the body, it may indicate external rotation of the knee, hip, and shoulder and extending of the back. Forces of gravity and the stance phase of gait tend to bring your body into pronation, and ground reaction forces and the push-off phase of walking tend to bring your body more into supination. For more discussion of phases of gait, see chapter 13.

BASIC ANATOMY

The musculoskeletal system includes the muscles, bones, joints, tendons, ligaments, cartilage, and fascia.

A *tendon* is found at the end of a muscle and connects the muscle to the bone.

A *ligament* connects bone to bone. It is a structure that helps to stabilize a joint.

A *joint* is the site of a junction between bones.

Joint cartilage covers bone surfaces to allow for smooth gliding of joints.

Fascia is a connective tissue.

Muscles that work with opposing forces around a joint or body region are called *agonists* and *antagonists*.

The illustrations in this chapter should be used as a reference to identify muscles, bones, and joints discussed in chapters 10–24.

INJURIES

Injuries common to outdoor athletes include muscle *strains*, tendonitis, ligament *sprains*, and *bursitis*. The following definitions will help you understand the injuries mentioned in each chapter.

Tendonitis is inflammation of the tendon, or the structure that connects muscle to bone.

Muscle strains are tears in the muscle belly or tendon and are also known as pulled muscles.

Ligament sprains are tears to a ligament.

Bursitis is inflammation of the bursa, which is a flat, pancakelike, fluid-filled sac. Bursas are located in places of the body affected by high amounts of movement, in order help reduce friction and allow the parts to slide and glide more freely. Bursitis commonly occurs in the shoulder, elbow, lateral hip, and kneecap regions.

PREDISPOSING FACTORS AND PREVENTION

Muscles and ligaments may overstretch and tear when they are subject to excessive mechanical loads that create undue tension. All tissues have a length tension curve of response to loads, which determines whether they will simply lengthen or tear given a certain load. There are many factors that may contribute to whether a sprain, strain, or joint injury will occur. A number of the factors are due to muscle imbalance, which is lack of balance in strength of muscles within a body region or between regions. Specific imbalances are covered in the body region chapters. The following factors may contribute to injury development.

Patterns of tight and weak muscles. Tight muscles usually activate quickly. They may pull joints into misalignment and lead to inhibition of their antagonists. Tight muscles may be a result of pain, joint motion problems (excessive mobility or less-than-normal mobility), or stress and central nervous system issues.

Inhibited muscles are weaker and activate more slowly. They withstand loads less well and are more likely to be strained or to lead to sprains or joint damage due to their inability to control motion. Muscles can be inhibited if antagonist muscles are tight, if there are postural problems, if they are stretched too much and overlengthened, as well as due to neurological problems (nerve pressure, disease, or autonomic nervous system dysfunction). Muscles can also be inhibited if joints are out of alignment, especially in the neck and low back. Muscles most prone to being weak or inhibited

FIGURE 18a

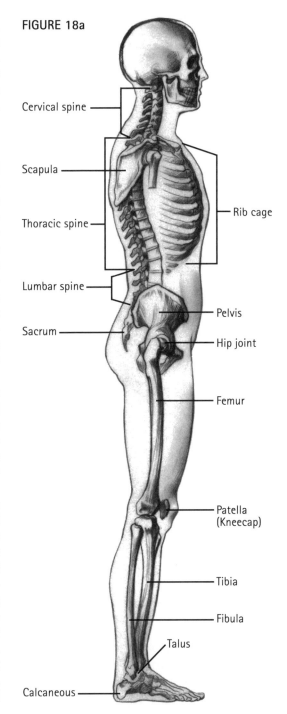

Cervical spine

Scapula

Thoracic spine

Lumbar spine

Sacrum

Rib cage

Pelvis

Hip joint

Femur

Patella (Kneecap)

Tibia

Fibula

Talus

Calcaneous

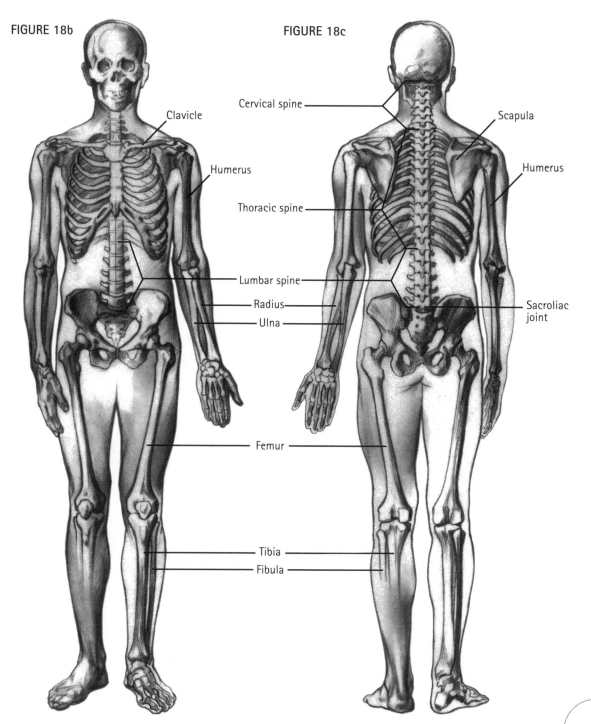

FIGURE 18b

FIGURE 18c

Clavicle

Humerus

Cervical spine

Scapula

Humerus

Thoracic spine

Lumbar spine

Radius

Ulna

Sacroiliac joint

Femur

Tibia

Fibula

141

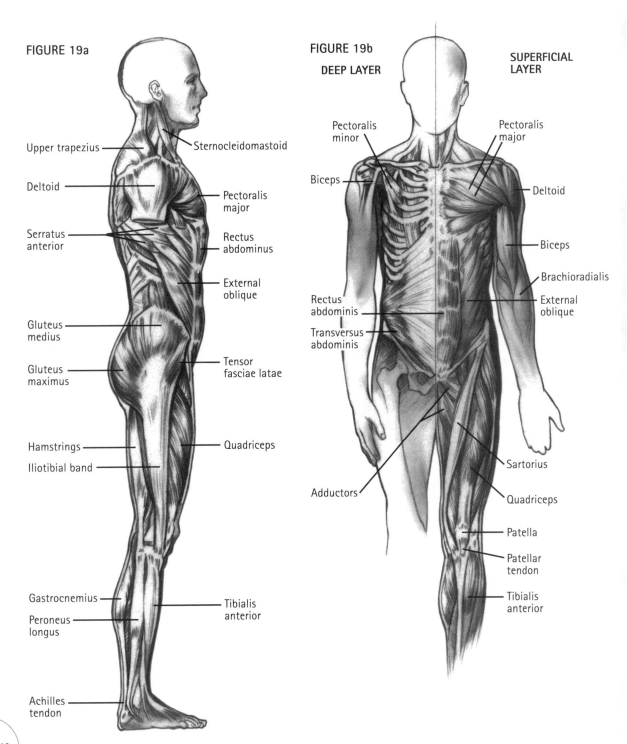

FIGURE 19a

Upper trapezius

Sternocleidomastoid

Deltoid

Pectoralis major

Serratus anterior

Rectus abdominus

External oblique

Gluteus medius

Gluteus maximus

Tensor fasciae latae

Hamstrings

Quadriceps

Iliotibial band

Gastrocnemius

Tibialis anterior

Peroneus longus

Achilles tendon

FIGURE 19b

DEEP LAYER

SUPERFICIAL LAYER

Pectoralis minor

Pectoralis major

Biceps

Deltoid

Biceps

Brachioradialis

Rectus abdominis

External oblique

Transversus abdominis

Sartorius

Adductors

Quadriceps

Patella

Patellar tendon

Tibialis anterior

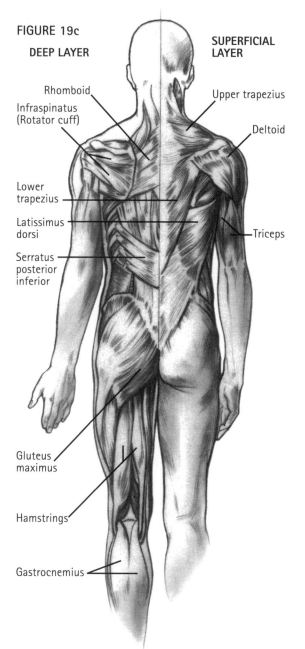

FIGURE 19c

DEEP LAYER

SUPERFICIAL LAYER

Rhomboid

Infraspinatus
(Rotator cuff)

Upper trapezius

Deltoid

Lower
trapezius

Latissimus
dorsi

Triceps

Serratus
posterior
inferior

Gluteus
maximus

Hamstrings

Gastrocnemius

are: the wrist extensors, rotator cuff, mid- and lower trapezius, abdominal obliques, gluteus maximus and gluteus medius, vastus medialis obliques, and the tibialis posterior. See chapter 4 for more information on tight muscles. Consider spending more time stretching your tight muscles and strengthening your weak muscles. Consider stress reduction techniques if you have chronic neck, shoulder, or upper-back tightness or pain. If you feel generally weak or you injure easily, consider consulting a health care professional.

Overuse. Excessive use of a muscle or muscles can lead to tendonitis or a strain. This may be from doing an activity or exercise with too much speed, duration, or resistance before your muscles are strong enough to handle the load. Build up gradually in your exercises and activities.

Inadequate equipment can lead to muscles having to work excessively. Footwear must be stable enough to support and control your body's motion. Orthotic supports may be useful in addition to good footwear.

Poor postural habits over prolonged periods may be due to inadequate knowledge of proper posture or to tight or weak muscles or joint misalignment. It can lead to shortened or lengthened muscles as well as joints functioning off of their normal axis of motion. See chapters 8 and 14 as well as the other body region chapters.

Improper recruitment of muscles during joint motions. When body regions move, more than one muscle is usually recruited. If one muscle is not doing its job, another muscle may have to overwork and get strained or develop tendonitis. For example, an inhibited *gluteus maximus* (buttock) can lead to hamstring problems during hip-extending activities such as climbing, backpacking, and running. Many functional exercises in this book work on recruitment pattern issues.

Improper movement patterns during exercise or activities. Form is important in exercise or activities so as to use muscles and joints properly with the least likelihood of injury. Make sure you understand the movement pattern of an exercise or activity before increasing resistance or speed.

Poor balance and agility can lead to injury of the extremities or spine from falling or excessive demands on muscles. Try to incorporate balance and agility exercises (from chapter 5 and the body region and activity chapters) into your program within 6–8 weeks of starting your activity.

Inadequate training and strength to control deceleration. Most musculoskeletal injuries are considered deceleration injuries because your tissues are exposed to quicker and more demanding forces during deceleration than acceleration. The demand for deceleration control is related to the pull of gravity as well as the need to control joint motion while a muscle is lengthening (eccentric contraction). Injuries occur when you cannot slow down and stop motion before failure. Many of the functional exercises address deceleration demands. See chapter 11 for details.

Inadequate strength training at longer muscle length, when muscles are normally weaker. Depending on your activity, you may need to train muscles when they are lengthened. This is especially true in climbing and certain boating activities. See the activity chapters for exercise advice for your activity.

Inadequate muscle training at the highest speeds that will be used during an activity. Do some of your exercises at higher speeds to simulate the speed demands of your activity.

Poor nutrition. Muscles, ligaments, and cartilage require certain nutrients for optimal function as well as for healing after exercise and activities. See chapter 3.

Inadequate attention during a task or activity. Focus your attention on your activity as well as the surface you are on, especially in steep or rough conditions.

INJURY PHASES AND HEALING

Different phases of tissue healing occur when you have injured a musculoskeletal structure. If you are doing a strength training program, take these injury phases into account to modify your strength training that involves an injured area.

Acute phase occurs immediately after an injury, lasting 24–72 hours. There may be pain, swelling, limited joint motion, muscle weakness, and muscle spasm. Minimize swelling utilizing ice or cold water; compression with bandages, braces, or tape; and elevation of a limb above the level of the heart. In addition, protect the joint from further injury, by limiting or modifying exercises or activities. Bracing, splinting, crutches, or slings may be used for more severe injuries. As soon as possible, restore pain-free range of motion. On day 2 or 3, pain-free range-of-motion exercises should help reduce swelling and restore tolerance for weight bearing or lifting.

Subacute (fibroblastic/repair) phase may last 14–21 days after onset of the injury. In this phase, there is clearing of swelling and cellular debris, and production of new cells and collagen to strengthen the area. Caution should be taken during this time and during the remodeling phase to limit exercises and activities so as to prevent worsening of the original injury. Remember that the pain will resolve much sooner than it takes to regain full strength and function. An injured tissue may only be 15%–20% strong at the end of this phase.

Exercises involving the injured body region should be done in pain-free ranges of motion and with minimal resistance to improve blood flow and decrease swelling. After acute pain and swelling have subsided an exercise may be done with 12–15 reps in a set for 2 sets. If no worsening occurs, progress to 3–5 sets of 20–30 reps. If there is pain at the time or within 24 hours of the exercises, they should be modified to involve decreased resistance. Exercises that involve other body regions away from the injury may be done with less resistance than used prior to the injury. This is important when exercising your arms and shoulders after a neck injury, or your legs after a low-back injury. You will find many balance exercises in chapters 5, 8, 10, and 11.

Other goals during this phase include regaining full joint motion, muscle, length, as well as balance and coordination. Gentle flexibility work can begin in this phase, but remember, injured areas can be injured more from aggressive stretching, so don't hold stretches in painful ranges and limit them to 20–30 seconds. Easy balance exercises can begin early in this phase. Functional strength and coordination exercises can begin in the middle of this phase, but should usually be modified to decreased ranges and decreased speeds.

Remodeling phase may begin within 2–3 weeks of the original injury and may last for many months (up to 1 year). In this phase, collagen in the scar tissue is being organized and aligned and the scar is strengthening, depending upon the exercise and activity stresses. An injured area may only be 40%–50% strong after 6 weeks, and thus caution should still be used in exercise and activities. Goals during this phase are to develop strong scar tissue and maintain cartilage; increase strength, flexibility, and balance; maintain aerobic capacity; and rehabilitate toward the functional demands of your activity.

In this phase, continue flexibility exercises and gradually increase the resistance of your strength training. Two to 3 sets of 12–15 reps are appropriate. Eight to 12 weeks into this phase, you may add a set of 6–8 reps of higher resistance to develop maximum strength, if you are training for activities that require quick bursts of activity or working against higher loads. Continue your functional exercises in this phase and incorporate more gravity and balance challenges. As you master the movement patterns, you can add speed to these exercises.

Outdoor activities should initially be done with less intensity, distance, and difficulty. Simulate and demonstrate competency in the motion, strength, and balance demands of your activity in a controlled environment before starting your activity. You can start getting back to your activity when you meet the following criteria:

1. You have normal lengths of muscles that have been injured.
2. Injured muscles and ligaments do not hurt when you simulate your activity for short duration.
3. You have good balance and coordination.
4. You have good muscle strength balance and recruitment in the injured and adjacent areas.
5. The joints of your spine have normal motion.
6. The joints in the injured or compensating areas have normal motion when compared to the noninjured joint on the opposite side of your body.

THE ABDOMINAL REGION

BY CARRIE HALL, P.T., AND MARK PIERCE, A.T.C.

▶ **THIS CHAPTER WILL HELP YOU:**
- Understand the function of your abdominal muscles.
- Perform a self-assessment of your abdominal strength.
- Learn new exercises that dynamically strengthen your abdominal muscles to meet the challenges of your sport or activity.

Your abdominal muscles are the core stabilizers of your trunk (torso). Essentially, your abdominal muscles are controllers and initiators of motion in rotation, forward and backward bending, and side-to-side movements. Functional abdominal strength provides dynamic control for these movements along with decelerating your body against changes in direction, speed, and surface.

All forms of outdoor activities require your body to be in an erect, semi-erect, or seated position relative to the ground and the forces of gravity. To develop optimal balance, coordination, and total body strength, perform functional abdominal exercises in standing and sitting positions, which are designed for dynamic abdominal function and injury prevention.

Understanding the anatomical and functional roles that your abdominal muscles play during activities will help you make educated exercise choices specific to your sport or activity and enable you to condition your abdominal muscles appropriately to meet those demands.

FUNCTION AND ANATOMY

There are four abdominal muscles positioned in specific layers covering the front, sides, and part of the back of your torso. Along with your back muscles, they form a link between your rib cage, spine, and pelvis. (See chapter 9 for illustrations of the muscles.) As a result, normal abdominal muscle length and strength is critical for proper torso alignment. With their attachments to the rib cage, spine, and pelvis, they provide a solid foundation for movement of your upper and lower extremities.

The first, and deepest, of the abdominal muscles is called the *transversus abdominus*. This muscle has fibers that run horizontally. Therefore, it functions like a girdle to provide support to your abdominal organs and spine.

The next layer is called the *internal oblique*, followed by the *external oblique*. These muscles have fibers that run diagonally to each other and cover primarily the sides and part of the back of the torso. They share the function of providing the primary force to produce rotation of the torso, but also have very different functions with respect to the pelvis and rib cage, as discussed below. The final layer is called the *rectus abdominus*. This is a muscle that extends from the ribs to the pelvis and is strengthened in the typical "ab" crunch.

The rectus abdominus and the internal oblique curl the rib cage toward the pelvis as in a sit-up. The internal and external obliques, along with the transverse abdominus, provide stability for the spine and pelvis during motions of the extremities.

The terms *upper abdominals* and *lower abdominals* relate to the relative functions of these muscles. The internal oblique and upper rectus abdominus are referred to as the upper abdominals, and the lower external oblique is referred to as the lower abdominals. The upper abdominals have a greater function controlling movements of the torso on the pelvis (e.g., sit-ups), and the lower abdominals have a greater function controlling the position of the pelvis and spine during leg and arm movements (e.g., lifting the leg to hike up a slope).

COMMON MUSCLE IMBALANCES

It is important to maintain balance in muscle strength and length between all four abdominal muscles, as well as between the abdominal muscles and the back and hip muscles. The most common imbalance is between the rectus abdominus/internal oblique group and between the external oblique/transverse abdominus group. This imbalance also alters the alignment and function of the low back and leaves it vulnerable to numerous injuries.

Most abdominal exercises emphasize strengthening of the rectus abdominus and internal oblique with crunch type exercises, for example, the bent-knees crunch, oblique curl-up, and feet-in-the-air crunch, as well as the curl-down abdominal machine. Rarely do you see exercises for strengthening the external obliques and transverse abdominus, and if you do see

them, the exercises are usually far more advanced than the average person's muscle strength permits (e.g., double leg lifts and leg lowering). Also, rarely do you see exercises to functionally strengthen the abdominal muscles in standing and sitting positions.

Muscle length is rarely discussed with respect to abdominal muscles. The typical postural problem of forward shoulders, increased curve of the upper back, and slumped chest demonstrates shortening of the upper fibers of the rectus abdominus muscle and upper, front fibers of the internal oblique. With this type of posture, it is inappropriate to perform trunk curl exercises or any variations. These exercises will only further shorten the rectus abdominus and internal oblique and exaggerate the postural problem.

Another common postural problem is a forward-tilted pelvis (excessive lumbar extension curve). This type of posture demonstrates overstretching of the external obliques. Again, trunk curl exercises will not specifically address this problem. An exercise that promotes a stable neutral pelvic position during progressively more difficult leg motions will more specifically strengthen the external oblique at its optimal length.

INJURY PREVENTION

In order to exercise your abdominal muscles safely, you must not only choose a safe technique, but also be sure you are exercising at the correct level for your strength. It certainly makes sense that you would not lift 30 pounds with your biceps if you could only lift 10 pounds safely and with good technique. Why, then, do we expect all individuals to be able to perform the same abdominal exercises?

Poor abdominal muscle strength, and/or imbalances in strength and length, are risk factors for the development of numerous musculoskeletal injuries and pain syndromes. The most common injury linked to the abdominal muscles involves the low back. Typically, the rectus abdominus and internal obliques become relatively stronger than the external obliques. An injury resulting from trauma, such as a low-back strain resulting from a fall, can be more severe or more difficult to recover from if an individual has poor abdominal strength prior to the injury.

EXERCISES

You can begin strength training exercises with 15 repetitions unless otherwise indicated. Progress your reps and resistance according to the guidelines in chapter 5.

MUSCLE BALANCING EXERCISES

The following exercises provide a foundation for developing muscle balance. It may be advantageous for you to develop competency in the following exercises prior to moving into the functional exercises. This will help you perform the functional exercises with balanced muscle activation patterns while tuning your body's fine motor control.

56 | Lower Abdominal Progression

Equipment: Firm, comfortable surface.
Purpose: Build the foundation for control over the lower abdominal muscles and improve the balance between the upper and lower abdominal muscles (external oblique/transverse abdominus).

Technique: Once you can perform this exercise, you may progress to variation 56.1 and omit this exercise; continue progressing through the variations in this manner. In order to progress from an easier exercise to the next in this series, you must meet the following criteria: First, the abdominal muscles must be pulled up and in, as if to bring your belly button (*umbilicus*) toward your spine. This will

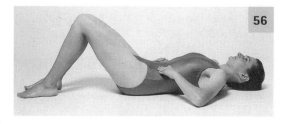

56

prevent a "pooched out" abdomen as increased strain is placed on the abdominal muscles from the progressively difficult leg movements. Second, the lumbar spine must remain in a neutral position with a slight extension curve, just enough to fit your hand between your back and the floor and not move into an exaggerated curve, or excessively flatten. The starting position is the same for this exercise and its variations. Lie on your back on a firm surface, such as the floor, with your knees bent and feet flat on the floor, with your shoes off. Place your little fingers on the bony anterior part of your pelvis to monitor pelvic motion. Your goal is to use your abdominal muscles to keep your pelvis from moving. Have your other fingertips on your lower abdominal muscles. Take a deep breath in, then exhale and pull your belly button toward your spine. Be sure to incorporate breathing to activate the transverse abdominal muscle. Do not concentrate on pushing your back flat but, rather, on lengthening your torso while pulling in your abdominal muscles. Start with 8–10 reps and gradually increase to 15–20 reps with each leg, an appropriate goal to reach before progressing to variation 56.1.

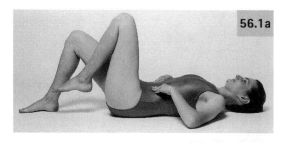

56.1a

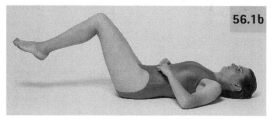

56.1b

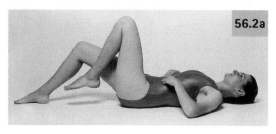

56.2a

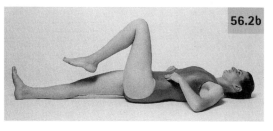

56.2b

Variations: 56.1. While keeping your abdomen pulled in (this occurs maximally at a full exhalation), slowly lift one leg so that the hip is at a 90-degree angle (56.1a). Breathe in while in the rest position; exhale as you lift your leg. Once you have completed the lift of the first leg, breathe in again, and then exhale while you lift the other leg to the same position (56.1b). Return to the starting position, one limb at a time. A good rule of thumb is to exhale as your legs are moving and inhale while they are resting. Remember that exhalation activates the transverse abdominus, which is required to stabilize your spine as you move your extremities. Alternate the starting leg with each subsequent repetition. Start each exercise with 8–10 reps and gradually increase to 15–20 reps with each leg, an appropriate goal to reach before progressing to variation 56.2. 56.2. Repeat variation 56.1, but instead of lowering the legs to the starting position, slide one leg down to a fully extended position while keeping the opposite leg elevated off the floor (56.2a and 56.2b). Breathe out as you slide the leg down. Breathe in while the leg is fully extended, and breathe out as you slide the leg back to the same position as the non-moving limb; repeat with the other leg. As soon as you are unable to stabilize the pelvis and lumbar spine and the abdomen begins to pooch

149

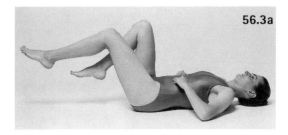

56.3a

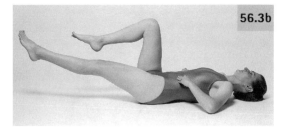

56.3b

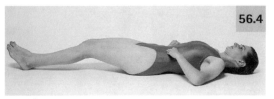

56.4

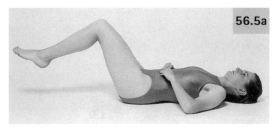

56.5a

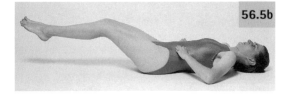

56.5b

out, stop and rest for a minute before continuing. Start each exercise with 8–10 reps and gradually increase to 15–20 reps with each leg, an appropriate goal to reach before progressing to variation 56.3. *Note:* If your hip flexors (front thigh muscles) are short, you will not be able to fully extend your leg without moving your spine out of neutral. In this case, stop sliding your leg when you notice your back moving from its neutral position. Eventually, your hip flexor muscles will lengthen as your abdominal muscles shorten and become stronger. 56.3. Repeat variation 56.2, but instead of sliding your leg, glide your leg down and back while keeping your heel 6–12 inches off of the floor. The non-moving leg should remain in a flexed position off of the floor (56.3a and 56.3b). Breathe similarly to variation 56.2. Perform 2–3 sets to develop endurance of these muscles. In preparation for functional exercises, achieve a minimum of 1 set of 20 repetitions. *Note:* It is easy to transition from a flat abdomen to a pooched abdomen in this variation. Keep your lower abs tight to avoid this problem. 56.4. From the starting position, lift both legs off the floor at the same time to the 90-degree position. Breathe in once both legs are elevated. Return to the starting position by lowering both legs at the same time. Breathe out as you move both legs down. Then, slide both legs simultaneously (while maintaining heel contact with the floor) to the fully extended straight-knee position, and breathe in as both legs are fully extended. Slide both legs back to the starting position; breathe out as you slide both legs up. Perform 2–3 sets to develop endurance of these muscles. In preparation for functional exercises, achieve a minimum of 1 set of 20 repetitions. *Note:* Variations 56.3 and 56.4 are similar in difficulty. You may find that sliding one leg at a time is more difficult than sliding two legs simultaneously, particularly if you have difficulty stabilizing against rotational forces. Choose the variation that is appropriate for you. Variations 56.3 and 56.4 are appropriate goals for the average person. 56.5. Repeat variation 56.4, but instead of sliding your heels, keep them 6–12 inches above the floor (56.5a and 56.5b). Slowly return them to the 90-degree position. Breathe as in variation 56.4. Perform 2–3 sets to develop endurance of these muscles. In preparation for functional exercises, achieve a minimum of 1 set of 20 repetitions. **Note:** Only the most fit individuals should try this variation. This is a difficult exercise and takes a high level of strength to perform properly. Don't do variation 56.5 if you have an active back problem.

57 | Upper Abdominal Strengthening

Equipment: Firm, comfortable surface.
Purpose: Strengthen your upper abdominals (internal oblique and rectus abdominus) to flex your torso.

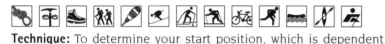

Technique: To determine your start position, which is dependent upon the length of your hip flexors, lie on the floor on your back with your legs out straight. If you can flatten your back against the floor with your legs out straight, this is your start position. If not, place a pillow or pillows under your knees until you can flatten your back against the floor. With your arms straight in front of your body, curl your chin to your chest. Once you have completely curled your chin to your chest, continue to curl your trunk (57a). As you raise your upper body to a sitting position, allow your neck to return to a neutral, relaxed position (57b; note the use of a support under the knees for tight hamstrings). To return to the start position, reverse your movement pattern. The start and finish position is the same for all variations of this exercise. If your hamstrings are tight, you may need to bend your knees to achieve a full sit-up position. If you are unable to curl upward through a full sit-up, just lift your head and shoulders off the floor. Start with 8–10 repetitions; 20 repetitions are an appropriate goal to reach prior to progressing to variation 57.1.

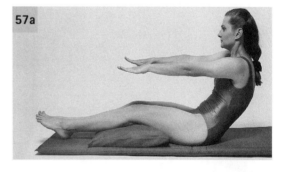

57a

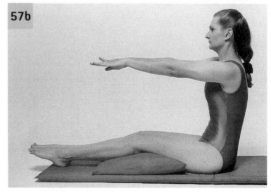

57b

Tips and Precautions: You should be able to perform a complete flexing of your torso before you flex (pivot) at your hips. You may notice that once you have completed the curl phase, your feet will want to lift upward. At that point you can secure your feet with a partner, under a couch, or under the bar of a sit-up board. The purpose of securing your feet is to counteract the fact that in order to sit up, you must contract your hip flexors. Without securing your feet, your hip flexors will attempt to lift your legs. If you find the need to secure your feet earlier in the trunk curl phase, it indicates that your abdominal muscles are fatigued and your hip flexors are taking over the motion. Stop and rest at this point. This is your maximum number of repetitions for this set. You must also be able to lift your upper body smoothly, without jerking, to the full sit-up position. Jerking movements indicate that your abdominal muscles either are not strong enough or have fatigued and your hip flexor muscles are trying to take over.

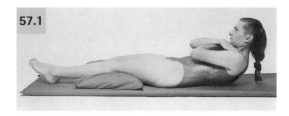

57.1

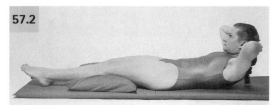

57.2

Variations: 57.1. With your arms folded across your chest so that your hands are on opposite shoulders, curl your chin toward your chest. Once you have completely curled your chin to your chest, slowly curl your trunk as you come to a sitting position. Maintain the curl throughout the movement. 57.2. With your hands supporting the back of your neck, curl your chin toward your chest. Once you have completely curled your chin to your chest, slowly curl your trunk as you come to a sitting position. Maintain the curl throughout the movement. Perform 2–3 sets of 20 repetitions to maintain the endurance of your abdominal muscles and progress safely to the functional exercises.

FUNCTIONAL ABDOMINAL EXERCISES

The majority of people continue to exercise the abdominal muscles with crunches, sit-ups, leg raises, and using various machines. This type of training is excellent for developing strength and muscle balance. Unfortunately, these exercises alone do not address all of the real-life functional requirements of the abdominal muscles during activities. To enhance performance in activities, train your abdominal muscles in the same way you wish them to perform. Functional abdominal exercises are designed to dynamically strengthen and challenge your abdominal muscles with movement patterns and balance challenges most commonly encountered during activities. These exercises are appropriate for many outdoor activities, icons for which are shown under the "purpose" heading (see Figure 1 in the Introduction). They are performed in sitting and standing positions and may involve additional equipment.

These exercises are non-traditional and very challenging. Make each exercise safe and pain-free. Start each exercise slowly and in a range of motion that you can control before increasing your speed or range of motion. Most of these exercises should be performed in a neutral zone of low-back alignment to prevent injury (see chapters 6 and 14). In addition, bring your belly button up and under your rib cage to initially activate your abdominal muscles. Make sure you breathe during the exercises. When you first try an exercise, begin with 8–10 reps in a set for just 1 set, and gradually increase the reps and the number of sets.

If you have a back problem, consult a health care practitioner skilled in biomechanics and musculoskeletal injuries before starting the following exercises. You should achieve competency in exercises 56.3 and 57.2 before progressing to the functional abdominal exercises.

58 | Beach Ball Shake

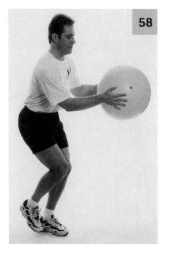

Equipment: Medium-sized beach ball (pour 4–6 cups of water into the ball and inflate).

Purpose: Strengthen the abdominal muscles in the transverse plane (rotation) and improve their ability to react in shortened rotational ranges of motion and changes of direction. Also condition the neck, shoulders, arms, hips, and legs and improve their ability to coordinate quick motions in association with the abdominal muscles.

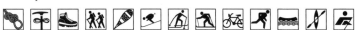

Technique: Hold the ball so that your hands face each other. Keep your elbows close to your sides and stand with your feet shoulder-width apart, knees slightly bent, and your low back in the neutral zone. Shake the ball vigorously side to side and non-stop for 30–60 seconds. Try this with one foot firmly on the ground and one foot just touching the ground. Perform 2–3 sets of 30- to 60-second intervals. Rest an equivalent amount of time between sets.

Tips and Precautions: Do not *roll* the water around the sides of the ball. Make sure the water is actually *hitting* the sides of the ball. Move as quickly as you can in a range of motion that does not cause pain. Make this exercise safe by maintaining your low back in the neutral zone.

Variations: 58.1. For an additional challenge, try balancing on one foot and perform the same time interval while shaking the ball. 58.2. After you have mastered that challenge, balance on one foot, shake the ball, and reach the ball toward the floor, then overhead. Keep the ball shaking through the entire movement.

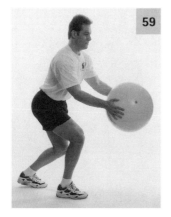

59 | Beach Ball Shake with a Forward Lunge

Equipment: Medium-sized beach ball (pour 4–8 cups of water into the ball and inflate).

Purpose: Improve the dynamic strength and flexibility of your abdominal muscles, mid to low back, and legs. Improve your functional leg and abdominal strength for forward, backward, and rotational motions.

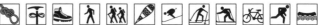

Technique: See Exercise 72 for basic lunge technique. Repeat the starting position of Exercise 58. While shaking the ball vigorously, lunge forward, then return quickly to the starting position. Make sure that the water in the ball is hitting the sides of the ball at all times through the lunge motion. Lunge again with the opposite foot and return to the starting position. One rep is a lunge done on first the right and then the left foot. Perform 2–3 sets of 15 reps.

Tips and Precautions: To begin, start your lunge motion slowly in order to determine a safe range of motion. Once you have developed your safe range of motion, increase your speed of movement. Keep the motions fluid, and react as many muscles and joints as necessary to facilitate the movement.

Variations: 59.1. Do as many reps as you can within 45–60 seconds. 59.2. When you become successful at Exercise 59, try reaching the ball toward the lunge foot. Remember to flex at your hips and knees and maintain a neutral low-back posture while reaching toward your lunge foot.

60 | Squat to Double-arm Overhead Diagonal Wall Reach

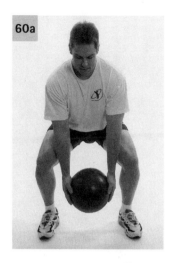

60a

Equipment: 3- to 5-pound medicine ball or any soft object weighing 3–5 pounds.

Purpose: Strengthen your abdominal muscles' ability to decelerate your body during backward bending and sideways rotational motions, such as in reaching, moving suddenly in a boat, or pushing off from a rock behind you.

     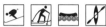

Technique: Stand with your back to a wall and take a step forward about 1 foot from the wall. Place your feet shoulder-width apart. Grasp the medicine ball, with your hands facing each other. Lower the ball down toward the floor and between your feet while bending your hips, knees, and ankles (60a). Squat down to a comfortable level, then return to the standing position while bringing the ball past your chest and raising it over your left shoulder and above your head until the ball touches the wall behind you (60b; note that this exercise should be done near a wall). Once you have touched the ball to the wall, return the ball toward the floor in a squat motion. Then repeat this motion to the right side. Perform 2–3 sets of 15 reps on each side of your body.

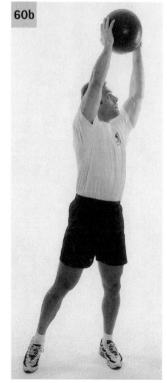

60b

Tips and Precautions: Follow the ball with your eyes through the complete range of motion. This will challenge your neck and upper back as well as your abdominals and legs. Allow your hips to translate forward as you reach overhead to the wall. This will help you maintain balance and add to the demands placed upon your abdominal muscles. Try to reach the ball as high as possible over your shoulder. Maintain your low-back neutral zone while flexing primarily at your hips. This will help limit the flexing of your mid and low back.

Variations: 60.1. Try balancing on one leg or changing the surface on which you are standing (for example, a soft, thick mat). 60.2. Try Exercise 60 while kneeling or half kneeling (one knee and one foot on the floor). Simulate the same stance you would normally assume during your sports activity. This is good for boating and cycling activities.

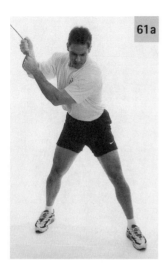

61a

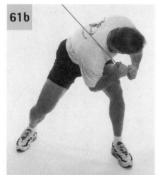

61b

61 Staggered Stance Abdominal Crunch with Rotation

Equipment: 3- to 5-foot piece of medium to heavy tubing and a door or high, immovable object.

Purpose: Increase the functional and dynamic strength of your abdominal muscles in forward and rotational movements. Coordinate this abdominal challenge with your legs to help you develop balance and functional strength for most outdoor activities.

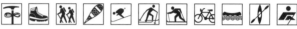

Technique: Attach tubing to a door or immovable object 2 feet above your head. Grasp the tubing with both hands. Stand sideways with your right shoulder facing the door. Step away from the wall until tension is developed in the tubing. Stagger your stance so that your left foot is in front of your right foot and your feet are wider than shoulder-width apart. Pull the tubing close to your chest and maintain this hand position during the exercise (61a). Simultaneously flex your hips and knees while rotating your mid back and hips. At the same time, bring your hands down toward your left knee, so that you end within 1 foot above your left knee (61b). Perform the same sequence in the opposite direction. Perform 2–3 sets of 15 reps on each side.

Tips and Precautions: Try to make this exercise smooth and continuous. Coordinate your arm, trunk, and legs through the entire range of motion. Avoid excessive forward positioning of your shoulders. Limit the flexing and rotating of your low back and maintain a low-back neutral-zone posture.

Variations: 61.1. Use a parallel foot stance, with your feet wider than shoulder-width apart. 61.2. Bring your hands down to touch your knee.

62 | Single-leg Stance Trunk Sidebend with Medicine Ball

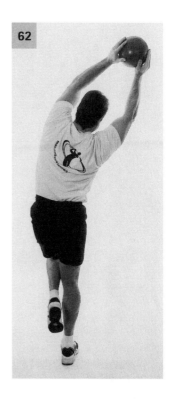

62

Equipment: 3- to 5-pound medicine ball or dumbbell.

Purpose: Strengthen the abdominal muscles and improve your ability to function in side-to-side motions while developing balance and coordination.

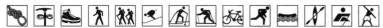

Technique: Grasp the medicine ball or dumbbell with your hands facing each other. Balance on one leg, knee slightly bent, with your toes 8–12 inches from a wall. Reach the medicine ball or dumbbell over your head. In an arc over your head, move the ball or weight toward your right side while bending your trunk to the right; then move the ball or weight to your left side while bending your trunk to the left. (Note that this exercise should be done near a wall.) Try touching the wall with the ball or weight randomly at clock positions of 10:00, 11:00, 1:00, and 2:00. Keep your low back in the neutral zone. Perform 2–3 sets of 30- to 45-second intervals.

Tips and Precautions: If you need to assist your balance, touch the floor with the opposite toes. Do not increase your speed or range of motion until you can balance for a full 30 seconds on either foot without assistance from the opposite foot.

Variation: 62.1. Change the surface you are standing on. (Stand on a mat or a half foam roll—start with the roll lengthwise parallel to your body, with the curved side up. Progress to placing the foam roll perpendicular to your body with the curved side up and then down. Be very careful with the roll in the curved-side-down position.)

63 | Standing Single-leg Abdominal Challenge with Dynamic Partner Resistance

Equipment: 8-foot belt and a partner.

Purpose: Develop your balance and abdominal strength with a strong base of support against a variety of directional changes experienced during any outdoor activity.

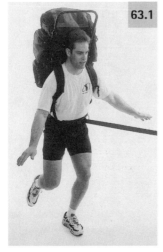

63.1

Technique: Both you and your partner should be in the standing position. Place the belt around your waist or chest and under your armpits, running the belt through the buckle but not fastening it. Have your partner take the end of the belt and supply just enough pull on the belt to challenge your ability to stay rooted to the floor. You will find yourself recruiting your abdominal muscles in order to stay upright. The object is to keep your feet fixed in one place and not let your partner pull you off balance. Also try this in a stride position, as if you were walking on a log. Have your partner apply tension to the belt for about 3–5 seconds, then change location. The partner can move around the exerciser to various locations, making the tension and location unpredictable. To become successful at this exercise and derive benefit, the partner should not overwhelm the exerciser with too much tension or apply the tension too quickly. Each set should focus pulls from quadrants of 10:00–2:00, 2:00–6:00, and 6:00–10:00 around an imaginary clock. Perform 2–3 sets of 15 pulls in each quadrant.

Variations: 63.1. Try this with a full pack on or while balancing on one foot. Beginning skiers can use ski poles, with their partner using gradual, slower pulls. Intermediate/advanced skiers can have their partners use very quick pulls in variable directions. 63.2. Do this while standing on a foam roll that is flat side up.

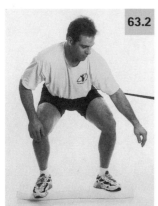

63.2

64 Single-leg Balance Overhead Double Arm Tubing Challenge

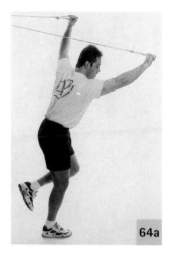

64a

Equipment: 2 pieces of tubing about 3–4 feet long and a door or high, immovable object.

Purpose: Functionally strengthen your abdominals in all three planes of motion, along with developing your abdominal muscles' ability to coordinate trunk stability with your upper and lower extremities.

    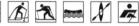

Technique: Anchor both pieces of tubing to a door or immovable object above your head. Face away from the door. Grasp one piece of tubing in each hand, with your elbows slightly bent and your arms overhead and in eyesight. Step away from the door until a mild amount of tension is developed in the tubing. This is your starting position. Balance on one foot with your knee slightly bent. Alternately move your hands forward, keeping your elbows still. When one hand moves forward, the other moves backward. Make sure you use your upper trunk and abdominal muscles to create the motion. Repeat this exercise on the other foot for the same time interval. Perform 1–2 sets of 30–60 seconds on each foot, moving as quickly as you can.

Tips and Precautions: Perform this exercise on both feet if you are uncomfortable with your balance. Start with short arm and shoulder motions until your strength and coordination develop. If you have a history of shoulder problems, keep the level of your elbows below your eyes during all shoulder movements.

Variations: 64.1. Gradually progress by beginning with your arms in a more overhead position. Once you are experienced with this, do sets with different arm starting positions. 64.2. Try balancing on a less stable surface, such as a thick mat.

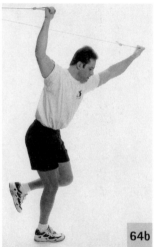

64b

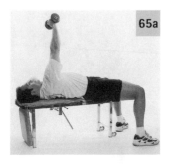

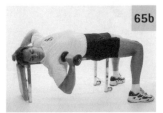

65 | Supine Single-arm Press with Trunk Rotation

Equipment: Bench and a 5- to 10-pound hand weight.
Purpose: Develop flexibility and strength of your abdominal muscles in coordination with your upper body. Enhance your ability to push and turn with improved confidence and strength.

Technique: Grasp the hand weight in your right hand. Place your back on the bench and position your torso so that your right shoulder blade is off of the bench. This will require you to maintain balance with your right foot and leg, along with your left hand (which will need to grasp the left side of the bench). Press the hand weight as far as you can over your chest. This is your starting position (65a). Next, bring the hand weight down toward your right side near your chest. Your hand weight should now be parallel to the front of your right armpit (65b). This movement will involve some rotation of your mid back. Make sure you follow the hand weight with your head and eyes through the full range of motion. After you have completed a set, repeat this exercise on the other side. Perform 2–3 sets of 15 reps on each side. Rest for about a minute between sets.
Tips and Precautions: Avoid excessive forward or upward motion of your shoulder joint. Primarily use rotation of your mid back to increase your range of motion.

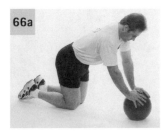

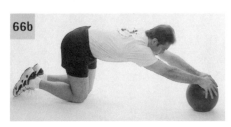

66 | Kneeling Ball Roll

Equipment: Medium-sized medicine ball or physioball.
Purpose: Functionally develop abdominal strength and upper-body coordination in all three planes of motion.

Technique: Kneel on the floor and place the ball out in front of you. Place your hands on the ball and lean on it (66a). Keeping one hand on the ball at all times, walk the ball away from your body as far as you can (66b). Walk the ball to your left, in front of you, and to your right. Make sure you stay in control of the ball and maintain balance. Return the ball to the starting position by rolling it back to your body. Start carefully with 1 rep in a forward direction. Work gradually to perform 2–3 reps in 3–4 different directions.

Tips and Precautions: Your center of gravity will move forward in the direction you travel. This will place a strain on your abdominal muscles, so do not overdo it by moving too far. Try not to let your low back arch. Maintain your low-back neutral zone as much as possible.

Variation: 66.1. Try this with one hand or in a half-kneeling position.

67 | Supine Crunch on Physioball

Equipment: Large physioball.

Purpose: Strengthen the abdominal muscles in the forward (sagittal) plane of motion and increase your mid to low back's ability to bend and extend. Also challenge your balance in a supine to seated position.

Technique: First, sit on the physioball and find your balance point. Slowly walk your feet away from the ball until your shoulder blades are on the surface of the ball and you are looking at the ceiling. Your hips should now be off the ball and your feet on the floor. Place your arms across your chest and allow your back to slightly extend over the surface of the ball. Curl your chin toward your chest and rise to a semi-upright position, maintaining balance and control over the ball. Perform 12–20 reps for 2–3 sets, resting about a minute between each set.

Tips and Precautions: Start slowly! Exercise in a pain-free and successful range of motion. Do not overextend your back. As you reach the top of the crunch, try bringing your hips toward your rib cage. This will put additional work on your lower abdominal muscles.

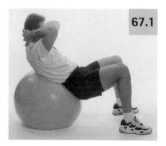

67.1

Variation: 67.1. You may wish to bring your hands behind your neck for added resistance and neck support. Don't jerk on your neck or head. Do not rely upon your arms to raise your body; use your abdominal muscles.

68 | Supine Ball Toss with Partner

Equipment: 3- to 5-pound medicine ball and a partner.
Purpose: Improve the abdominal muscles' ability to react, decelerate (slow down), and accelerate (speed up) the trunk against multi-directional external forces.

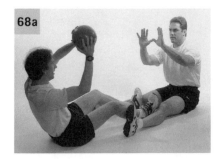

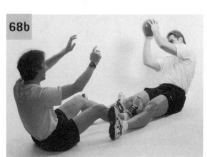

Technique: Both you and your partner should sit on the floor with your legs straight or knees slightly bent and the soles of your feet facing each other. With the medicine ball in your hands and your arms overhead (68a), lower yourself, back down, completely to the floor, then sit up and toss the ball at various angles to your partner. Your partner will receive the ball and lower him/herself toward the floor, back down with arms outstretched and overhead (68b). Repeat the motion by having your partner toss the ball back to you; play catch with each other. Toss the ball in different directions to make this exercise challenging in all planes of motion. Perform 2–3 sets of 12–20 reps or until fatigued.

Tips and Precautions: Before attempting this exercise, you should be successful at Exercise 56.2. Keep your feet in contact with the floor at all times. Toss the ball to the left and to the right of your partner. Keep the ball within reach while making it challenging.

Variation: 68.1. Try elevating one foot off the floor, or try bending your knees.

69 | Seated Physioball Boaters/Cyclist Reaction Challenge

Equipment: Large physioball.
Purpose: Strengthen your abdominal muscles' ability to react to changes of direction in a seated position.

Technique: Sit on a large physioball with your toes barely touching the ground. Pick one foot up off of the ground and try to balance. Work toward balancing with both feet off of the ground. Also try pushing off of one foot with the other foot on the ground, to challenge your balance. You can use ski poles or dowels as a stabilizing aid. To increase the challenge, perform this exercise with a partner and have him/her push randomly on the ball. Use your poles for safety. This exercise especially benefits boaters. Spend 2–3 minutes on the ball per set, for 3 sets 2 times per week.

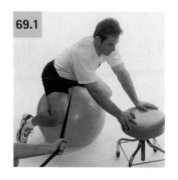

Variations: 69.1 (for cyclists). The object of this variation is to develop strength and balance control over directional changes. Sitting on the ball, move your feet behind you, making contact with the floor with the balls of your feet in a position similar to how your feet would be placed on your bike pedals. Put your hands on the seat of a chair, bench, or stool, gripping the edges the way that you would grip your bike handlebars. If you have a moving stool, move the stool farther away in front of you and from clock positions of 10:00–2:00. Place an 8-foot-long belt around your waist or upper torso and under your armpits, passing the end of the belt through the buckle but not fastening it. Plant your feet firmly on the floor for balance. Have a partner take hold of the end of the belt and try to pull you off balance while changing the pulling direction frequently. Your partner should pull just enough to challenge you, giving tugs in clock quadrants of 10:00–2:00, 2:00–4:00 or 2:00–6:00, and 6:00–10:00 or 8:00–10:00. Perform 2–3 sets of 10–15 pulls in each quadrant. 69.2. When you become successful at variation 69.1, try it with one foot off the floor. You will only need minimal resistance from your partner.

Tips and Precautions: The partner should not administer an overwhelming force to the exerciser. Allow the exerciser to develop the coordination and strength to meet each challenge.

GENERAL CONDITIONING PROGRAM

The exercises below are recommended for establishing a basic abdominal program for the average person desiring good functional abdominal strength and tone. You can add any of the other abdominal exercises in this chapter to your basic program to prepare for specific activity challenges.

Exercise 56.3 (2–3 sets of 15 reps)

Exercise 58 (2 sets of 30- to 45-second intervals)

Exercise 61 (2 sets of 12–15 reps on each side)

Exercise 62 (2 sets of 12–15 reps to each side of your body)

Exercise 67 (2 sets of 12–15 reps)

The Knee, Thigh, Hip, and Buttock Region

By Mark Looper, P.T., Mark Pierce, A.T.C.,
and David Musnick, M.D.

▶ **THIS CHAPTER WILL HELP YOU:**
• Understand how this critical region functions.
• Do basic functional exercises such as squats, lunges, step-ups,
  hops, and jumps to improve your functional strength.

Your hip, buttock, and knee allow you to position your foot where you want it to go. They allow you to move pedals, run or climb on rocks and trails, and move or stabilize yourself in boats. They also help you to decelerate so that you can control your speed going downhill. They are very important, along with your lower leg and abdominal muscles, in controlling balance.

FUNCTION AND ANATOMY
The muscles described below basically work as movers and decelerators of motion, depending on whether the foot is on or off of the ground or how you are using your hip and knee if you are sitting. See chapter 9, Anatomy, Muscle Balance, and Musculoskeletal Injury, for illustrations.

The *psoas* muscle flexes your hip (placing your knee in front of your body and closer to your chest) and works in conjunction with the hip extenders. The hip abductor (*gluteus medius*) moves the foot and knee away from the body when your foot is off of the ground. When your foot is on the ground, it slows down side-to-side motion of your pelvis. The abductors work in conjunction with the groin muscles (adductors).

They bring the thigh and foot closer to the body or stabilize your leg from going away from the center of the body. The *iliotibial band* (ITB) on the side of the hip assists the abductors in slowing down your pelvis from moving sideways when your foot is on the ground. When your foot is off of the ground, the ITB assists your abductors in moving your leg away from the midline of your body.

The *quadriceps* (quads), the muscles on the front of the thigh, extend your knee if your foot is off of the ground, or decelerate the knee from flexing and collapsing if the foot is on the ground. They work in conjunction with the *hamstrings*, which flex the knee if the foot is off the ground, or decelerate knee and hip flexion if the foot is on the ground.

If you are sitting in a crew boat or on a bicycle, these muscles work more to initiate motion in flexing and extending the knees and hips. If you are walking, especially downhill, these muscles work more to decelerate or control your body and keep you upright. This explains why your quads and kneecaps may hurt more after downhill hiking or running.

Muscle function is often broken down into either open (foot is free to move) or closed (foot is fixed on the ground, a pedal, or a platform, for example) kinetic chains of motion. In order to better understand muscle function in a closed kinetic chain environment, imagine yourself descending fairly steep terrain. When your foot makes contact with the ground, a strong inward rotational force is generated as your foot moves from an arched position (*supination*) and begins to flatten (*pronate*). Your knee and hip then bend to absorb the force of your body weight. This requires muscles that catch you or decelerate your leg's internal rotational force and your hip and knee during flexion. Without proper muscular deceleration, we may overstrain or injure the leg, or accelerate down the hill faster than we can control.

Once we have decelerated, we need our muscles to propel our body over the foot, muscles that externally rotate the hip as well as extend the hip and knee. Thus, the cycle continues, from deceleration to propulsion to deceleration. Exercises in this chapter work on both these functions.

The *patellofemoral joint* consists of the *patella* (kneecap), which is imbedded in the center of the quadriceps tendon and slides up and down in the groove on the *femur* (thigh bone) as the knee is bent or extended. The knee joint consists of cartilage and many ligaments. When you are bearing weight, tension from the quadriceps muscle group is present in all knee positions, thereby firmly fixing or stabilizing the front of your knee. Knee motion is primarily flexing and extending. The knee joint is much more susceptible to injury than the hip joint. The hip is a very stable joint that can move in many directions. Hips may have tendon problems, but the joint is rarely injured. The hip can become problematic due to adjacent joints, such as the back, that compensate for the lack of hip motion.

COMMON MUSCLE IMBALANCES

One of the most common muscle imbalances at the hip is weakness of the *gluteus maximus* (buttock muscle). This often coincides with weaker abdominal muscles. This results in the pelvis being tilted forward, increasing the arch in the low back (*lordosis*). The hip flexes and the thigh rotates inward. Hiking or exercising in this position can stress and strain the low back and lead to hip and knee strains, tendonitis, or bursitis.

The gluteus maximus and *tensor fasciae latae* (lateral hip muscle) both connect to the iliotibial tract. A common imbalance is that the gluteal muscles are underutilized and underdeveloped, and the tensor fascia lata gets tighter, resulting in shortening of the ITB. This can translate into increased friction over the bony surfaces at the hip and knee, leading to hip and knee bursitis. The hamstrings on many people are tight or weak and thus are prone to "pulling." They can also place more strain on the back or knee. At the knee, a common imbalance is a weaker inner quad muscle (VMO).

STRATEGIES FOR STRENGTHENING

Your exercise program for this region should address your muscle imbalances and use your muscles in a functional manner. When strengthening your hips, buttocks, and thighs, it is important to do the majority of your exercises in ways that mimic the function of your activity. If you are sitting during your activity, do most of your exercises while sitting as well as some while standing. If you are standing during your activity, do most of your lower-extremity exercises while standing. If you don't have any current goals but simply want to stay fit, follow the Basic Strengthening Program.

OBJECTIVES

1. Maintain flexibility in your hip joint, hamstrings, calf, and ITB to lengthen the

commonly tight areas. Use stretching Exercises 1–9.

2. Develop strong buttocks, hamstrings, and inner quads to strengthen these commonly weaker areas. Use Exercises 20, 22–25, 28, 29, 31, and 32. (Exercises 26, 27, and 30 are advanced exercises for your buttocks, hips, and balance.) Use Exercises 70–74. (Exercises 75 and 76 are advanced.)

3. Develop and challenge your balance to improve your muscles to work dynamically. Choose from Exercises 20.1, 27, 28.1, 30, 31.1, 37–40, 59, 62–64, 69, 70.2, 73, 75, and 76.

BASIC STRENGTHENING PROGRAM

This program will give you a basic functional strength foundation for this body region based on the above objectives. You can add any of the other exercises listed above to meet specific activity goals.

1. Do stretching Exercises 1, 3, 5, 6, 8, and 9.
2. Do Exercises 23.3 and 23.4 or 24, 72, 72.3, and 73.
3. Do Exercises 38.1 and 62.

EXERCISES

The exercises below are basic versions of the squat, lunge, step-up, and jump, and should be practiced before going on to the combination exercises in chapter 5, Strength and Balance Training, and the more advanced jumps in chapters 8, Creative Use of the Outdoors in Training, and 20, Snowboard and Ski-Specific Training. The exercises in this chapter are considered closed kinetic chain exercises (except for Exercise 71) and are well suited to the outdoor enthusiast. All of the exercises can be done in sets of 15–20 reps except for the hops and jumps; build up your strength and balance before doing hops and jumps.

Note: All of the exercises in this section except Exercise 71 use your hamstrings in a functional manner.

70 | Squat

Equipment: Level surface to start; may progress to hills or balance equipment (see chapter 5).
Purpose: Establish basic buttock, quad, and calf deceleration strength. The squat is also the basis for jumping and plyometrics.

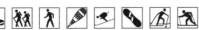

Technique: Beginners should start with mini- to half squats. Start on flat ground with your weight evenly distributed side to side and front to back. Stand with your feet shoulder-width apart. Lower your buttocks until your knees are at an angle of about 60 degrees. Keep your back in a neutral position to avoid excessive flexion. Be sure that your knees are aligned with your first and second toes. It isn't necessary to go lower than having your thighs parallel to the ground. If your knees hurt with a squat, you can reduce the depth or unload part of your body weight with ski poles. Try 15 reps and do 2–3 sets slowly, then gradually increase speed.

Variations: 70.1. Hold free weights or use a pack while squatting. 70.2. Do a squat on one leg. Do not increase the depth of your squat until your balance has improved and you can do it pain-free. 70.3. Try doing squats on a hill. 70.4. Squat machines are another alternative. The best ones are upright or at a 45-degree angle. For rowing athletes, it makes sense to use a sitting leg press machine. 70.5. *The Squat and Clean*, excellent for crew and climbing, is a difficult lift requiring precise spine positioning and technique. Refer to an Olympic lifting text or have a trainer in a gym demonstrate it to you. Don't do this if you have any active spine problems.

71 | Hamstring Curls

Equipment: Ankle weights and vertical surface (such as a wall), or hamstring curl machine (seated).

Purpose: Increase the strength of your hamstring to flex your knee, especially for cyclists and crew.

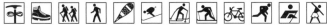

Technique: Attach an ankle weight to one ankle and stand on the opposite foot with your knee slightly bent. Stabilize yourself by touching a wall. Maintain both thighs in a vertical position while bringing your heel to your buttock. To use a hamstring curl machine, refer to the instructions on the machine or consult a trainer for technique. Do 15 reps for 2–3 sets with each leg.

Tips and Precautions: Keep your back in a neutral spine position to avoid excessive low-back stress. Try to limit excessive upper-body motion during the exercise.

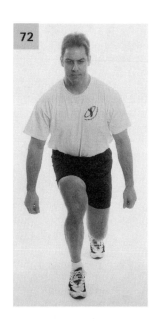

72 | Lunges

Equipment: Level indoor or outdoor surface, hills.
Purpose: Improve your ability to handle your body's weight in a deceleration mode, landing on one foot.

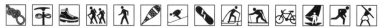

Technique: For a forward lunge, start in a standing position with your feet parallel to one another and 1–2 shoe widths apart. Place one foot about 1½–2 feet forward and allow your front knee to bend. The *excursion* of the lunge is the length from where your toe begins in the start position to where your heel makes first contact with the surface after you lunge. If you are shorter than 5 feet, 5 inches, you may want to start with a 1-foot excursion. Progress your lunge excursion gradually. Perform most of your lunges within a 1½- to 2-foot excursion. You may do some of your lunges past this range if your activity requires longer lunge movements. Before progressing to longer lunges, follow these guidelines:

1. The movement should be pain-free.
2. Wobbling or swaying of your knees or torso should be minimal.
3. Keep your low back in a neutral position and allow minimal forward or side-to-side motion of your back with the lunge.
4. Before increasing the excursion of the lunge past 2 feet, try increasing the speed of your lunges while maintaining good control of motion.

Control the speed of knee flexion and stop at about 55–60 degrees. Allow your back knee to bend and your back foot to lift up at the heel. Try to align your forward knee over your first and second toes. Return to the start position by pushing off of your front foot. Try alternating the lunge foot that you put forward. (See also Exercise 23.3, lunge with weights.) Try a set with 15 lunges on each foot. Try to increase the speed of your lunges to see how many you can do in 30–45 seconds, especially if you are a skier or climber.

Tips and Precautions: If the forward lunge is painful, try decreasing the depth of the knee flexion and add lunges in different directions, especially to the sides. If a lunge is still painful, try unloading it as in variation 72.1. In any lunge, make sure your knee is in line with your foot.

Variations: 72.1. Unload a lunge to decrease kneecap pain by using ski poles or dowels to support part of your body weight as you bend your knee in the basic lunge. 72.2. If you are a telemark skier, increase your lunge excursion as your ability allows, simulating your skiing. 72.3. *Sidestep (lateral) Lunge*: Lunge to one side and then the other while keeping your feet facing forward. Measure your lunge excursion from the inside of your non-lunging foot to the inside of your lunging foot. Try to avoid leaning your shoulder toward your lunge foot. Perform most of your lunges with an excursion of 1½–2 feet. If you are a cross-country or telemark skier or a mountaineer, some of your lunges should have excursions of 2–2½ feet. You can do lateral lunges with hand weights held at your sides or with ski poles. (A more advanced version of this is a sidestep lunge on stairs. You can do this up 2–3 stairs at a time to simulate sidestepping up a hill in cross-country skiing.) 72.4. Perform a sidestep lunge while shaking a partially water-filled beach ball or a body blade vigorously side to side. This is excellent training for snowboarders. 72.5. Try a walking lunge by stepping forward with each lunge instead of returning to the start position. 72.6. Try doing variation 72.5 with hand weights as in Exercise 24 while doing a lunge walk. 72.7. Do a walking lunge with a partially filled beach ball or a body blade. Shake it side to side vigorously, to increase the balance and abdominal challenge (see Exercise 59). 72.8. Do a walking lunge in a sidestepping motion. 72.9. Perform variation 72.8 while shaking a ball or body blade. 72.10. Doing a lunge with a biceps curl is an excellent way to exercise your arms, back, and legs simultaneously (see Exercise 23). 72.11. Doing a lunge with an opposite knee reach is excellent for telemark skiers (see Exercise 24). 72.12. Lunge with a combined shoulder elevation (see Exercise 25). 72.13. The lunge matrix is a dynamic whole-body lunge combination exercise (see Exercise 26). 72.14. Try lunges on outdoor terrain, especially hills (see chapter 8). Add resistance or balance challenges by holding hand weights or wearing a backpack. 72.15. *Rotational (transverse) Lunge*: Position yourself in the center of an imaginary clock and locate 3:00, 4:00, and 5:00 (to your right and slightly behind you) and 9:00, 8:00, and 7:00 (to your left and slightly behind you). Start by lunging toward 3:00 with your right foot while pointing the toes of your right foot at the 3:00 position. Remember to pivot on your non-lunge foot so that you don't stress your knee. The guidelines for lunge excursion are the same as for the forward lunge. Once you have lunged to a safe range, return to the start position in the center of the imaginary clock and face 12:00. Repeat this lunge maneuver toward 4:00 and 5:00 with your right foot, then switch to your left foot and lunge to 9:00, 8:00, and 7:00 (see Exercise 26c).

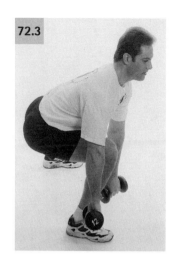

72.3

73 | Step-ups

Equipment: 4-inch step on a step platform, or stairs or bleachers with a 6- to 8-inch step.

Purpose: Improve your leg's ability to go up steep inclines, steps, rocks, or logs, which is essential to the hiker, climber, or mountaineer.

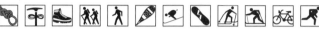

Technique: Start with your feet shoulder-width apart, about 6–12 inches from the step. Lift and place one foot onto the step surface and then shift your weight forward, keeping your back in a neutral

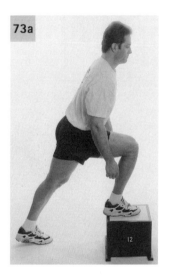

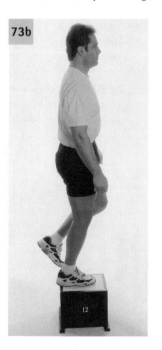

position. Shift your weight forward until you feel your back heel lifting off the ground, or until about three-fourths of your weight is on your front foot (73a). Then push off of your back foot and straighten your front knee (73b). Place both feet on the step and return to the start position with your knees slightly bent. You can repeat the step-up with the same knee each time in 1 set, or alternate the stepping-up foot. Increase the height of the step gradually. You can use a staircase and step up 2–3 stairs at a time. Backpackers and climbers should gradually increase step height to simulate the highest step up that you might have to take in the outdoors. This may be as high as 2–3 feet. When doing a high step, weight shifting is very important. You may want to use ski poles to assist you on a high step to simulate a handhold. Do 2 sets of 15 reps. Try to do one set of 4–6 high step-ups if you are a scrambler or a climber.

Variations: 73.1. Do a step-up with an overhead press (see Exercise 31). 73.2. Do a step-up with resisted shoulder extension (see Exercise 32).

74 | Anterior Step-down

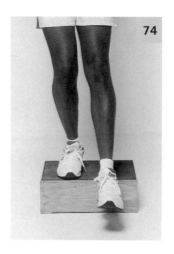

74

Equipment: 4-inch step on a step platform, or stairs or bleachers with a 6- to 8-inch step.

Purpose: Improve your ability to control gravitational forces while moving downhill.

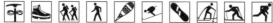

Technique: Stand with both feet on the step, facing "downhill." Balance on one foot and with the other foot reach to the floor in front of you. Allow both knees to bend and try to keep your back in a neutral position. During this initial phase of the step-down, try not to transfer your body weight over the descending foot. Touch your heel to the floor and then return back to the start position. Use the foot and leg on the step to raise yourself back to the start position. Do 2 sets of 15 reps.

Variations: 74.1. Increase the step height, especially if you are a scrambler or climber. You can use 2–3 stairs. 74.2. Increase the distance from the step to the ground touch area to 10 inches away, etc. 74.3. Add resistance by wearing a backpack or holding hand weights. 74.4. On stairs, do connected step-downs of 2–3 stairs for 30–240 seconds.

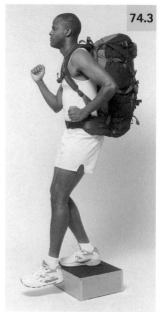

74.3

JUMPS AND HOPS

You can begin adding jumps and hops to your program after you have established a good aerobic and strength base. You should be able to do Exercises 27, 30, 37, 38.3, 40, and 70–74 before doing hops and jumps. You should not do these if you have any ongoing musculoskeletal injuries.

Vertical jumps are appropriate for rock climbers. Hopping (or leaping) and landing on the opposite foot is more functional for mountaineering and snowshoeing. For glacier mountaineering, emphasize hopping with side-to-side and forward leaping motions. Try this both up and down a hill. Do side-to-side hopping on level ground first, then progress to a hill and vary the angle and distances of the hopping motion. Occasionally try a longer leap if you anticipate having to jump over a crevasse, etc. You may begin with a short run before some of your hops. For downhill skiing and snowboarding, in general, a mix of more jumping than hopping is appropriate and should be practiced on a level surface before doing them on a downhill slope. Jumps are also functional for crew preparation.

A hop is performed by leaping and landing on one foot. Hops can begin and land on the same foot or begin on one foot and land on the opposite foot. In general, a hop requires more balance and strength than a jump. A jump begins and finishes on both feet. Try basic jump exercises prior to hop exercises.

Your hops and jumps can start out small and progress to longer distances to simulate the motions of your activity. You can vary the amplitude, direction, and slope with your jumps. You can do your hops and jumps in sets of 3–8 reps initially in the same direction and distance. As you increase in your general strength, perform your hops and jumps with greater distances and speeds.

Hops and jumps engage the torso and the arms to propel weight off the ground, so they are considered total body movements. Do an aerobic warm-up and some lunge or squat exercises before doing hops and jumps. After performing jumping and hopping exercises, cool down with an aerobic period of 5–10 minutes consisting of a brisk walk, cycle, or run.

Proper form is imperative while hopping and jumping. Don't allow your knees to bend more than 90 degrees when you land. Protect your back by doing most of your bending from your hips, knees, and ankles. Hops and jumps should not be done if you have limited motion in your ankle or if you have a knee, back, or foot problem. If you have sore knees or any other problems that make landing from jumps uncomfortable, try the same routine but use water jumps or uphill jumps to soften the impact.

75 | The Basic Jump

Equipment: Level floor or ground; progress to using hills, snow, and/or a backpack.

Purpose: Improve your ability to balance while decelerating and propelling your body in an explosive manner, such as in activities on snow, on climbing walls, and in the mountains. Also improve power in runners.

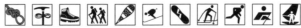

Technique: Stand with your feet slightly farther than shoulder-width apart, with your arms in a relaxed position at your side. Wind up by bending your knees and hips (75a). Allow your trunk to move forward while you bring your arms behind you. Simultaneously push off with both of your legs while swinging your arms forward, and let your entire body extend completely to maximize the full power that

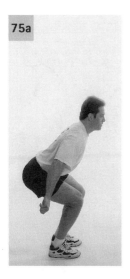

75a

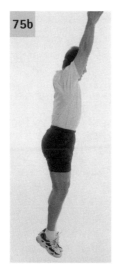

75b

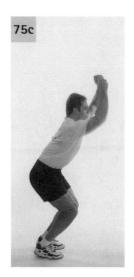

75c

you are generating (75b). Land on both feet. When landing, think of yourself as a shock absorber as your feet, ankles, knees, and hips share the impact of contact. Your feet must land in the same direction as the start position with no loss of balance (75c). When learning a new jump, practice 2–4 of them and gradually build to 8–12 in a set. The more explosive the jump, the fewer you should do in a set. **Variations:** 75.1. *Vertical Jump*: Start with more knee bending and less hip flexing. Thrust your arms overhead and upward. This is good for climbers. 75.2. *Squat Jump*: This emphasizes the lower body and does not use the arms for momentum. From a half squat, jump straight up for maximum height. Do this as described for exercise 75.1, but place your hands behind your neck. 75.3. *Double Leg Forward, Uphill and Downhill Jump*: Jump forward and land on both feet. Rest 3 minutes between sets. Going uphill, try for maximum height, land softly, and absorb landing forces with your legs. Try 4–8 repetitions. Try these backward, sideways, and at an angle (75.3a). These are specifically designed for snowboarders. In downhill jumping, be careful and keep your back from flexing excessively. Use your hips, knees, and ankles to absorb the impact rather than your low back. To simulate skiing, alternate turning your body to the left and right with each jump. Try this with lower-amplitude jumps before increasing the height of your jumps (75.3b). 75.4. *Rotational Jump*: Start with your feet shoulder-width apart, jump, and rotate 90 degrees to your right or to your left. Upon landing, jump and return to your initial starting position. As your balance and strength improve, increase your rotational jump to between 90

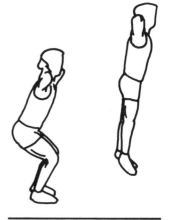

75.2

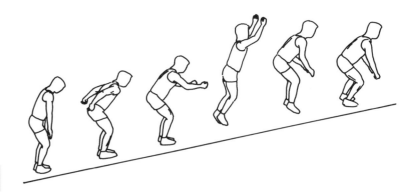

75.3a

and 180 degrees in both directions. As you land your jump, reach across your body with your left hand to hip level. Repeat the same jump-and-reach motion to the opposite side. Perform this motion for 8–12 reps on each side. For an additional balance and strength challenge, progress your left-hand reach from hip level toward your right foot. Repeat this in the opposite direction. These are excellent for snowboarders. 75.5. *Lateral Jump*: Follow the directions for exercise 75.2, but take off and land on both feet. You can do this over a step or a log to make it more challenging (see exercise 49.2d). These are good for snowboarders, windsurfers, and alpine skiers.

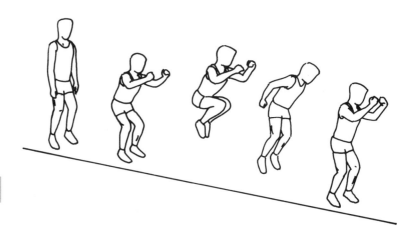

75.3b

75.6. *Lateral Jump with a Ball Toss:* Do exercise 75.5, and have a partner throw a ball to your side in the direction that you are jumping. These are good for snowboarders, windsurfers, and alpine skiers. 75.6. *Loaded Jump:* Increase the jump challenge by using ski poles or wearing a loaded backpack while performing the previous jumps. Use your ski poles to help during the push-off phase. Pole-assisted jumps are most appropriate for telemark and downhill skiers. Pack-loaded jumps are most appropriate for backcountry snowshoers, telemark skiers, and mountain climbers.

76 | The Basic Hop

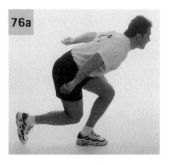

76a

Equipment: Level floor or ground; progress to using hills, snow, and/or a backpack.

Purpose: Improve your ability to balance while decelerating and propelling your body in an explosive manner, such as in activities on snow, on climbing walls, and in the mountains. Also improve power in runners.

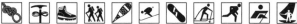

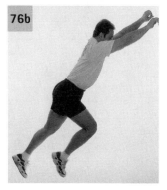

76b

Technique: Balance on one leg with your stance leg slightly bent. Lift your opposite foot off of the ground with your knee flexed. Your trunk should be forward and your arms hanging freely by your sides. Wind up by bringing your arms behind you, allow your trunk to flex further forward, and bend your stance knee further (76a). Then simultaneously push off of your stance foot and bring your arms forward (76b), and land on your opposite foot. You can add resistance or a balance challenge by wearing a backpack.

Variations: 76.1. *Vertical Hop:* Perform exercise 76, but don't flex your trunk as much in the wind-up phase. Bend your knee further and propel yourself upward. This is useful for climbers. 76.2. *Lateral Hop:* Stand on your right foot. Sidebend your torso toward your hop direction (left, in this case) while you move your standing hip to the opposite side (to the right) to load and maintain balance. Wind up your arms to the right in front of your body. Push off from your right foot, swinging your arms to the left, and land on your left foot. This is useful for skiers and snowboarders. 76.3. Try a very short run and a hop (good for runners, mountain climbers, hikers, and backpackers). 76.4. Try a forward hop while shaking a partially water-filled beach ball or a body blade side to side to increase the balance and abdominal challenge. 76.5. Hop up or down a hill or incline (good for skiers and climbers).

The Ankle and Leg Region

BY JOHN RUMPELTES, P.T.

▶ **THIS CHAPTER WILL HELP YOU:**
- Understand the function of and learn a few basic exercises for your ankle/leg region.

The ankle joint is essentially a hinge joining the foot with the lower leg. The foot must alternately absorb shock and become a rigid lever to propel the body forward. The muscles of the lower leg contribute significantly to balance, as well as propulsion (as in walking uphill) or deceleration (walking downhill or stepping down). Shock absorption requires the muscles to decelerate forces from above in a controlled manner so as to transfer these forces smoothly. With propulsion, the muscles affecting the foot hold it relatively rigid, so there is adequate leverage to push the body forward. The ankle joint moves primarily in *dorsiflexion* (the movement of the ankle that pulls your foot and toes up to your shin) and in *plantar flexion* (the movement of the ankle when standing on your toes or in the push-off phase of walking or running).

SELF-TESTS

Many activities require advanced balance ability. An ankle injury may contribute to a loss of balance ability. If you have had a serious ankle injury or feel unsure of your balance abilities, try these self-tests and some of the balance exercises in chapter 5.

Note: If you have pain with these self-tests or are not able to increase your motion with the exercises suggested, consult a health care provider.

1. *Dorsiflexion Tightness.* While standing with your feet parallel and shoulder-width apart, squat slowly, keeping your heels on the ground, until reaching the first barrier to further motion (your back should stay straight). Now look down directly over your kneecaps toward the floor. If mobility is restricted, your toes will be in view under the kneecaps. The further you can move your knees out over your toes without lifting your heels, the better your mobility is in dorsiflexion. Now repeat this self-test, noting the arch position at the beginning and end range of the squat. If the arch flattens and the knee moves inward, this is a sign of your body compensating for restricted motion. If you are restricted in your motion, do Exercises 9, 10, and 77.

2. *Plantar Flexion Tightness.* Start in a standing position and rise up on your toes. Your heel should rise at least 2–3 inches

above the floor and you should bend at least 45 degrees in your first (big) toe joint. If this is tight, do Exercise 78.

3. *Joint Looseness.* Sit in a chair and cross one leg so that your ankle is on your opposite knee. Hold your heel and gently try to move it upward. If your heel and sole of your foot move upward excessively on one side compared to the other side, you may have loose ligaments. If there has been a history of ankle injuries and repeated rolling of your ankle, you also may have loose ligaments. A person with this problem should wear more stable shoes and do functional exercises that emphasize balance. (See chapters 5 and 8.)

FUNCTION AND ANATOMY
The two bones of the lower leg, the *tibia* and *fibula*, run parallel and contact each other as they sit on and cradle the *talus bone*, thus forming the ankle joint. The muscles of the lower leg play a major role in balance, deceleration, and propulsion, linking the supportive foot to the leg and body above. The muscles can be divided into two groups: the *plantar flexors* (calf, etc.) and the *dorsiflexors* (*tibialis anterior*, etc.). The dorsiflexors decelerate the toes and foot moving toward the ground just after heel contact. This allows for controlled lowering of the foot. The dorsiflexors also lift the foot and toes as they swing forward, to assure clearance with the ground. The plantar flexors help with balance by maintaining the body's center of gravity over the foot. They also support the arch of the foot. When walking or moving, the plantar flexors propel the body forward or decelerate the body moving forward over the fixed foot.

See the illustrations in chapter 9.

COMMON MUSCLE IMBALANCES
Calf muscle shortness or tibialis anterior weakness is common in the lower leg, which alters ankle and foot function. Balance abilities are frequently not very good, resulting from weakness or ligament laxity in the foot, leg, or torso/hip/buttock region. Calf and Achilles stretching should be essential components for the outdoor enthusiasts' fitness program. Entire hip, thigh, lower leg, and ankle muscle training can be incorporated for optimal balance and strength using the balance exercises in chapter 5 and the lower extremity exercises in chapter 11.

INJURY PREVENTION
Problems in ankle/leg function can lead to inefficient hiking, running, etc., and can predispose an active individual to injuries. The most common problems in lower leg or ankle function are due to decreased motion in the foot or ankle or increased motion due to foot type or ankle ligament looseness. Tight calf muscles and Achilles tendons (see Self-Test 1, Dorsiflexion Tightness, above) are more common than tight ankle joints, but both may be loosened up with stretching and functional exercises such as a squat or lunge (see chapter 11). These changes can result in compensations that include increased flattening of the foot during movement and/or increased mechanical tension within the muscle-tendon tissue of the calf group and Achilles tendon.

Ankle joints may be loose as a result of bad sprains that did not heal well. With joint looseness, there can be problems in the foot, knee, hip, or back, and balance abilities may be compromised.

EXERCISES

Many of the exercises in chapters 5, 8, and 11 use the muscles of this region for strength and balance. Exercises 9 and 10 are good for flexibility. The following are additional exercises for this region. You can begin strength training exercises with 15 repetitions unless otherwise indicated. Progress your reps and resistance according to the guidelines in chapter 5.

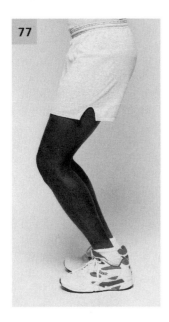

77 | Partial Squats for Improved Ankle Motion

Equipment: None.
Purpose: Facilitate range of motion as well as increase general strength.

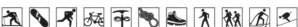

Technique: Stand with your feet shoulder-width apart. Bend your knees approximately 30 degrees, keeping your heels on the floor and making sure that your knees are over your first and second toes. Make sure to keep your chest up and your back flat, flexing at your hips. If you can keep in good alignment, try to increase the squat depth. Your goal is to complete 2 sets of 15 reps with no pain, to lead to an improvement in motion in conjunction with an Achilles stretch.

Variation: 77.1. *Single Leg Squat:* Stand on one leg and go into a squat as described above; this increases motion or improves balance on one leg.

78 Three-way Calf Raises

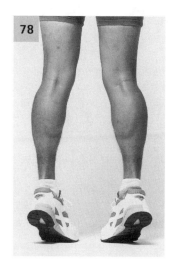

Equipment: Flat surface or stair edge.

Purpose: Strengthen the calf group and increase stability during the more strenuous portions of the calf raise motion used in all standing activities, especially climbing motions.

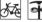

Technique: Stand on a flat surface, near an immovable object for balance support if necessary (or with your heels over a stair edge, for more of a stretch). Elevate your body over your toes as high as you can raise your heels; do this in three different foot positions: feet facing forward, toes pointing in, and toes pointing away from each other. Try to complete 10 reps per foot position, for a total of 30 repetitions per set. Complete 2–3 sets. Try to do this without holding on or with very little support.

Variation: 78.1. To make this more challenging, hold free weights or wear a backpack.

The Foot Region

By Katrina Sullivan, D.P.M.

▶ **THIS CHAPTER WILL HELP YOU:**
• Understand foot function.
• Learn about footwear and orthotics.

The foot acts as a dynamic foundation for the body during standing and movement. It is helpful to understand what happens to the foot during walking to understand how alterations in foot support can affect the rest of your body.

FUNCTION AND ANATOMY

The walking cycle (the gait cycle) has a few phases. At *heel strike* the heel of the foot (or shoe) makes initial contact with the ground. During the *stance phase* the foot is on the ground bearing weight. It must be flexible enough to adapt to various surfaces and be able to *pronate* (flatten) somewhat to accomplish this. The foot has two important roles during contact with the ground; it is a mobile adapter to uneven surfaces and a shock absorber. As we walk or run, we load more weight on the foot until the *toe-off* (*push-off*) *phase*, when the foot has to be more stable and go into an arch-up position (*supination*) to propel the body forward. Those same joints that allowed movement now need to lock tight for proper function.

The foot is comprised of 28 bones and numerous joints, muscles, tendons, and ligaments.

The foot is divided into three regions: heel area (*rearfoot*), arch area (*midfoot*), and ball of the foot with toes (*forefoot*). See Figure 20.

COMMON MUSCLE IMBALANCES

Excessive relaxation of the arch and rolling in of the ankle (*pronation*) during contact with the ground can place the ankle, knee, or leg in a position of internal rotation stress while that structure is trying to accept the body's weight. This contributes to overuse injuries. A tight, high arch can lead to shin splints and stress fractures, since the full impact stress of loading is transmitted directly up the leg. A tight arch may not relax during Self-Test 1, Body Rotation Foot Arch (later in this chapter).

INJURY PREVENTION

Function of the foot can influence function of the ankle, leg, knee, hip, back, and even upper body. Foot, ankle, knee, hip, or back pain may result from inadequate foot support. Balance and agility may also be compromised by inadequate foot support. This is why proper foot position or posture can be key for exercise and

FIGURE 20

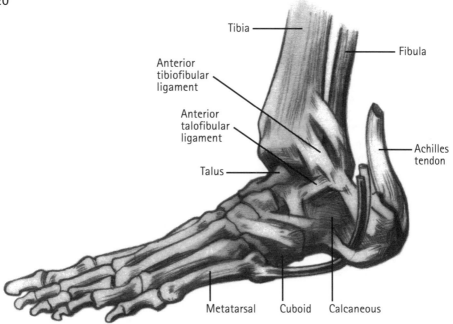

Tibia

Fibula

Anterior tibiofibular ligament

Anterior talofibular ligament

Achilles tendon

Talus

Metatarsal   Cuboid   Calcaneous

activity participation. How does one tell if one's arch is working properly? The inner arch usually maintains a moderate air space between the skin and the ground during standing. There should be minimal callus formation on the bottom of the foot and the toes should remain straight. Hammertoes and bunions are a sign that the arch is not maintaining proper posture during gait. In addition, try Self-Test 1, Body Rotation Foot Arch.

FOOTWEAR FOR ACTIVE PEOPLE

There is no one shoe that will fit all people or perform best for all activities. In shoe gear selection, two main categories must be considered: fit and function—the right shoe for the right activity, with a proper fit. Today's athletic shoes are designed with particular activities in mind.

Shoe fit takes the primary role in this equation. Adequate width in the ball of the foot and toe region is very important for the foot to function within the shoe properly. The shoe needs to be long enough, a thumb's width from the end of the longest toe. Make sure you have both feet measured for width and length before you buy shoes. If you have orthotics, bring them with you when you try on shoes and make sure the shoes you purchase come with a removable insole. The shoe needs to have a firm heel counter to provide support to the foot. The arch placement or lack of arch is the least important feature, since that is the easiest to modify with ready-made arch supports or custom orthotics.

High-arched individuals do better with a curve-lasted shoe (inflared near the big toe) as long as they do not overpronate. (The *last* is the shape that the shoe is built around.) People with flat feet and people who are overpronators (the arch sags and the ankle rolls inward) do better with a semi-curved- or straight-lasted shoe.

For running, you should have a running shoe. For hiking, there are a variety of shoe options in regard to lightness and stability. In general, if you pronate excessively, you likely would benefit from a more stable shoe that has more support in the heel counter and arch.

To choose footwear, understand the activity and your needs for stability and support. Learn your foot type: high arch vs. low, narrow vs. wide, good function vs. injury prone, and any abnormal shape or idiosyncrasies. Once you have determined your needs, learn about the current shoes being offered that meet those requirements. Many magazines carry seasonal shoe reviews, and reputable outdoor stores have knowledgeable staff that can teach you about the brands that they carry. Try shoes on after doing activity on your feet (they will be slightly larger) and wear the same socks that you would use for that sport. If you are unsure about your foot type or needs, seek medical advice prior to shopping. Also try Self-Test 2, Shoe Stability (below), on any new shoe before you purchase it.

SELF-TESTS

1. *Body Rotation Foot Arch.* Stand with your bare feet flat on the ground. If the inner side of the middle of your foot is almost touching the floor, you likely have pronated (flatter) arches. Next, rotate your upper body to the left as far as you can go while keeping your feet flat on the floor. Your right arch should flatten and your left arch should rise up. If this does not happen, you might have high-arched feet. See chapter 12, Self-Test 1, Dorsiflexion Tightness. If your ankle and

Achilles tendon are tight, this is very commonly associated with a high-arched foot.

2. *Shoe Stability.* If you have feet that pronate, it is desirable to have a stable shoe or boot to wear. The following method will help you find shoes that are very unstable. In one hand, hold one of your shoes where the sole material meets the heel, and with your other hand hold the sole in the widest part of the forefoot. Attempt to twist the shoe, first from the forefoot and then from the heel. A slight twist is OK, but if you can twist it more than 25 degrees, it is probably not very stable. Also try pinching the material 1½ inches above the superior part of the heel counter. If you can pinch it and touch your thumbs together, it is likely not very supportive.

ORTHOTIC USE AND SELECTION

To understand the indications for when to use an orthotic versus an arch support, it is important to understand the difference between these two devices. A functional biomechanical orthoses (*orthotic*) works by realigning the foot to its correct posture. The foot is balanced in relationship to the ground and the leg it supports. The goal is to restore the major joints of the foot to their best position and to control excessive motion during gait. The functional orthoses is custom-made for the individual. It can be extremely helpful to support alignment of your feet and lower extremity in all weight-bearing activities, including hiking and skiing.

Arch supports act by supporting the foot under the arch. Peculiarities of the individual are not necessarily addressed. Many people can derive benefit from a good-quality arch support at a fraction of the cost of a custom device. When choosing an arch support, look for firm material in the arch region. Soft, squishy devices cannot change the posture of the foot sufficiently.

If you have flattened arches, there are a number of generic arch supports that may work reasonably well. It makes sense to try these on in a store and see if they are comfortable and support your feet. Generic arch supports are relatively inexpensive inserts that may be very useful for hikers, skiers, runners, and climbers. They can help the feet relax and can support the feet in relation to the rest of the body. Using an arch support or orthotic can often improve balance and athletic performance.

If you have foot, ankle, or knee pain, consider consulting a podiatrist or sports medicine specialist to see if orthotics might help you.

The Neck and Mid and Low Back Region

By Kim Bennett, P.T., and David Musnick, M.D.

▶ **THIS CHAPTER WILL HELP YOU:**
- Learn neutral spine alignment.
- Develop protective strategies to observe during exercise and outdoor activity to prevent injury.

Protection and proper positioning of your neck, mid back, and low back are essential for injury-free exercise and outdoor activities. These regions contain discs, bones, joints, and nerve tissue and can be injured or become painful from poor posture or lifting motions. Pain in any part of your spine can make your activities less enjoyable and decrease your abilities to move quickly, lift or pull, and make appropriate balance adjustments. This chapter is helpful to anyone who wants to ensure the safety and preservation of one of our most important pieces of equipment, the spine.

FUNCTION AND ANATOMY

For illustrations, see chapter 9.

Your spine is composed of vertebral bones stacked in a column with discs in between. These discs act as shock absorbers and controllers of motion. Nerves exit at openings formed by the facet joints (which join adjacent vertebral levels) between the vertebral bones. Your spine must protect these structures and allow for movement to help you position your head, arms, and legs.

Your low back (*lumbar spine*) has five levels of vertebrae connected to a triangular *sacrum*

bone, which is connected to your pelvis through your *sacroiliac* (SI) joints. See Figure 21, Low Back Detail. The low back has a normal, slightly arched/extended curve. It contains the nerves that go to your legs. The low back has limited movement compared to the other spinal areas. Its lower discs can become painful from flexed sitting and standing postures as well as from improper lifting. Your sacroiliac joints have a role in transferring forces from your legs to your upper body. The stability of the SI joint and strength of surrounding muscles are very important for spine and lower-body function. There are anatomical variations in the structure and ability of the SI joint to fit together in a stable manner. The most stable joints are S-shaped. The less stable joints are more C-shaped or straighter. People with less stable joints or weaker muscles may have pain in the SI joint (buttock pain) or even weakness or giving way of a leg. The muscles that lead to a tightening around the SI joint include the latissimus dorsi (on the opposite side of the joint), the spinal extensors, deep hip rotators, gluteals (especially gluteus maximus), and hamstring muscles. In addition, strong abdominals are important for low-back stability. If you have

FIGURE 21

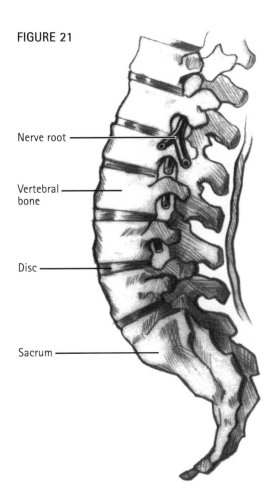

Nerve root

Vertebral bone

Disc

Sacrum

Your mid back (upper back or *thoracic spine*) contains ribs and must be flexible to rotate and bend in many directions. It has a normal, flexed curve. It contains many muscles related to spinal rotation and bending. It is important to do some flexibility work to maintain your mid-back motion. Exercises 17, 18, and 21 are good to do on a regular basis for this purpose. A rotary torso machine may be used in a health club or you can do Exercise 80 if you have special needs for enhancing your back rotation.

Your neck (*cervical spine*) encloses your spinal cord and nerve supply to your arms. Its primary function is to position your head and eyes. Neck, shoulder, and arm pain and headaches can occur from joint and disc problems. Muscles in this region control the movements of your head and neck. Your neck is closely related to your shoulders, and tight shoulder muscles can pull on your neck. Getting your low back into good alignment can help with alignment of your neck. In the neck region it is more important to maintain flexibility and to practice good lifting and posture habits than to work on pure strength.

INJURY PREVENTION

Problems in one area of the spine can lead to problems in another area. Problems can be due to acute injuries or to wear and tear from poor posture over many years. It is important to be aware of good posture while you are exercising and while you are engaging in your outdoor activities. Back and neck problems are more likely when you are subjecting your spine to lifting, prolonged sitting, and carrying packs. Injuries can occur during lifting, falling, and abrupt shifts in a boat. For safety during lifting, refer to Posture and Lifting later in this chapter.

The postural deviations most people have include a head too far forward of the shoulders, the shoulders slumped forward and turned in, the back of the skull resting too close to the back

sacroiliac or low-back problems or you would like to generally strengthen your back, consider doing Exercises 27, 28, 29.1, 30, 32, 56, 57, 58, 61, 62, 67, 70, 71, 80, 81, 91, 102, and 103. If you have low-back and especially SI problems, be careful with Exercises 27, 28, 29.1, 30, 32, and 102.

Your low-back discs, facets, and SI joints are the most commonly injured from improper lifting and abnormal movement patterns. Consider consulting with a health professional competent in assessing and treating (with exercise and other methods) SI and low-back problems if you have persistent low-back problems.

of the spine, and the mid and low back excessively rounded. Postural patterns such as those can lead to disc or joint problems and shortened muscles.

COMMON MUSCLE IMBALANCES

The most common muscle imbalances in the spine are due to tightened or weakened muscles. Tight hamstrings can cause excessive flexing and more stress on the discs of the low back. Very tight quadriceps can cause excessive arching of the spine and more stress on the joints. Tight abdominal and chest muscles affect mid-back position. Tight and/or weakened upper neck and shoulder muscles can lead to poor neck alignment. Weaker gluteal and abdominal muscles can contribute to low-back problems. Weaker neck flexors can contribute to neck problems.

NEUTRAL ALIGNMENT

Knowing what neutral alignment is, and knowing how to balance the muscles acting around your neck and back, are both important in protecting this vulnerable region.

There are obvious curves in the normally aligned spine when it is viewed from the side. The neck and low back have a slight arch backward and the midback has a flexed curve. Normal curves indicate correct vertebral stacking designed to protect the component parts of the spinal system.

In adults the normal curves of the spine result in an alignment that, when ideal, brings the ear over the shoulder, the shoulder over the center of the hip joint, and the hip joint slightly in front of the center of the knee and ankle joint. This is called a "neutral alignment."

Neutral alignment indicates that the individual joints of the spine are in normal alignment with one another, which is necessary for good maintenance of joint structure. When there is good alignment at each vertebral segment,

joints are in their most balanced position, with weight distributed over the vertebral bodies and two facet joints. Muscles, ligaments, and bony structures are arranged so motion can occur most freely in each direction the joint moves. Muscles and ligaments are balanced (adapt) in length and strength to allow this to happen, and pairs of adjacent joint surfaces are held parallel and spaced apart, with forces equally distributed across their cartilage liners. Exercise 79 will help you assess your alignment. See chapter 6 for discussion and illustration of neutral alignment in sitting and standing postures, and for exercises to experience them.

APPLYING THE CONCEPT OF NEUTRAL IN EXERCISE AND ACTIVITY

The following examples give you an idea of what to look for in achieving neutral alignment and what to avoid. Once you have the idea, apply this to other settings and activities.

When you are ready to lift, stop and take a minute to find neutral back and neck alignment, then contract your abdominal muscles (pull them up and in slightly) enough to provide support for this alignment but not to pull you out of it. Then lift the weight, trying to maintain a neutral spine alignment. Note that in some of the functional exercises in this book, you may be moving in and out of a neutral alignment.

Bending your neck forward under pressure stresses the facet (intervertebral) joint and places ligaments and the back wall of the disc at risk. You might see this happening to someone who is doing abdominal crunches and beginning to pull himself up using his head as a handle as he fatigues, rather than lifting his upper body with his upper abdominal muscles. Use your hands behind your neck to support it in crunch exercises. Doing squats with a bar across the shoulders with the neck held flexed will result in muscle contraction across these flexed segments, compressing them out of alignment. Latissimus pull-downs are frequently done with excessive forward neck posture and low-back flexing. See Exercise 91 for pictures of good and improper neck positioning during this exercise.

These examples illustrate cases where the stack of vertebrae in poor alignment are subject to brief episodes of fairly high levels of pressure, sometimes with quick thrusting motions. Because of poor alignment, joint structures are not protected, placing disc, ligaments, muscles, and joint surfaces, including their cartilage linings, at risk.

In exercise during which joint loading may be less but forces are constant for prolonged periods, static poor alignment can lead to similar joint irritation and discomfort and may ultimately lead to injury. In the case of biking, for example, in an attempt to create less wind resistance, riders often bend forward in the mid back and round their shoulders forward. This creates a sharp, extended angle in the neck and forward head and compresses the space into which the lungs should be expanding. Bending at the hips, keeping the back flat (chest slightly raised), and keeping shoulders and neck tucked slightly back creates less stress on the back of the neck and the mid back as well as opens up the area of the chest cavity.

Another example of static loading out of alignment occurs while hiking with a top-heavy backpack. A backpack loaded so a bulky object is perched at the top, forcing the head forward, will result in compression at the back of the vertebral segments. Reloading the pack so there is room for the neck to move back into its neutral alignment and making sure that weight is distributed to the hip strap reduces these forces.

POSTURE AND LIFTING

Certain postures and motion patterns are likely to lead to spine pain and injury. In general, it is safer when lifting to be close to the object that you are lifting and do most of your lifting with your legs and buttocks.

LUMBAR SPINE (LOW BACK)

Posture: In general, sitting or carrying things with a flexed, slumped low back can put excessive pressure on your discs. It is best to sit with a neutral posture.

Lifting: Try to avoid lifting with your back flexed and rotated when your knees are relatively straight. (See Figure 22, Improper Positioning During Lifting.) Many people pick up their packs, skis, or even boats in this position. You should position yourself and lift with your hips and knees flexed (bent) and your back in a neutral position. It is important to face the object and position it close to your center of gravity (torso area), if it is heavy (see Figure 23, Proper Positioning During Lifting). You may want to do the initial lift with your elbows straight. Once you have the object positioned, use your legs and buttock muscles to straighten your knees. Avoid extending your back too much during the lifting. Your thigh and buttock muscles are much stronger than your back

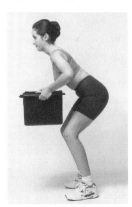
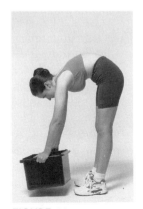

FIGURE 22   FIGURE 23

muscles. The joints and discs are also safer using this positioning. (See chapter 17 for details on lifting packs.) Remember that proper positioning and lifting is important no matter how light something looks.

THORACIC SPINE (MID BACK)

Posture: Good thoracic posture in neutral is with a normal flexed curve and avoids excessive flexing, extending, or sidebending.

Lifting: Avoid lifting while reaching behind you, or while you are extending and rotating your thoracic and lumbar spine. This can injure your ribs, along with surrounding joints.

CERVICAL SPINE (NECK)

Posture: Neck pain and problems are most likely to occur in a forward head position. When sitting, standing, or carrying a pack, try to position your neck in a neutral position. Avoid having something on your back that pushes your head forward.

Lifting: Your neck muscles are involved with lifting. Avoid excessive head and neck flexing with lifting. Be careful when you are lifting an object with an elevated arm that is away from your body. If you feel pain in your neck with weight lifting, decrease your resistance and make sure your form is good.

EXERCISES

You can begin strength training exercises with 15 repetitions unless otherwise indicated. Progress your reps and resistance according to the guidelines in chapter 5.

79 | Finding Neutral

Equipment: A large wall mirror and a hand mirror.
Purpose: Find neutral alignment in a standing position.

Technique: Stand sideways to a wall mirror, looking straight ahead. Hold a hand mirror in front of you so that you can see your head and upper back in the wall mirror. Keeping your nose and chin parallel to the floor, gently slide your head backward on your neck so that your earlobe is lined up over the center of your shoulder joint. At the same time lift your *sternum* (breastbone) slightly, but be careful not to arch your back. Your shoulders should line up over your hips. Once you know what this feels like, do it without looking, but check with the mirror periodically to be sure alignment is correct. Hold 3 seconds, repeat 5 times. (You won't need the mirror long.)
Variations: Do Exercises 43 and 45 to find neutral in your lower back while sitting and standing.

80 | Spine Rotation

Equipment: 10- to 45-pound Olympic plate or 5- to 10-pound hand weight; rotary torso machine (for Variation 80.1).
Purpose: Improve your stomach and back strength and ability to rotate.

   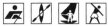

Technique: Stand with your knees slightly bent and hold an Olympic weight or hand weight to your chest with both hands. Focus your eyes on a point directly in front of you and maintain a neutral spine position. This is your starting position. Begin twisting slowly to the right, then the left, in a short arc. As you develop your motion pattern, increase your speed and range of motion. Perform 2–3 sets of 15 reps in each direction.
Variations: 80.1. Use a rotary torso machine to do resisted trunk rotations. Do Exercises 21, 60, 61, and 65 for spine rotation, and do Exercise 62 for spine sidebending.

81 | Waiter's Bow

Equipment: None.
Purpose: Improve your ability to bend at your hips while maintaining your spine in good alignment.

        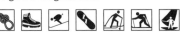

Technique: Stand with your knees slightly bent with your low back in neutral and your head held level. While maintaining a neutral spine, flex at your hips until your hips and low back are at a 45- to 60-degree angle with the floor, or you feel the pull of your hamstrings. Allow your hips and buttocks to translate backward as you flex your hips. Keep your chest up and mid back extended. Maintain your neck in a neutral position and avoid hyperextending your neck. Do this 6–8 times slowly until you have the motion pattern down, then progress to bending your knees while you are bending at your hips. Do this with progressively deeper knee bending to simulate positions that you will have to lift in.
Precautions: This exercise can aggravate an active back problem and should be stopped immediately if you have any back pain.

15

The Shoulder, Upper Torso, and Arm Region

By Carrie Hall, P.T., Sara Meeker, P.T., and Mark Pierce, A.T.C.

▶ **THIS CHAPTER WILL HELP YOU:**
- Understand the function and anatomy of the shoulder, upper torso, and arm region.
- Learn exercises to functionally strengthen and provide balance to this region.

The shoulder is a highly mobile joint, which allows you to move your arm and position your hand. This joint has the largest range of motion of any joint in the body, and must be a stable structure that can provide a base from which your arm and hand can function. This versatility of function is made possible by a balance in muscle forces around the shoulder joint and the shoulder blade.

Each muscular force, which acts to move the arm, must be countered by another force, which keeps the ball stable in the socket. Common overuse injuries are usually a result of an imbalance between the dynamic muscular forces around the shoulder joint.

FUNCTION AND ANATOMY
For illustrations, see chapter 9.

The shoulder joint is a "ball and socket" joint. The socket component is a part of the shoulder blade (*scapula*) and the ball is the top end of the arm bone (*humerus*). Muscles around the shoulder girdle have a number of different functions. They may primarily act as decelerators, stabilizers, and movers. Muscles often play multiple functional roles, depending on the activity and motion patterns of the shoulder. Scapular muscles move the shoulder blade upward and downward to coordinate the motion of the blade with the arm. They also act to track the shoulder blade over your posterior upper rib cage to provide a mobile base of support for arm and hand activities.

The rotator cuff (also called simply cuff) muscles primarily stabilize the ball in the socket against excessive upward and forward migration during arm movements powered by the deltoid and other larger mover muscles. The cuff muscles also help to rotate the arm inward (internal rotation) and outward (external rotation).

The shoulder blade muscles include the *upper, middle,* and *lower trapezius* (traps), *rhomboid major* and *minor,* and *serratus anterior.* Their functional role involves keeping the shoulder blade in proper relationship to the upper back during arm motions. Since the shoulder blade creates the socket half of the shoulder joint, the shoulder blade must rotate upward as the arm rises, in order to maintain the relationship of the socket to the ball. These muscles must also control blade position on the upper back while the arm is lowered. A weakness or lack of coordination of the scapular muscles may lead to altered shoulder joint function and could lead to excessive use of the cuff muscles and possibly strains and tendonitis. The scapular muscles are often overlooked in strength training but their function is paramount. These muscles should be exercised with some sets using lower weights and many repetitions due to their endurance role. Exercises 82–86, 88–91, 93–95, and 99–105 strengthen the scapular muscles.

Several muscles cross the shoulder joint and connect the arm bone (humerus) to the shoulder blade (scapula), collar bone (*clavicle*), or trunk. They generally fall into two groups. The first group is deep and close to the joint, and travels a short distance. They create a cufflike structure that acts to keep the ball pulled into the socket and helps to stabilize the joint. These muscles include the *supraspinatus*, *infraspinatus*, *teres minor*, and *subscapularis*. They have some mover function in that they can rotate the ball in the socket and thus are strengthened with internal and external rotation motions. Most people do not specifically and functionally exercise the cuff muscles. Use Exercises 27.1, 92, 92.1, 102, and 102.1 to strengthen your cuff.

The second set of muscles that cross the shoulder joint are more superficial. These are the ones that you can see on body builders. Their primary function is to move the arm. They tend to be longer muscles than the rotator cuff and attach lower on the arm bone. Because they attach farther from the shoulder joint, they have a good mechanical advantage to move the arm but are not good at stabilizing the ball in the socket. They work with the cuff and scapular muscles to raise and lower the arm. These include the *deltoid*, *pectoralis major* (pecs), *latissimus dorsi* (lats), *triceps*, and *biceps*. The deltoid, along with the biceps, helps to move your arm in

front or to the side and over your head. The lats and pectorals help to bring your arm closer to your body.

Strengthening of the elbow flexors (biceps, *brachioradialis*, and *brachialis*) and extensors (triceps) is important, because they are both movers and stabilizers. A primary role of the elbow flexors and extensors is to move objects. Examples include lifting a pack, putting an ice ax in the snow or ice, paddling a kayak, etc. Training for this function is important if you frequently will be lifting heavy or lighter objects. Exercises to train for this function are dynamic exercises including biceps curls, triceps extensions, and rows with free weights, pulleys, or tubing. This can also be done with machines, but there is less coordination training accomplished.

Shoulder muscles also can work to control movement of all or part of the body's weight through space as in pulling, lowering, and pushing. Examples include climbing on rock walls, boulders, or ice; paddling or rolling a kayak; etc. You may train for this function by doing pull-ups, dips, or push-ups. Free-weight biceps elbow flexion exercises (curls) and triceps elbow extension exercises are useful for building a strength base for these functions.

When the hand is performing strong resisted tasks, the elbow works as a "brace" to transfer the forces from the hand to the shoulder girdle and torso. The arm and hand are then used in weight-bearing positions. Four examples of this dynamic are isometric hanging by your fingertips from a ledge or bar, keeping bicycle handlebars steady on a long ride, holding an ice ax in an arrest position, and bracing a paddle in whitewater kayaking. Exercises that train for this type of function are push-ups including use of an isometric hold at various elbow ranges, dips in a gym or outdoors, or using climbing walls. Exercises 66, 69, 86, 98.1, and 101 work on this function.

The shoulder region frequently functions

with the abdominal, hip, and leg regions. See the activity chapters for training programs that incorporate these concepts. Some of the most important functional relationships and applicable activities are:

Arm elevation related to hip, low-, and upper-back extension; mountaineering, backpacking, kayaking, snowboarding, snowshoeing, scrambling, gym or rock climbing.

Same-side hip extension/flexion with internal rotation related to external shoulder rotation, while the opposite hip relates to internal shoulder rotation; mountaineering, gym or rock climbing, downhill skiing, snowboarding, scrambling.

Hip extension related to arm push-off or pull-down; mountaineering, gym or rock climbing, scrambling.

Elbow and shoulder extension with hip flexion and extension, during any activity using poles, especially uphill; downhill skiing, telemark skiing, cross-country skiing, showshoeing.

Right shoulder/arm, left hip (gluteal area), spinal extensors, and rotators, along with oblique abdominals, in deceleration of torso flexion and rotation; windsurfing, telemark skiing, cross-country skiing, snowboarding, snowshoeing, canoeing, kayaking.

COMMON MUSCLE IMBALANCES

Since the shoulder joint depends so heavily on muscles to maintain its integrity and proper joint mechanics, it is particularly vulnerable to injuries resulting from muscle imbalances. An imbalance between the superficial and deep muscle groups that surround the shoulder joint, or an imbalance within a group, are common causes of shoulder injury.

Muscles that commonly become tight, strong, and overused are the latissimus dorsi, upper trapezius, pectoralis major, and rhomboid major and minor. Muscles that tend to be weak or underused are the rotator cuff and the middle and lower trapezius. When performing exercises to strengthen the weak muscles (cuff and lower traps), some attention should be paid to exercises that isolate the muscles in less functional positions (Exercises 88 and 92, this chapter). If one were to load up the weights in an attempt to strengthen the subscapularis (internal rotation), one could expect to recruit pectoralis major, latissimus dorsi, and teres major. The goal of the exercise is to find and work at the threshold where subscapularis can internally rotate the shoulder alone without the help of the bigger, stronger muscles. This may mean that one is working with much smaller amounts of weight. Since the weak, underused muscles tend to be stabilizers, they must not only be strong, they must be resistant to fatigue. Thus, endurance training with higher reps and lower weights is an important component of the strengthening program of the cuff and traps (Exercises 88, 92, 94, and 95, this chapter).

The shoulder and upper back work functionally together with the buttock, hip, and leg region during many sitting and standing activities. Performing some exercises that functionally integrate these regions can improve your ability to lift, reach, pull, push, and maintain your balance.

INJURY PREVENTION

Injuries of the shoulder are quite common and usually involve the rotator cuff (supraspinatus and infraspinatus) and the long head of the biceps. These are prone to injury, including strains and tendonitis, because they are easily frictioned and frequently loaded excessively. The injuries in this region may also heal slowly because of poor blood supply, frictioning, and associated neck problems. Motions that may load them excessively are straight-arm elevations to the front or to your side. Exercises 94 and 95 and other arm elevations should be done with much less weight than biceps curls (start with one-fifth the weight and gradually work your way up). Be careful to keep heavier loads (packs, boats, windsurfing boards, climbing gear, etc.) closer to your body and lift them in front or to your side.

Balance and agility are important in preventing shoulder sprains and bruises due to falling. If you work on balance and perform some of your shoulder training in unison with your abdominal, hip, and leg regions, you can decrease the risk of shoulder injuries.

The strengthening program in this chapter can help prevent these injuries. This program is designed to maintain balance between all of your shoulder muscle groups. It includes exercises for the rotator cuff and shoulder blade upward rotators (mid and lower trapezius and serratus anterior) that typical upper-body programs do not include. Many of the functional exercises include shoulder, torso, and hip combinations. Careful attention to form is also critical to promote muscle balance and optimal joint motions.

ISOLATED UPPER-BODY EXERCISES

For Exercises 82–99, pictures are included only for a few exercises that are less commonly known. The other exercises are commonly done in health clubs and are well known to most trainers. The terms *hand weights* and *dumbbells* refer to free weights and are used interchangeably. You can begin strength training exercises with 15 repetitions unless otherwise indicated. Progress your reps and resistance according to the guidelines in chapter 5.

CHEST

The various bench presses are done to strengthen your chest, shoulders, and triceps, which will increase your ability to push. For these press exercises, start with 12–15 reps in a set. Progress to 1–2 sets of 6–8 reps to work toward maximum strength.

82 | Dumbbell Flat Bench Press

Equipment: Bench and dumbbells.
Purpose: Challenge your ability to coordinate your arm motions while gaining strength in your chest, shoulders, and triceps. By using a pair of dumbbells instead of a regular barbell, the challenge of balance and coordination increases. Target muscles: middle pectorals, serratus anterior, anterior deltoid, and triceps.

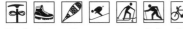

Technique: Grasp a pair of dumbbells and lie back on a bench with your knees bent and feet resting on the bench. Pull your abdomen up and in to ensure your back remains stable throughout this exercise.

Extend your arms so they are perpendicular to the ceiling, with the dumbbells directly over your shoulders and palms facing your feet. Lower the dumbbells, while allowing your elbows to bend, until the dumbbells meet the level of your chest. Return the dumbbells to the start position while lifting them in the same path. Perform 2–3 sets of 15 reps.

83 | Dumbbell Incline Bench Press

Equipment: Incline bench and dumbbells.
Purpose: Put more emphasis on your upper chest and anterior shoulder. As you change the angle of the bench to an incline, the workload is placed on different parts of the target muscles: middle pectorals, serratus anterior, anterior deltoid, and triceps; emphasis on the upper pectorals.

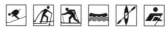

Technique: Hold a pair of dumbbells with your palms facing forward. Lie back on an incline bench with your knees bent and feet resting on the floor. Pull your abdomen up and in to ensure your back remains stable throughout this exercise. Extend your arms vertically toward the ceiling while positioning the dumbbells directly above your shoulders. Lower the dumbbells with an outward semicircular motion while allowing your elbows to bend until the dumbbells meet the level of your chest. Return the dumbbells to the start position in the same path. Start with 2–3 sets of 15 reps.

84 | Dumbbell Decline Bench Press

Equipment: Decline bench and hand weights.
Purpose: Increase your strength and ability to push your body in an upward direction. Target muscles: middle pectorals, serratus anterior, anterior deltoid, and triceps; targeting lower pectorals.

Technique: Lie face up on a decline bench and grasp a pair of dumbbells with your palms facing forward. Lower the dumbbells in an outward semicircular motion while allowing your elbows to bend, until the dumbbells meet the level of your chest. Return the dumbbells to the start position while lifting them in the same path. Start with 2–3 sets of 15 reps.

85 | Barbell Flat, Incline, or Decline Bench Press

Equipment: Bench and barbell.
Purpose: Develop sheer power and strength for pushing; however, the limitations on versatility and range of motion inherent with barbells make them a second choice after dumbbells. Target muscles: pectorals, serratus anterior, anterior deltoid, and triceps.

Technique: Use a spotter if possible. Lie face up on a flat, incline, or decline bench, with your knees bent and feet resting on the bench or floor. Pull your abdomen up and in to insure your back remains stable throughout this exercise. Extend your arms so they are perpendicular to the ceiling, with the barbell directly over your shoulders. Grip the barbell with both hands and lower the barbell to your chest. Push the barbell straight above your chest to a point of balance. Perform 2–3 sets of 15 reps.

86 | Push-Up

Equipment: None.
Purpose: Develop upper-body strength and coordination. Improve your ability to push while using your entire body. Target muscles: serratus anterior, pectorals, anterior deltoid, triceps, and abdominals.

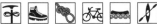

Technique: Lower yourself to the floor and position yourself on your hands and knees. Place your hands a little wider than shoulder-width apart, with your elbows straight. Next, move your feet backward until you are balanced on your hands and the balls of your feet. Your body, arms, and legs should be relatively straight and your abdominals tight. You are now in position and ready to perform a push-up; remember to keep your back straight during the entire exercise. Start by bending your elbows, in control, and lower your chest toward the floor until your elbows reach a 90-degree angle. Once you have lowered yourself to this position, immediately extend your arms and raise yourself back to the start position. Do 2 sets of 5–15 reps.

Tips and precautions: A good rule of thumb is that if you cannot perform 5 regular push-ups in a row with good form and back positioning, start with knee push-ups (see variation 86.1). When you can perform 10 knee push-ups in a row, advance to regular push-ups.

Variations: 86.1. *Knee Push-Up*: This is a good place to start if you have any doubts about your ability to perform regular push-ups.

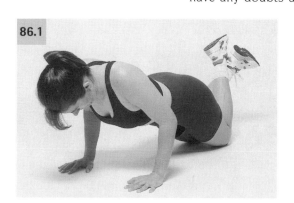
86.1

Kneel on your hands and knees with your hip angle halfway between 90 degrees and lying on the floor. Position your hands so that they are under your shoulders, with your fingers facing forward. Lower yourself toward the floor and try to touch your chest to the floor, then push up to a straight-elbow position. Do a set with your hands in this position, then do another set with your hands wider than shoulder-width apart and with your shoulders and hands rotated inward. 86.2. You can strengthen your ability to push from standing and angled standing positions by standing near a wall and doing a regular push-up, leaning and pushing at various angles. This is a good osteoporosis prevention exercise.

87 | Flat Bench Dumbbell Flies

Equipment: Bench and a pair of 5- to 20-pound hand weights.
Purpose: Enhance your strength for motions that involve moving your arms inward. Target muscles: pectorals, anterior deltoid, biceps, and triceps.

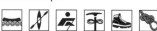

Technique: Grasp a pair of hand weights with your palms facing each other and lie face up on a bench with your feet resting on the bench. Extend your arms completely so that the hand weights are positioned directly over your chest and touching each other, with your palms facing inward. This is your starting position. Next, lower the hand weights in an arc and out to your sides, while allowing your elbows to bend. When the hand weights reach the level of your shoulders, return them in an arc to the starting position directly over your chest. Start with 2–3 sets of 15 reps.

UPPER BACK/SCAPULA STABILIZERS

In Exercise 88, you must begin with the standard exercise and progressively build to variation 88.6. Do not progress to the next variation until you are able to complete 15 repetitions of the current level with correct technique. When learning the exercise motion pattern, do not use any weights. Gradually advance to using a light weight (2–5 pounds).

88 | Stomach Lying Elbow Lift

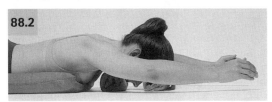

88

Equipment: Pillow, towel.

Purpose: Strengthen the different parts of your trapezius and provide balance for your shoulder blade. Target muscles: middle and lower trapezius, posterior deltoid.

Technique: Lie on your stomach with a pillow under your abdomen and chest. Roll up a towel lengthwise and place it (or a face cushion) under your chin and forehead to support your head. Place your hands on the back of your head. Barely lift your elbows. Keep your neck muscles (upper trapezius) relaxed, and contract the region between your shoulder blades (lower trapezius). Keep the contraction just enough to lift your elbows so as not to use your rhomboids to excessively squeeze your shoulder blades together. Hold the contraction for 5 seconds. Lower your elbows and repeat up to 20 times. Stop when your neck muscles become tense.

Variations: 88.1. *Stomach Lying Elbow Lift with Arms Extended*: Start as in Exercise 88, above. Slowly extend your elbows so that your arms are straight. Do not move your shoulders during this exercise. Bend your elbows so that your hands return to the position behind your head. Lower your elbows to the floor. Repeat 15 times. Stop when your neck muscles become tense, as this is an indication that the middle and lower trapezius are fatigued. 88.2. *Stomach Lying Elbow Lift with Arm Extension Overhead*: Start as in Exercise 88, above. Straighten your elbows while extending your arms to meet in front of your head. Be sure not to tense your neck muscles (upper trapezius) during this variation. If you are unable to keep your neck muscles relatively relaxed, you are not ready for this

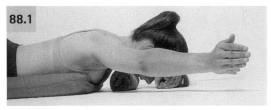

88.1

88.2

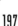

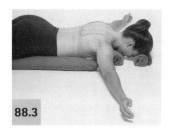
88.3

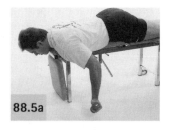
88.5a

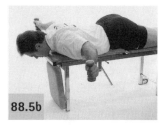
88.5b

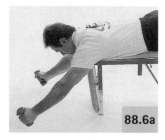
88.6a

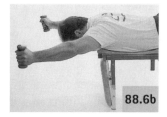
88.6b

level of exercise. Return your hands to your head, then lower your elbows and relax. Repeat 15 times. 88.3. *Stomach Lying Horizontal Arm Lifts*: This isolation exercise strengthens your middle trapezius muscle. Set up the pillow (or cushion) and towels as in Exercise 88, above. Position your arms straight out from your sides at slightly more than a 90-degree shoulder angle. Rotate your forearms so that your thumbs face upward and front elbow crease faces forward. Barely lift your arms off the floor. Hold your arms up for 3 seconds. Lower your arms and then relax. Repeat for 15 repetitions. 88.4. *Stomach Lying Diagonal Arm Lifts*: This isolation exercise strengthens your lower trapezius muscle. Set up the pillow (or cushion) and towels as in Exercise 88, above. Position your arms midway between straight out from your sides and straight up in front of your head. Bend your elbows slightly. Rotate your arms so that your thumbs face upward. Barely lift your arms off the floor. Be sure to lift your entire arm, not just your elbow. Hold your arms off the floor for 3 seconds. Lower your arms and then relax. Repeat for 15 repetitions. (The end position is the same as in Exercise 88.1 above.) 88.5. *Stomach Lying Reverse Horizontal Fly*: This isolation exercise strengthens your middle trapezius and posterior deltoid muscles. Lie on your stomach on a weight bench. Bend your knees if they extend too far off the bench. Pull your abdomen up and in. Your head should be slightly off the bench and in line with your spine with your chin tucked. Hold a pair of dumbbells with your palms facing forward and thumbs up. Your arms should be relaxed at chest level and resting on the floor, or against the bench if the bench is tall. Keep your elbows slightly bent (88.5a). Raise the dumbbells in a semicircular motion directly out from your sides, with your thumbs pointing up toward the ceiling; raise your arms to just below chest height (88.5b). Do not lift beyond chest level. Lower to the start position using the same path. Exhale in the up position and inhale in the down position. Do sets of 15 repetitions. 88.6. *Stomach Lying Diagonal Reverse Fly*: This isolation exercise strengthens your lower trapezius muscles. Lie on your stomach on a weight bench. Bend your knees if they extend too far off the bench. Pull your abdomen up and in. Your head should be slightly off the bench and in line with your spine. Hold a pair of dumbbells with your palms facing inward and thumbs up. Your arms should be resting on the floor, or against the bench if the bench is tall. Keep your elbows slightly bent (88.6a). Raise your elbows in a semicircular motion diagonally upward toward your head to just below the level of your head. Your shoulders and arms should be at approximately a 135-degree angle. (88.6b). Do not lift your elbows above the level of your head. Lower to the start position using the same path.

89 | Pulley/Cable Row

Equipment: Pulley cable row machine.

Purpose: Strengthen your upper back for rowing and pulling activities. Target muscles: rhomboids, trapezius, lattisimus, erector spinae, biceps, and posterior deltoid.

    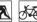

Technique: Grasp the handles of the low pulley with your palms facing inward while maintaining a neutral low back position. Straighten your knees until they are slightly flexed and bring your back to an upright position with your arms extended. Keeping your back straight, bend at the hips and reach the handle toward the pulley. When your hands are just past your knees, return your back to the upright position and pull the handle to your ribcage. Make sure you end the pull with your chest up and your elbows slightly behind you and to your sides. Do 2 sets of 15 reps.

Variations: 89.1. Do the above exercise with a pulley or tubing and one arm while sitting on a bench or a ball. Position your knees so that your feet are flat on the floor. 89.2. *Cross Body Row Arm Extension*: Use less weight for this variation than you would use for a standard row. Position the left side of your body so that you are standing perpendicular to a high pulley. Grasp the handle with your right hand so that your arm is across your face, and bear most of your weight on your right leg with your knee bent. Simultaneously pull the handle toward and past your right hip while pushing off of your right leg and transferring your weight to your left leg. Then let the pulley go back to the starting position, transferring your weight to your right leg.

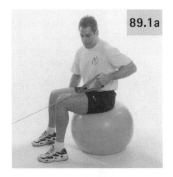

89.1a

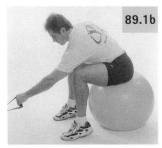

89.1b

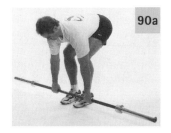

90 | Bent Barbell Row

Equipment: Barbell and bench.
Purpose: Gain balance while strengthening your entire back, rear shoulders, and biceps. Some outdoor activities require your upper body to be in a bent-over posture while pulling with either one or both arms. This exercise will benefit your balance and strength to meet those requirements. Target muscles: posterior deltoids; upper, mid, and low back; trapezius; and biceps.

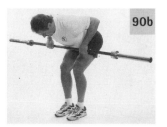

Technique: Squat and grasp a barbell with your palms facing toward your body and slightly wider than shoulder-width apart (90a). Once you take hold of the barbell, stand up straight and place your feet shoulder-width apart. Next, bend your hips and knees and assume a position in which your back is parallel to the floor with your low back in a neutral position. At the same time you are getting into position, lower the barbell toward the floor. Keep your back straight and stable, and row the barbell to your chest, allowing your knees and hips to flex slightly to assist your back during loading (90b).
Precautions: Don't attempt this exercise if you have a history of low-back problems unless you are supervised. Try Exercise 89 or 102 instead.

91 | Latissimus (Lat) Pull-downs to the Front and Rear

Equipment: Lat pull-down machine.
Purpose: Strengthen your arms, shoulders, and upper back for pulling and climbing activities. Target muscles: latissimus, teres major, and biceps.

         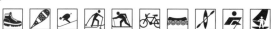

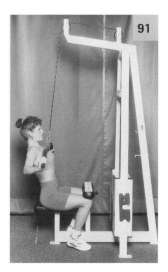

Technique: Select a comfortable weight and start by gripping the bar with your hands apart a distance about 6–10 inches wider than your shoulders. Sit on the bench and allow your arms to extend over your head. Maintain a safe posture in your neck and low back. Once you are seated and gripping the bar, keep your head level and pivot backward at your hips until you have the overhead pulley in sight. You should now be in a semi-reclined position. Pull the bar to your upper chest. Return the bar to the starting position with

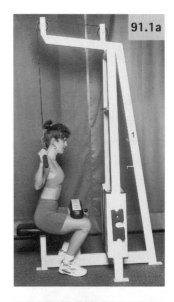

91.1a

your arms in front of you and overhead. You may allow a small amount of forward and backward motion to occur with your upper body during this exercise. Do not bend forward while pulling down. Perform 2–3 sets of 15 repetitions.

Tips and Precautions: Pull the bar down toward the top of your chest and at the same time exhale and raise your chest up to meet the bar. This will create a slight amount of extension in your upper and mid back during the pull-down portion of this exercise. This will also prohibit you from rounding your upper back and overextending your neck. If you need to translate your body forward during the pull-down, pivot from your hips. Try not to bend forward with your upper back and neck.

Variations: 91.1. *Pull-down to the Rear*: Assume the same starting position as a pull-down to the front. Maintain a safe posture throughout the exercise by keeping your head level, stomach tight, and low back in the neutral zone. Pull the bar down to meet the top of your shoulders (91.1a), without bending forward with your neck or upper back (91.1b, poor neck posture). Return to the starting position in control of the weight and allow your arms to extend overhead.

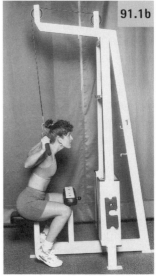

91.1b

The following variations are good for boating, climbing, and mountaineering activities. 91.2. *Single Straight Arm Lat Pull*: You will need a high pulley and a handle for this variation. Tubing can be substituted for the cable if pulleys are unavailable. Attach a single handle to the cable and stand so your body faces sideways to the cable. Position your arm so that it is halfway between parallel to the floor and overhead, and slightly forward from the side plane of your body. Once your arm is at the top of the motion, return your straight arm to your side. This can also be done with both arms simultaneously. 91.3. Start in the same position as variation 91.2, but position your arm halfway between straight ahead and directly out to your side. Pull the cable down across your body to your opposite leg. 91.4. Do variation 91.3 with a bent elbow so that the ending position is with your elbow at your side and your palm facing outward. 91.5. Do Exercise 30, Standing Lat Pull-Down, which uses your legs and shoulders simultaneously.

SHOULDERS

92 Rotator Cuff Rotations

Equipment: Bench and 1- to 5-pound dumbbell.

Purpose: Provide balance for your shoulder and strengthen the usually weak rotator cuff muscles. Target muscles: supraspinatus, infraspinatus, teres minor, subscapularis, and posterior deltoid.

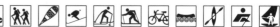

Technique: Kneel and position your upper body lengthwise alongside a bench with your shoulder and upper arm supported on the bench. Position your arm to extend out from your side, with your elbow bent down at 90 degrees. Your arm should hang from your elbow down, not from your shoulder. (You can also do this lying on your stomach on a bed, adjacent to the edge of the bed.) Place one or two rolled towels beneath the front of your shoulder. Keep as much of your shoulder supported on the bench as you need. Grasp a light dumbbell in your hand. Slowly rotate your shoulder externally so that your forearm is raised parallel to the floor, and the back of your hand faces the ceiling (92a). Then rotate your shoulder in the opposite direction (internally) so that your palm is facing the ceiling (92b). Do not let your shoulder displace into the towel roll. Think of keeping your shoulder pulled "away" from the towel roll. Your range of motion will be more limited in internal rotation versus

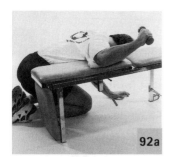

92a

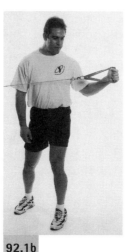

92b

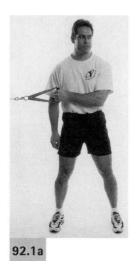

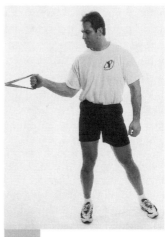

92.1a

92.1b

92.2a

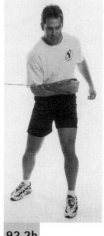

92.2b

external rotation (possibly only about 10–20 degrees' difference). Do 2–3 sets of 15 reps.

Variations: 92.1. Stand sideways next to a pulley that is at armpit level, grasping the pulley with one hand so that it crosses your torso, with your elbow flexed to 90 degrees (92.1a). Rotate your arm externally and weight-shift in the same direction as your hand is moving. Allow your torso rotation to occur naturally (92.1b). Do a set of 15 reps. 92.2. Turn your body 180 degrees (92.2a) so that you are rotating the pulley toward your chest (internally); weight-shift in your legs in the same direction as your hand is moving. Allow your torso rotation to occur naturally (92.2b). This can also be done with pulleys at different heights.

93 | Dumbbell Overhead Press

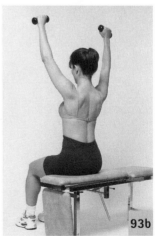

93a

Equipment: Bench, mirror, and dumbbell.

Purpose: Improve your ability to press objects overhead. Target muscles: deltoid, supraspinatus, triceps, and trapezius.

    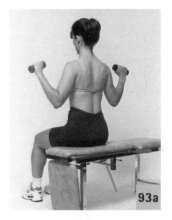

Technique: Sit at the edge of a flat bench (or stand up), facing a mirror if possible. Hold a dumbbell in each hand. Place your feet hip-width apart and sit with your back erect, looking directly into the mirror. (If standing, be sure your pelvis and spine are in neutral.) Hold the dumbbells at shoulder height, palms facing forward (93a). Extend your arms upward until your arms are fully extended (93b). As you extend your arms, be sure your upper trapezius relaxes after the half-way point, and you squeeze your lower trapezius to finish the motion. At the end of the motion, your shoulders should not be up around your ears, but relaxed, with your elbows fully extended above your head. Your arms, however, should be in line with your ears, not in front of your head. Exhale in the up position and inhale in the down position. Perform 2–3 sets of 15 reps.

93b

94 | Lateral Dumbbell Raise

Equipment: 3- to 8-pound dumbbells.
Purpose: Strengthen your rotator cuff and provide more balance to your traps. Target muscles: deltoid, supraspinatus, and trapezius.

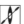

Technique: You can perform this exercise standing or sitting. Standing is more challenging to balance, and therefore requires more trunk and lower-extremity control. Grasp a pair of light to moderate-weight dumbbells, holding them with your palms facing each other. Raise the dumbbells to your sides in a large arc until your hands are over your head. Try to do most of the raises with your arms at approximately 30 degrees in front of your body. In the end position, your palms should be facing forward. Slowly return to the start position, reversing your hand position back to facing each other. Exhale in the up position and inhale in the down position. Perform 2–3 sets of 15 reps.

95 | Front Dumbbell Raise

Equipment: 1 pair of 3- to 10-pound hand weights.
Purpose: Improve your ability to elevate your arm over your head and provide more balance to your traps. Target muscles: deltoid, supraspinatus, trapezius, and serratus anterior.

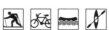

Technique: This exercise may be more beneficial when done with your back against a wall to monitor the position of your shoulder blades. Grasp a dumbbell in each hand. Hold the dumbbells so that your thumbs face upward. Have your abdomen pulled up and in. With your elbows slightly bent, raise the dumbbells, one at a time, in a semicircular motion to arm's length overhead. As you raise your arms overhead, relax your upper trapezius at the halfway point and squeeze your lower trapezius to complete the motion. Return to the start position, maintaining your shoulder blades against the wall while you lower your arms. Exhale in the up position and inhale in the down position. Perform 2–3 sets of 15 reps.

BICEPS

96 | Alternate Dumbbell Curls

Equipment: 1 pair of 3- to 20-pound hand weights.
Purpose: Strengthen your arm flexors. Strong biceps are helpful for pulling, lifting, and climbing activities. Target muscles: biceps, brachialis, and forearm flexors.

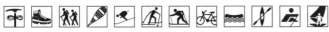

Technique: Stand holding the dumbbells, with your knees slightly bent. Have your palms facing inward at the start and toward your chest at the finish position. A variation is shown in Exercise 23 with a biceps lunge combination. Perform 2–3 sets of 15 reps.

TRICEPS

97 | Triceps Extensions

Equipment: Barbell, dumbbells, or a high pulley weight machine.
Purpose: Isolate the triceps muscles and develop strength for arm extension and shoulder-arm stability. Target muscles: triceps and serratus anterior.

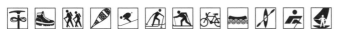

Technique: This exercise can be performed with free weights or various machines. If you choose free weights, lie face up on a bench and place your feet on the bench. Grasp the dumbells and position them over your chest with your hands about 10 inches apart (with your palms facing each other). Once you feel balanced and in control of the weights, slowly bend your elbows and lower them toward, then past, your forehead; then return the weights to the starting position. Perform 2–3 sets of 15 reps.

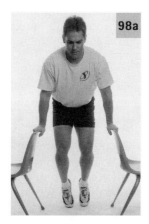

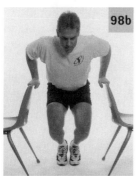

98 | Dips

Equipment: Dip machine that will unload body weight, or 2 chairs.
Purpose: Improve your ability to push your body vertically and push yourself with poles. Target muscles: triceps and pectorals.

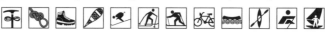

Technique: Use a setting on the dip machine that will unload about half of your body weight. Lower yourself and then raise yourself up with your chest and arms. Do 12–15 dips in a set and decrease the amount of weight assist if you are not fatiguing by the end of the set. To do a dip with chairs, place them facing away from each other and start by balancing on your toes, holding onto the backs of the chairs while in a semi-upright position (98a). Lower yourself between the chairs until your chest meets the level of your hands (98b). You can assist with your legs to make this easier. Perform 2–3 sets of 15 reps.
Tips and Precautions: Unloading part of your weight during dips and chin-ups can be accomplished using a number of machines, including the Gravitron® and the Cybex®. These machines allow you to reduce the workload of the exercise until you are able to perform the exercise safely.
Variations: 98.1. Try isometric holds of 3–5 seconds at various locations during the dip. This is a good exercise for climbers. 98.2. See chapter 8 for outdoor dip variations.

99 | Chin-ups

Equipment: Assisted chin-up machine or chin-up bar.
Purpose: Develop the strength and muscular endurance required to pull yourself up on climbs. Target muscles: posterior deltoid, biceps, trapezius, rhomboids, and serratus anterior.

Technique: With an assisted chin-up machine, unload your body weight by about 50% and place your feet or knees on the platform. Use a handhold of palms facing each other and palms forward. Raise yourself up until your hands are at the level of your chin. Lower yourself to the start position. If you can do a chin-up without any unloading of your body weight, you can use a chin-up bar about 6 inches higher off the floor than you can reach with arms extended overhead. Jump up or climb onto a stool and hold the bar with your hands slightly more than shoulder-width apart, with your hands facing forward. Pull up and try to touch your chin to the bar. After you have pulled yourself to the top, lower yourself slowly and return to the start position. Perform 2–3 sets of 15 reps. Gradually work up to a set of less weight unloading at 6–8 reps.

Tips and Precautions: Try to prevent your back from hyperextending by keeping your abdomen pulled up and in. Tighten your stomach muscles throughout this exercise. Try not to swing back and forth. Make sure to exhale on the way up, and inhale on the way down. If you are having trouble completing a full chin-up, have an exercise partner assist you. For example, while you are hanging on the bar, bend your knees and allow your partner to grip the front of your ankles. This will give you a foundation from which to push. You may then govern the amount of assistance suitable for your needs, without having your partner lift you.

Variations: 99.1. Try changing your grip width or the position of your hands. Occasionally grip the bar with your palms facing you, or use an alternate grip. 99.2. Climbers and scramblers should do this exercise with palms facing away.

FUNCTIONAL SHOULDER EXERCISES

Chapter 5 contains numerous functional shoulder exercises that integrate the upper- and lower-body regions. (See Exercises 20–27 and 29–35).

The following exercises are functional exercises, which focus primarily on the upper-body region. Not well known in health clubs or discussed in other texts, they are described in detail here.

Target muscles are not listed for these exercises because these exercises integrate multiple muscle groups and body regions. Some of the exercises are better simulations of certain activities but still have applicability for the others listed. See how you feel in relation to your activity after you have given an exercise a few weeks of practice.

100 | Single-arm Dumbbell Press

Equipment: Bench and one 5- to 20-pound hand weight.
Purpose: Improve the dynamic strength and function of the muscles surrounding your chest, shoulders, arms, neck, and anterior torso.

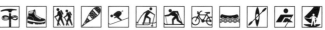

Technique: Hold the hand weight in your right hand and lie face up on the bench. Next, slide your body to the right, so that your right shoulder blade and right buttock are off the bench. Your right foot and leg will need an adequate purchase on the floor to help support your body from falling off the bench. Your left hand may grasp its same side of the bench for additional support. Press or push the dumbbell in your right hand directly over your chest and reach it toward the ceiling (see photo 65a). Next, bring the hand weight down toward your right armpit and allow your upper body and neck to slightly rotate to the right. Follow the hand weight through its path with your eyes and head (see photo 65b). This will enable your upper body and neck to move in coordination with your arm. Repeat this motion with the other side. Start with 1–2 sets of 12–15 reps, then move up to 2–3 sets of 15–20 reps.

Tips and Precautions: Follow the motion of the hand weight with your head and eyes. Move slowly at first and develop your most efficient path in which to move the hand weight from over your chest, then toward the floor. Allow gravity to assist you during the downward phase, and try not to let the hand weight drift outside the plane of your shoulder. Move quickly and in control through the full range of motion.

101 Variable-level Push-ups

Equipment: Staircase (or any other series of multilevel steps).
Purpose: Increase the synergistic and functional strength of your chest, shoulders, abdominals, and arms. Improve coordination between your upper and lower body by varying the style of a push-up.

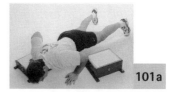

101a

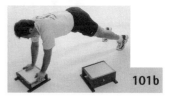

101b

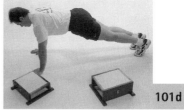

101c

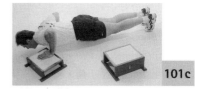

101d

Technique: Once you have mastered the push-up (see Exercise 86), make it more challenging by placing your right hand on an elevated surface, such as a 4- to 8-inch step, while keeping the other hand on the floor. Now, perform a push-up (101a). While you are in the "up" position, with your arms straight, step the left hand up from the floor to the same level as the right hand (101b). Again, perform another push-up, then step the right hand down to the floor while the left hand remains on the step, and perform another push-up (101c). Finally, bring the left hand down to the floor to match the level of the right hand and perform a push-up (101d). Repeat this sequence by leading with your left hand and traveling to your left. Each time you relocate your hand, perform a push-up. Perform 2–3 sets of 15 repetitions of this exercise with any combination of surface or elevation challenges.

Tips and Precautions: When attempting this exercise for the first time, limit your hand positions to a shoulder-width apart, and lower yourself only as far as you feel comfortable. If you have any recent history of shoulder or neck problems, this exercise could aggravate it. Always exercise in a pain-free range of motion. Be careful and move slowly at first, then increase your speed while maintaining your control.

Variations: 101.1. Push-ups can also be performed by leaning against a bench or boulder at various angles. This is good for climbers (who should wear a pack) as well as for individuals wishing to prevent osteoporosis. 101.2. Try elevating your feet on a 2- to 4-inch step, then proceed with the push-up sequence from left to right and from right to left.

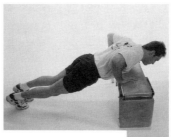

101.1a

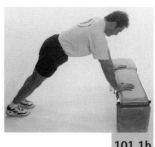

101.1b

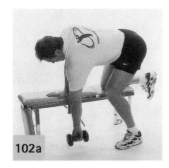

102a

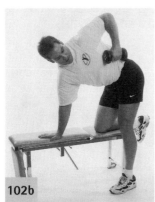

102b

102 Single-arm Dumbbell Row

Equipment: Bench and one 5- to 30-pound hand weight.

Purpose: Increase your strength, flexibility, and muscular coordination of your back, posterior shoulder girdle, arm flexors, and abdominals. Combine complementary body regions with respect to their functional unity.

     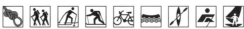

Technique: While holding the hand weight in your left hand, step to the left side of the bench. Place your right hand and right knee on the bench so that your right shoulder is over your right hand and your right hip is over your right knee. Your left foot remains on the floor for support and balance. Now you are in position and ready to start. Reach the hand weight in your left hand toward the floor while turning your hand so that your palm faces outward when you have reached the bottom. Make sure you follow the hand weight with your head and eyes, and allow your upper body to rotate in unison with your left arm (102a). Next, pull the hand weight toward your left rib cage while rotating the hand weight so that your palm is facing inward when you have reached the top. Again, make sure you follow the hand weight with your head and eyes, and allow your upper body to rotate in unison with your arm (102b). Repeat this sequence on the opposite side by bracing yourself on the bench with your left hand and left knee. Perform 2–3 sets of 15 repetitions on each side.

Tips and Precautions: If you have a history of neck or low-back problems, find a comfortable start position and move only in a pain-free range of motion.

Variations: 102.1. To strengthen your shoulder external rotators, use a lighter weight and rotate your shoulder at the top of the row portion of this exercise. Make sure that your elbow is close to your side when executing the external rotation. 102.2. Try this exercise with one end of the bench elevated 2–4 inches. This will create either an incline or a decline, depending on which side you are facing.

103 | Single-leg Hip, Knee Extension/Pull-down

Equipment: High pulley machine or 4-foot length of tubing.

Purpose: Challenge your balance and strength, as well as coordinate the muscles that are responsible for pulling you up a hill or climbing a rock face.

       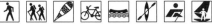

Technique: Stand tall with your right arm extended overhead. Balance on your left leg with your knee bent, and touch the floor with your right forefoot for a balance assist. While pulling the pulley handle or tubing to your chest, push off with your left leg and buttock and come to a balanced stance with your left leg straight. After you have completed a set balancing on your left leg, repeat the same maneuver while balancing on your right leg. Perform 2–3 sets of 15 repetitions on each leg, 2–3 times a week.

Tips and Precautions: If you have a history of knee or neck pain, reduce the depth of the squat portion of this exercise. Make sure that you don't extend your neck too far, and remember to move in a pain-free range of motion and only as far as you can balance. Keep your assist foot directly next to the balancing leg throughout the entire motion of this exercise. When your balance has improved, keep your assist foot up in the air until you can complete a full set without touching your assist foot to the floor.

Variation: 103.1. Try the pull-down while balancing on a thick foam pad, or change your grip on the bar or tubing; for example, use an underhand grip or a grip that allows your palms to face each other. This changes the loads on various muscle groups responsible for pulling and rowing.

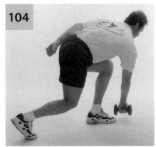

104 Staggered Stance Cross Diagonal Row with Dumbbells

Equipment: One 3- to 20-pound hand weight.
Purpose: Increase the strength and coordination of your shoulders, arms, back, and legs in unison and in all directions of motion.

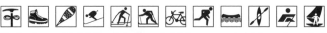

Technique: Hold the hand weight in your right hand and stand with your left foot one stride length ahead of your right foot. While bending your knees, hips, and low back, reach the hand weight toward the left foot and twist your right hand inward. Once you have reached as far as you feel comfortable, stand back up while "rowing" the hand weight toward your right hip. You may wish to transfer your balance onto the right leg at this point and prepare yourself for the next repetition. Perform 2–3 sets of 15 repetitions on each side.

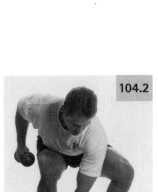

Tips and Precautions: Make sure to use your legs and hips during this exercise. Follow the hand weight with your head and eyes through your full range of motion. Avoid this exercise if you have a recent history of low-back problems.

Variations: 104.1. Try moving your feet farther apart or into a wide parallel stance. 104.2. Try balancing on a foam roll with the curved side down and your feet perpendicular to the long axis of the roll. When beginning this variation, start without hand weights and reach only to waist height and across your body while maintaining your balance on the foam roll. When this becomes easier, perform the cross-body reaches toward the floor while holding your hand weights.

105 Seated or Half-kneeling Reach/Row

Equipment: Bench and 3- to 8-pound hand weight.
Purpose: Strengthen the muscles of the upper back and lats in patterns common to rowing and oar sports.

Technique: Start by holding the hand weight in your right hand and place your left hand or elbow on your left knee. Sit on the front of the bench with your right foot (toes) slightly behind your right knee and your left foot positioned under your left knee. Bend and twist at your waist while reaching the hand weight forward to straighten your elbow (105a) until the dumbbell approaches the floor ahead

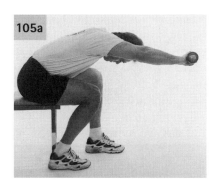
105a

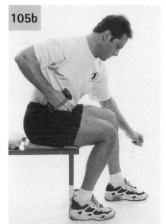
105b

of your left knee (your right shoulder should be between your knees). Your low back should be in a neutral position, although slightly rotated. Your right palm should be facing the floor, with your arm straight and upper body nearly touching your left thigh. Next, simultaneously pull the hand weight toward your right hip while returning your upper body to a semi-erect position (105b). Once you have completed a full repetition, repeat this motion in a smooth and controlled fashion, without stopping in the middle, for a full set. Perform this motion pattern on the opposite side for an equal number of sets and repetitions. Perform 2–3 sets of 15 repetitions on each side.

Tips and Precautions: If you have a history of low-back or shoulder problems, avoid this exercise.

106 Single-leg Stance Floor Reach to Overhead Press Combination

Equipment: Two 3- to 8-pound hand weights.
Purpose: Challenge your balance while increasing the strength and coordination of your upper and lower body to function as a unit. Develop strength and balance to move objects from overhead to the floor.

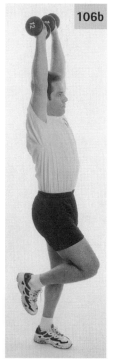
106b

Technique: Hold the hand weights close to your chest with your palms facing inward. Balance on your left leg, with the toes of your right foot touching the floor behind the heel of your left foot. Reach the hand weights toward your left foot while bending your left knee, hip, and back (106a). While you are reaching the hand weights toward your left foot, allow your right foot to slide across on the floor, directly behind you or to your left. This will aid your balance and control while maintaining most of the work on your left leg. Once you have reached the hand weights to a safe level, return to a standing

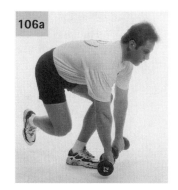
106a

position. Then press the hand weights over your head while maintaining your balance through the full range of motion (106b). The motion from floor to overhead should be one fluid motion without stopping. After you have performed a set of this exercise while balancing on your left foot, repeat the same coordinated motion while balancing on your right foot. Perform 2–3 sets of 15 reps, balancing on each leg.

Tips and Precautions: When first starting this exercise, make sure to use your assist leg as much as you need. Allow it to slide across the floor or assist you in regaining your balance. Use your knees as much as possible to decrease the involvement of your back. Reach toward your balance foot only in a pain-free and safe range. If you cannot control the full motion from floor to overhead with your hand weights, you are not moving in a safe range. Either decrease your range of motion toward the floor, or perform this exercise without hand weights. When you can complete a full set of 12 reps without hand weights, try the exercise with weight.

Variation: 106.1. Try varying the direction you move your assist foot (the non-balance foot). This changes the load and activity of your balance leg and trains your muscles to adjust to various directional challenges. For instance, if you are balancing on your right leg, allow your assist leg and left foot to slide toward your right instead of behind you. This changes the dynamics of the exercise considerably.

107 Standing-weight Shift Triceps Press

Equipment: One 5- to 25-pound hand weight.

Purpose: Enhance the coordination of your arms and improve their ability to work together as a unit during elbow extension and side-to-side motions. Stress your triceps, shoulders, and thighs.

Technique: Hold the hand weight overhead with your fingers laced together and your arms extended. Place your feet shoulder-width apart, with your knees slightly bent. Start by squatting to a shallow depth and lowering the hand weight behind your neck. Your elbows should now be pointing toward the ceiling. Next, shift your body weight onto your right leg, then simultaneously straighten your right leg and extend your arms, raising the hand weight above your head. Allow your left foot to raise off the floor so that you are balancing on your right leg when your arms are fully extended over your head. Return to the start position by lowering the hand weight behind your head and repositioning your balance over both feet, with your knees slightly bent. Now, shift your weight onto your left leg and simultaneously straighten your left leg while raising the hand weight over your head by extending your arms. Repeat this motion, shifting your body weight from side to side and keeping your elbows pointing toward the ceiling while extending your arms overhead. Perform 2–3 sets of 15 reps. Try to achieve 15 repetitions over each side during a 30- to 45-second interval.

Tips and Precautions: Try to make the transitions from left to right smooth and congruous, and be sure to include your squat in the middle of the transition with your hand weight behind your neck. When you have shifted your body weight, you should be balancing on that foot while extending your arms overhead. Do not hit the back of your head with the hand weight.

Variation: 107.1. Rise up on the balancing foot's toes while you are extending the hand weight overhead. This adds your calves into the exercise and increases the balance challenge.

THE BASIC UPPER-BODY CORE PROGRAM

These seven exercises are recommended for establishing a basic core strength program for this body region. You can add exercises to this program according to your physical and activity goals. All exercises can be done in 2–3 sets of 15 repetitions.

Try them in the order given: Exercise 88, 92, 86, 91, 96, 98, and 102. You might finish the sets for one exercise before moving to the next, or alternate from one exercise to the next for the first set, then the second, then the third, etc.

The Forearm and Hand Region

By Craig London, P.T.

▶ **THIS CHAPTER WILL HELP YOU:**
- Learn strengthening exercises for your wrists and fingers.
- Learn measures to prevent injuries, including taping.

The elbow, wrist, and hand contain structures that are relatively small that may be subjected to repetitive or very high loads. The fingers are very susceptible to injury, especially in climbers.

FUNCTION AND ANATOMY

See chapter 9 for anatomy illustrations. Also see Figure 24, Hand Detail, in this chapter.

The movements of the forearm are pronation and supination; that is, movement of the forearm from a palm-up position to a palm-down position (pronation) and vice versa (supination). The most powerful supinator muscle is the biceps. The pronator muscles are less powerful than the supinators. Exercises that are effective for these muscles consist of rotating weights in a controlled manner. One effective drill is to hold a hammer (or a light weight) at one end and rotate the forearm from palm up to palm down.

The wrist moves in controlled patterns that allow the hand to achieve the optimal position for fine movements. The movements of flexion and extension are each about 85 degrees. There are five *metacarpal* bones in the palm of the hand, and the fingers each have small finger bones (*phalanges*) with many muscles attached.

The anatomy of the finger flexor muscles have several unique features that support the important functions of the hand. Several muscles originate from the common flexor tendon, a site of frequent injury. The muscles quickly form into tendons that travel great lengths to their attachments. This enables a large and effective concentration of forces to produce movement in a very compact manner.

The tendons and a nerve pass through a bony arch and tunnel at the wrist (the *carpal tunnel*). There are several fibrous sheaths (*pulleys*) that keep the tendons coursing in their proper tracks. These sheaths are a site of injury from overuse and trauma. If the muscle contractions are very strenuous for prolonged periods, the tensile strength of the fibrous bands can be overwhelmed, creating irritation and fraying of fibers. This can also happen if the lines of force are altered when the fingers are twisted or laterally deviated. This places extra pressure on the ability of the fibrous bands to keep the tendons in place. Rock climbing often places both of these types of pressure on the hand and fingers. To avoid flexor tendon injuries, it is important to use good technique as well as to strengthen the flexor and extensor tendons and the muscles of the shoulder and upper back.

Many of the extensor muscles of the wrist

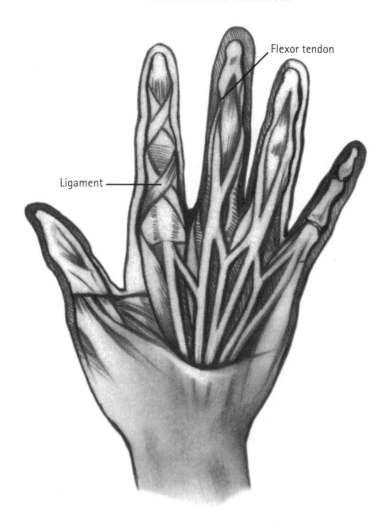

Flexor tendon

Ligament

FIGURE 24

and fingers originate from the same region on the outside of the elbow. Often these muscles are not strong enough in comparison to the overused flexors. To avoid injuries it is important to strengthen these extensors.

There are many muscles and tendons that move the fingers. The pulleys and the tendons are often injured with repetitive fingertip holds, especially if only one or two fingers are used with body-weight resistance.

COMMON MUSCLE IMBALANCES

The most common imbalance in this region is strong wrist and finger flexors combined with extensors that are relatively weak. This can lead to muscle tightness, pain, and overuse injuries. Another common weakness is the inability to lift our body weight, as in pull-up and triceps dip movements.

When considering the function of the hand, wrist, and elbow, the upper back, shoulder, chest, and upper arm are vital regions to exercise because they are important in positioning and stabilization (see chapter 15).

INJURY PREVENTION

Proper taping can add to the load tolerance of your fingers and wrist. The following techniques can be learned quickly and are often used by serious rock climbers.

Wrist taping: The goal of strapping the wrist is to help limit extension of the wrist joint. Excessive extension, especially while weight bearing, can sprain the two rows of carpal bones and the small cartilaginous disc in the wrist. Use 1½-inch-wide tape, and position your wrist in mid range with your fingers spread apart. Start taping on the back of the wrist where your wrist meets your hand. Wrap 2–3 times around the wrist, with appropriate tightness around the creases of the wrist. After taping, make sure that you can extend your wrist just slightly less than your range before you were taped.

Finger taping: If you have had a prior injury, tape a finger joint to support the sheaths and divert some of the forces off of the flexor tendons. Use ½- or ¼-inch-wide tape. Tape a figure eight pattern by starting the first piece on the palm side of the joint just below the joint crease. Tape a diagonal to the superior side of the joint. Continue the tape horizontally around once, and then cross over the joint to the inferior side. Make sure that the crossing occurs on the palm side of the joint. Tape 2–3 times around the joint. Make sure the joint can bend, that the skin is a normal color, and that you can feel the skin on your finger past where you have taped.

EXERCISES

You can begin strength training exercises with 15 repetitions unless otherwise indicated. Progress your reps and resistance according to the guidelines in chapter 5.

108 Finger Flexor Grip

Equipment: Spring-loaded grips, hand and finger putties and balls, elastic bands, and elastic sheets.
Purpose: Strengthen your fingers for better gripping.

Technique: Select one of the several tools available for finger drills, which come in various pressures, and squeeze it briefly for 15 reps in a set. Try a few out and see what feels best for you. Gradually increase the resistance on your fingers with more challenging putties and hand grips.

109 | Weight Roll-up

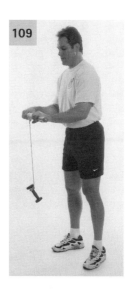
109

Equipment: A rope of shoulder height attached to a 1-foot-long, 1½-inch-diameter dowel on one end and to a weight on the other end.
Purpose: Strengthen and balance your wrist extensors.

Technique: With your arms in front of you and lower than parallel to the floor, and with your elbows bent, grasp the dowel on either side of the rope and slowly wind the rope up and down. Alternate the hand you are using to wind it up. The intensity of the drill is increased by the amount of weight attached to the rope and by the time it takes to complete. Start with 1 pound and roll at a comfortable pace. Progress from there by doing 4–5 reps and gradually increasing the weight. This exercise can quickly lead to forearm fatigue, so try not to overdo it.

110 | Dumbbell Palms-up Wrist Curl

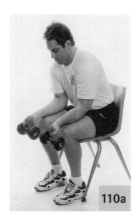 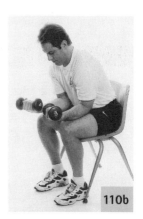
110a 110b

Equipment: Two 1- to 10-pound free weights and bench.
Purpose: Strengthen your wrist flexors.

Technique: Grasp a pair of dumbbells and sit on a seat or a bench with your forearms resting on your thighs. Hold the dumbbells palms up. Lower the dumbbells as far as possible (110a), and then curl them up as high as possible (110b). Do not let your forearms raise off your thighs. Do 2–3 sets of 15 reps.

111 | Dumbbell Palms-down Wrist Curl

Equipment: Two 1- to 10-pound free weights and bench.
Purpose: Strengthen your wrist extensors.

Technique: Begin as in Exercise 110. Hold the dumbbells with your palms down. Lower the dumbbells as far as possible. Do not keep a tight grip with your fingers. Curl the dumbbells upward as far as possible. Don't let your forearms raise off your thighs. Do 2–3 sets of 15 reps.

112 | Sitting Olympic Plate Hand Squeeze

Equipment: 5- to 25-pound Olympic weight plate (one with a ridge).
Purpose: Strengthen your finger flexors and the intrinsic hand muscles. This technique is most useful for climbing athletes.

Technique: Sit down with your feet spread apart; with one hand, hold an Olympic plate by the ridge. Lower the plate until your fingers are nearly extended (112a). Curl your fingers upward, raising the plate a few inches (112b). Continue raising and lowering the weight for 15 reps or until you fatigue.

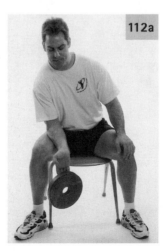
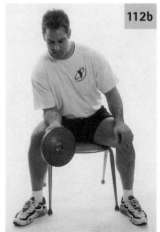

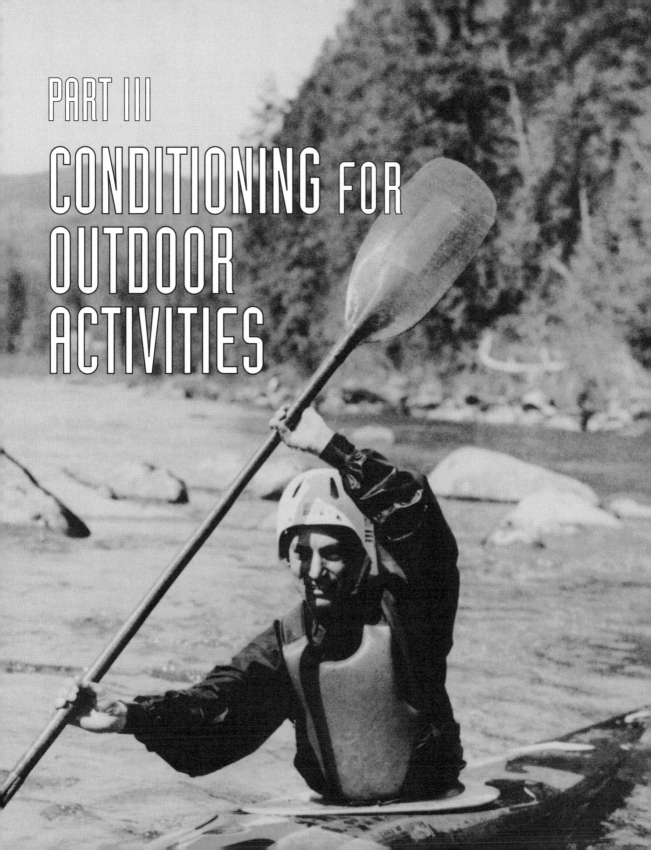

PART III

CONDITIONING FOR OUTDOOR ACTIVITIES

Conditioning for Hiking, Backpacking, and Snowshoeing

By David Musnick, M.D.

▶ **THIS CHAPTER WILL HELP YOU:**
- Understand the aerobic, balance, and strength demands of hiking, backpacking, and snowshoeing.
- Understand how to avoid common injuries from these activities.
- Develop a basic conditioning program to achieve goals of a full day of strenuous hiking, backpacking, or snowshoeing.

Getting in shape for hiking, backpacking, and snowshoeing consists primarily of improving your aerobic fitness both in town and on outdoor training days. Some basic strength and balance exercises can help, especially if you are doing steeper trails requiring handholds, areas with river or boulder crossings, or deep snow with uneven terrain. Common problems associated with inadequate conditioning are feeling easily winded, muscle soreness, kneecap area pain (especially with downhill grades), shoulder area discomfort, and falling. Occasionally, back and neck problems can develop if packs are lifted or loaded improperly or during a fall while snowshoeing. If you are in good condition, you reduce the likelihood of developing these problems and you enhance the possibility of enjoying your outdoor activity.

MUSCULOSKELETAL DEMANDS
Hiking and backpacking primarily involve your lower extremity from your hips to your feet. The demands on your knees are greatest in downhill hiking and in large uphill steps. Dynamic balance is important for river crossings. Adding a heavy pack can stress your shoulders, hips, neck, and back. The majority of people with mild back problems can tolerate a pack very well but have to be careful in how they lift the pack on and off their back, as well as how they position it for good neutral neck and low back positioning (see chapters 6 and 14).

Snowshoeing places similar demands on your knees but even greater demands on your ankles because of uneven snow surfaces. The muscles in your buttock, in your inner thigh, and all around your hips are used quite a bit and benefit from strength training. Snowshoeing gives you more frequent challenges to your balance than does hiking. Hiking on uneven terrain can put even more stress on your back. Strength training for snowshoers is similar to that for backpackers, but should have more balance, abdominal, buttock, and hip exercises.

MUSCLE IMBALANCES

The common muscle imbalances for hiking, backpacking, and snowshoeing are inadequate strength in the quadriceps and lower legs in controlling downhill motion. The hamstrings may also be somewhat weak in comparison to their much stronger quadriceps counterparts. The hip and buttock muscles are often not strong enough, especially the hip muscles on the front and inner groin in snowshoers.

WARM-UP

Warming up for these activities can be as simple as taking a brisk, 5-minute walk around the parking lot before doing some stretches. To prepare for backpacking over river crossings or for snowshoeing, add a short walking lunge and Exercises 38.1 and 40 (for the latter, use your car keys if you don't have a ball available).

STRETCHING

Do some stretching after you have warmed up during your midweek workouts and before you leave the trailhead (if it is not too cold).

Do Exercises 1, 3.1, 5.2, 7, 8, 9, and 19.

AEROBIC CONDITIONING

Hiking, backpacking, and snowshoeing are highly aerobic activities that are usually done for many hours at lower intensities, generally at 50%–65% maximum heart rate (max HR). They are often done on slopes of varying grades, on boulder fields or scree slopes, or off-trail, which can temporarily increase the aerobic demands to a higher level (often to interval levels). Snowshoeing in deep powder, in very cold weather, or on uneven snow increases the aerobic demands.

The minimum aerobic program (see chapter 2) should be modified in a number of ways to allow your body to more easily meet the aerobic demands of hiking, backpacking, and snowshoeing.

Do 4–5 short aerobic sessions each week at 70%–85% max HR.

Within 4–8 weeks of your first moderate hike or snowshoeing trip, begin increasing the duration of the aerobic period of all of your exercise periods to 35–40 minutes, not including warm-up and cool-down. Increases should be gradual, no greater than 10%–15% per week.

Six weeks before your first long hike or snowshoe trip, begin one low-intensity, longer-duration (LILD) activity per week at one-third to one-half your expected distance and elevation gain. Gradually increase the elevation gain, distance, and degree of difficulty every week.

In general, in your aerobic program it is good to achieve a distance and elevation gain that are within about 60%–75% of those expected during your planned outdoor activity. If you are not able to gradually work up to this amount of elevation gain or distance, you may still be able to do the hike or snowshoe trip. You might need to take more frequent breaks or go slower, and you might have more muscle soreness afterward. To preserve your knees, take adequate time and frequent breaks when hiking downhill.

SPECIFIC AEROBIC ACTIVITIES FOR HIKING, BACKPACKING, AND SNOWSHOEING

Indoor: Taking step classes, stair climbing on machines (the rotating stair machines are best) or actual stairs, using treadmills, and using EFX cross trainers (this and slide boards are excellent for snowshoers).

Outside: Cross-country skiing, walking, jogging, climbing stairs (see stair climbing options 5, 6, and 7 in the Modes of Aerobic Conditioning section of chapter 2), and snowshoeing. Stair climbing with single, double, and triple stairs is some of the best in-city training.

STRENGTH TRAINING

For the most part, you can hike, backpack, and snowshoe without a rigorous strength-training program. The program below, a basic one that can be done in a short period of time, can help keep you well toned and make your outdoor activity more enjoyable with less effort, less muscle soreness, and a lower likelihood of overuse injuries. You can do your exercises in 2–3 sets of 15–20 repetitions because you are working on the endurance aspect of your strength.

Upper-body strength of the shoulder girdle and the posterior back is useful for lifting your pack and for using handholds and ski poles. Strengthening your lower body is important for longer and more challenging trips and to be able to handle steep trails, uneven terrain, or deep snow.

HIKING AND BACKPACKING

The strength training program outlined below is the maximum suggested. You may want to start with a few exercises from each category and build up gradually to doing the entire group. Exercises that involve hops need only be added if you will be crossing rivers or boulder fields. Make sure you do squats and lunges for 4 weeks before adding hops. It is a good idea to vary the lunges you do at each workout.

Lower body: Exercises 48, 70, 72, 72.3, 72.5, 73, 74, 74.3, 74.4, 76, and 76.3.

Abdominals: Exercises 56 (or variations 1, 2, or 3), 60, 62, and 67.

Lower/upper body: Exercises 23 and 32 (optional).

Upper body: Exercises 88.4, 91, 92.1, 94, 95, and 102.

SNOWSHOEING

Do the strength exercises for hiking and backpacking, above, with the following modifications:

Lower body: Add Exercise 72.11.
Abdominals: Add Exercise 64.

Lower/upper body: Add Exercises 27, 30.1, 31.1.
Upper body: Add Exercise 98.

BALANCE AND AGILITY

Consider doing balance exercises within 4–6 weeks of beginning your outdoor activity, to improve your stability on boulder fields, logs, slopes, snow, and river crossings. You can do them twice a week for 5–10 minutes and make them part of your strength workout. Try doing them with a backpack after you have mastered them. If you have kneecap problems and you experience pain with balance exercises, try doing them with ski poles to decrease the weight on your knees.

HIKING/BACKPACKING

Do Exercises 37.1, 37.2, 38.1, 38.3, and 40.

SNOWSHOEING

Do the above plus Exercise 39.1.

WEIGHT-SHIFTING EXERCISES

Weight-shifting awareness and movement (see Exercise 47) are useful techniques for backpackers and snowshoers, especially on river crossings or on steep or unsteady terrain while using high stepping motions. Get an idea of how you can move your torso and body weight with more weight on the forward foot so there is optimum weight balance between your feet (and your hands, if there is a handhold or you are using ski poles or a walking stick), so that you can extend your forward knee and move onto that foot in the most stable way possible.

Experiment with weight-shifting while doing step-up Exercises 48.1, 48.2, 48.3, and 73 to find the amount of weight-shifting to the forward foot that gives you the optimum combination of momentum and balance. You can do this outdoors while stepping onto a rock or log or a high step on a trail. Too much weight-shifting forward can lead you to fall forward or cause too much flexing of your low back. In town, try this with a backpack to really notice the importance of weight-shifting. If you are a snowshoer you can use poles during the exercise.

PACK POSTURE

Many people with heavy packs overcompensate in their posture and get into positions of excessive flexion of their back, shoulders, and neck. This can lead to pain. It is more likely to happen when you are tired and on steep hills. It can also happen if the top of the pack or equipment is pushing your neck forward. Intermittently check your body to see that you are in a reasonable pack-carrying posture. Good pack posture means having your head aligned over your shoulders and looking out onto the terrain or out at the scenery. Have your low back in a neutral position and not slumped forward. Practice Exercise 45 without a pack. Then practice it with a pack or using only low back movement in a much more limited motion (avoid excessive flexing). It is also important to have well-padded hip straps and secure them on the crest of your pelvic bone so that you carry most of the weight there and not on your shoulders. Carrying excessive weight on your shoulders can lead to shoulder and neck pain, or tingling in the fingers.

In Figure 25a, notice the forward head and excessively flexed posture. In Figure 25b, the neck and low back are in a more neutral position.

PACK TYPES AND FIT

A pack should be large enough to carry your gear in a comfortable and balanced way. There should be enough room so you do not have to stuff gear in the top in such a manner that your neck is pushed forward. The pack should not sway very much from side to side when you bend slightly to the right or left; this will challenge your back and legs excessively. The waist

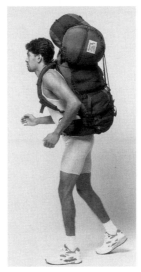 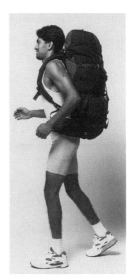

FIGURE 25a   FIGURE 25b

belt should be very well padded and rest comfortably on the crest of your hips.

PACKS: GETTING THEM SAFELY ON AND OFF

It is important to use proper body mechanics when lifting your pack. This is a time of increased risk for a back injury. Always bend with your knees rather than your back. When putting a heavy pack on, try squatting down in front of the right-hand pack strap, with your right knee in front of the left. Your right knee can either be on the ground or within 1½ feet of the ground, but should be close to the pack. Your back should be relatively straight.

Raise the pack up to rest on your right thigh, then put your right arm in the strap (see Figure 26a on next page). Stand up carefully using both legs, and minimize any extending in your back (see Figure 26b on next page). If you have back problems, place the pack on one knee and lean it against a tree trunk or a boulder to make it easier to get it on. Removing and lowering

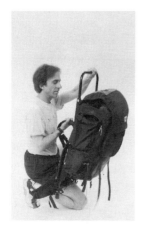
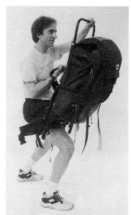

FIGURE 26a   FIGURE 26b

your pack requires care and is basically the reverse of this.

Avoid picking up your pack by bending forward and rotating at your low back and then extending your back. These are the positions most likely to lead to injury. A back injury is more likely with a heavy pack, but it can happen while lifting even a light pack improperly, so always use good lifting principles (see chapter 14 for further lifting details).

BOOTS AND STABILITY

The boots you wear can influence how stable you feel on a hike or a snowshoe trip. If you plan on crossing rivers, logs, scree slopes, or boulder fields, you need a full leather boot or a leather combination boot with reinforcement in the heel area. The sole should resist excessive twisting. If you can twist your boot more than 25 degrees (with the top of the boot as 0 degrees, use one hand to twist where the heel meets the sole and keep the other hand on the forefoot), your boot may not be stable enough for any significant backpacking. Try out a boot by doing this twisting test as well as by standing and

balancing on one leg and moving your arms in different directions to see how stable you feel. Boots can be too stiff or heavy if you are planning on light day hiking with few balance challenges. For snowshoeing, choose boots that are stable as well as warm. Refer to chapter 13 for further information on shoe fit.

WALKING UPHILL

Try to avoid excessively long strides or high footholds when hiking uphill. If you have kneecap pain going uphill, focus more attention on step-up exercises, such as Exercises 48 and 73, and practice weight-shifting with a step height of 6 inches or less. Gradually increase the step height to approximate the step reach you want to be able to do in the outdoors.

WALKING DOWNHILL

Walking downhill demands lower-extremity deceleration to counter the forces of gravity. The muscles that are most important are the quads, hamstrings, buttock/hip girdle, and calf muscles.

PRACTICAL POINT
It is very important to take breaks and not go too fast when you are walking downhill, even though it may feel less taxing aerobically. There are a lot of forces on your kneecaps when you walk downhill. You can decrease the likelihood of kneecap or thigh muscle pain by taking breaks every 1–1½ hours and by doing Exercises 74, 74.3, and 74.4.

GOAL PROGRAMS
Example 1. A 16-mile, 2- to 3-day backpacking trip with 4,000 feet elevation gain, or a day hike of 8–10 miles with 4,000 feet elevation gain.

In general, 8 weeks of preparation should be adequate. Do the aerobic program listed earlier in this chapter. Include the strength training program listed earlier in this chapter, 2 days a week with two sets of 15–20 repetitions. You can add a lower-repetition (8–12), higher-resistance set if you wish to build more strength. Try to incorporate some balance activities into your program during the last month. When you have achieved a 6-mile, 2,500-foot-elevation-gain hike, you will be ready for a longer day hike or backpacking trip. If you are already doing a minimum aerobic and strength program, preparation may take less than 6 weeks.

Example 2. A whole day of moderate snowshoeing, approximately 6 miles with a 2,000- to 3,000-foot elevation gain.

Proceed as in Example 1 above, but do more lower-body strengthening and balance work earlier. Use hikes, cross-country skiing, jogging, stair climbing, or snowshoeing for your lower-intensity, longer-duration (LILD) activity. If you use aerobic modes other than snowshoeing, begin shorter snowshoe training activities before your first long trip because of the unique hip and buttock demands of snowshoeing. When you are able to do 4 miles with 1,500–2,000 feet of elevation gain, you should be ready for your longer trip. Give this at least 8 weeks of preparation time.

Conditioning for Scrambling and Rock Climbing

By Dan Cauthorn

▶ **THIS CHAPTER WILL HELP YOU:**
- Understand the special muscle, joint, and movement demands unique to technical climbing.
- Do a dynamic strength training program designed to prepare you for a full day of climbing.
- Create a flexible, 4- to 6-month periodization planning program to develop specific climbing strength, endurance, and technique to achieve these following specific goals:
  1. A 10-mile-round-trip, strenuous Class 3 rock scramble.
  2. A multipitch (6–8 pitches) technical Class 5 rock climb.
  3. Thirty minutes of steep (vertical to overhanging) sport/gym climbing.

Scrambling and rock and sport climbing have unique and exacting strength, endurance, coordination, balance, and psychological demands. Overall strength, with special attention to the upper body, and especially the fingers, is a prerequisite to any climbing endeavor. In standard climbing classification, scrambling is basically an aerobic activity of off-trail hiking and mountain peak ascents that involves use of the hands and legs with nontechnical climbing. A scrambling ascent is rated Class 2 or 3 (see *Mountaineering: The Freedom of the Hills*, pp. 510–516).

Layered onto the physical demands are the complex movements and problem solving skills required for success on steep and exposed terrain. Improving your functional strength and balance can help decrease injuries and enhance performance, and help you achieve your climbing goals.

MUSCULOSKELETAL DEMANDS

In climbers, muscles increase in lactic acid, cramping, and swelling. Many climbers call this "getting pumped." Sport climbers often fail because their arms get pumped and they can no longer hold on. The muscles in the hand and forearm, along with the supporting muscles of the shoulder and back, can be strengthened so that one is less likely to get pumped and more able to continue climbing.

Upper Body
Climbing activities vary in their requirement for upper-body strength. Generally, the demand

increases as the angle of the climb gets steeper and the holds get smaller and farther apart. Scrambling involves a lot of pushing, dipping, rowing, and pull-up maneuvers at different angles but with large hand- and footholds. Technical climbing exerts similar demands on the upper body but usually on steeper pitches with smaller holds. There are more significant demands for strength in the shoulder, upper back, forearm, and fingers. The joints and muscles of these regions are often stressed at various lengths and disadvantageous angles.

Most climbing is done in the forearm pronated position, when the palm is facing the wall. Climbers should do most of their pull-ups in this position.

Core/Back

The back is involved in just about every climbing motion. Moves are performed in positions in which the neck and back are very extended, bent, or rotated. Then a climbing move is attempted while the core is twisted at the end of its motion range. Injuries to the back can occur, which may be quite debilitating and even dangerous if you are in the middle of a long climb. Tips to prevent such injuries include:

1. Avoid lifting heavy gear with your back; instead, lift with your legs and buttocks (see chapters 14 and 17).
2. Train your abdominal muscles.
3. Practice some weight-shifting climbing techniques so you move your core (torso, back, and abdomen) and center of gravity well, to preserve your strength. Avoid quick extending motions while hyper-extending, as well as quick flexed, rotated positions, especially with a loaded pack.

Lower Body

The buttocks, hamstrings, quads, and calves all play significant roles while climbing. Training for strength and muscle balance in the legs is

important. Good climbers raise their bodies with their powerful leg and buttock muscles, carefully conserving the strength in their arms. The lower body also must perform extreme ranges of motion, especially in the flexing of the hips and knees in high stepping on trails, snow, or walls with high footholds (see Figure 27). The climber

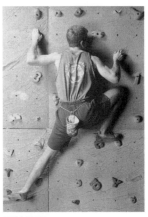

FIGURE 27

attempts to rise up from that position using muscles that are in a most disadvantageous position.

Hip and thigh strains can be minimized with proper training during a gradual progression of strengthening exercises to simulate using higher and higher footholds or step heights (if you are training for snow or non-wall terrain). Principles of weight-shifting are important to optimize your body position to make these moves more efficient and easier on your body. (See chapter 6 for information on weight-shifting.)

Practice stepping exercises (Exercises 48 and 73) using weight-shifting techniques.

MOVEMENT DEMANDS

Perhaps the most important element of all concerning the demands of climbing are the actual movement patterns. The ability to move your center of gravity and core in good coordination with your arms and legs is very important and can decrease the strength demands on certain muscles. Training, through climbing movement drills and exercises to memorize movement patterns (or develop "engrams"), is important. (Refer to Goddard's *Performance Rock Climbing* for more details on engrams.) There are many movement patterns or "moves" that can be practiced on boulders, on rock walls, or on indoor walls. These moves can be practiced by experimenting with hand, feet, and body positioning, and with weight-shifting, to find the technique that seems to be most efficient and require the least effort. It is better to move in ways that do not require putting joints in the end of their range, if possible. Practicing a move with efficient technique can help the climber integrate moves into a repertoire that can be used so that when similar climbing challenges are encountered, one can climb more efficiently and quickly. Good technique and accompanying strength gains are fostered by training specifically to develop balance, weight-shifting skills, and efficient and relaxed moves.

MUSCLE IMBALANCES

Muscle imbalances are common among climbers. The climbing muscles like the chest, lats, biceps, and forearm and finger flexors tend to get strong fast. Muscles that tend to be underdeveloped are the finger/wrist extensors, triceps, rotator cuff, and the lower to mid trapezius. Balancing these muscle groups with training can be important for avoiding injury.

WARM-UP

Try the Dynamic Warm-up Drills in chapter 4. Do all of them, or at least the aerobic and stretching components.

STRETCHING

Scramblers and both levels of climbers should do Exercises 1, 3.1, 3.3, 5, 7, 8, 9, 11, 13, 16, and 19.

CLIMBING-SPECIFIC AEROBIC CONDITIONING

The aerobic demands of climbing can be graded from the higher demands of scrambling to the lower demands of multipitch climbing to sport climbing. Aerobic training that is more specific for climbing includes running, hiking, using a treadmill, stair climbing and using stair-climber machines, using rotating climbing walls, using rowing machines, step or high-impact aerobics classes, and using cross-country ski machines. Other aerobic activities can be done intermittently, but are not well suited for training the climbing muscles.

SCRAMBLING

This type of climbing is primarily aerobic. The moves are lower strength, but must be sustained over a long period of time. Most scrambles are 8–12 miles with 3,500–5,000 feet elevation gain. The scrambler should follow and make modifications to the aerobic program in chapter 17. Start increasing your aerobic training within 3 months of your first scramble climb.

Do 4–5 short aerobic sessions per week with sport-specific activities (at least 2 of these sessions should be 40–50 minutes in length; the others could be 30 minutes). You can do a few aerobic activities in one session to add up to 50 minutes. Non-machine stair climbing is excellent aerobic training and should be done 1–2 times per week within 6 weeks of your first scramble. Vary your activity with running or fast-walking single, double, or triple stairs.

Start a low-intensity, longer-duration (LILD) activity within 6–8 weeks of your first scramble (this could be a hike or a snowshoe or cross-country ski trip). Each week increase the duration and elevation of your LILD trip until you have reached approximately three-fourths of the mileage and elevation of your first planned scramble. If you anticipate a scramble on snow, make sure some of your training trips involve some snow hiking.

Consider some Fartlek-type interval training 1–2 times per week within 6 weeks of your first scramble. Doing intervals of 30–120 seconds while on a training hike or on aerobic equipment could more quickly improve your aerobic fitness. (See chapter 2 for information on Fartlek interval training.)

MULTIPITCH CLIMBING

Follow the aerobic training schedule for scramblers, above, but your LILD trips can be shorter to simulate the distances of your approach to your climb. A climber should do training hikes or scrambles, beginning within 6 weeks of the first climb, with a climbing pack of similar weight as would be carried on the approach to the climb. It is important to have enough muscular endurance so that carrying a heavy pack does not drain you before the climb actually begins. The activity of climbing on a moderate (up to Class 5.8) multipitch climb can be aerobic if there are long, easy stretches on which a climber can move relatively quickly and the climbing moves do not seem very difficult to the endurance- and strength-trained climber. On more difficult terrain, the climber moves much more slowly, and strength and power are very important.

Don't forget how strenuous a descent can be in terms of aerobic, strength, and balance demands. Descending even simple terrain can be aerobically strenuous for a tired climber after a long, multipitch climb. Take it slowly and take intermittent breaks for rest, fluid, and food.

SPORT CLIMBING

Sport climbing is characterized by being steep, powerful, and short, and is not usually aerobic but primarily anaerobic. Much sport climbing is done in climbing clubs and requires only doing minimum aerobic conditioning. The approaches and descents from the climbing area itself present the aerobic challenges. These can vary greatly according to the climbing area.

Do the minimum aerobic program outlined in chapter 2, with climbing-specific modes of exercise.

Add a low-intensity, longer-duration (LILD) activity 1 time per week if your climbs involve a long approach hike.

STRENGTH TRAINING

The following exercises to help you develop strength can be done in conjunction with the climbing-specific exercises at the end of this chapter.

If you are short on time, you can do 1 set each of the abdominal (ab) exercises. Do 2 sets of the other exercises. Do them 2–3 times per week. Climbers and scramblers should start 8–12 weeks before their season. You can do all of your strength exercises on 1 day (2 longer strength exercise sessions per week) or do split sessions (4 shorter sessions per week).

LEVEL 1 CLIMBERS
Upper body: Exercises 23, 30, 86, 88 (all levels), 91, 92, 94, 98, 99.2 (gradually work up to a less assisted dip and chin-up), and 102.

Forearm and hand: Exercises 108, 109, 110, 111, and 112.

Abdominals: Exercises 50, 56.1, 56.2, 56.3, 61, 62, 63, 64 (with both feet on the floor), and 67.

Lower body: Exercises 30–32, 48, 70.2, 70.4, 72.3, 74, and 91. Alternate Exercise 31 or 32 with Exercise 48 and Exercise 30 with Exercise 91.

SCRAMBLERS
Upper body: Do the Level 1 program, above. Consider substituting Exercise 101.1 for 86. Add Exercise 91.3. Spend more time on your dips than on push-ups.

Forearm and hand (start within 4 weeks of your first climb): Exercises 108 and 109.

Abdominals: Do the Level 1 program, above.

Lower body: Do the Level 1 program, above, but omit Exercise 31 and focus on Exercise 48 for your step-ups. Add Exercises 26.1 or 26.2 and 76.3 after 1½ months of strength training.

LEVEL 2 CLIMBERS

These exercises are recommended for sport and more advanced outdoor climbing. Do the Level 1 program with the following modifications.

Upper body: Work up to fully unassisted dips and pull-ups. In some of your workouts, substitute Exercises 55 or 101 for 86, 103 for 91, and 104 for 102. Add Exercises 20, 83, 84, 91.2, 91.3, 93, 106, and 107.

Forearm and hand: Add fingerboard exercises (Exercise 118) after 6 weeks of a basic upper-body program.

Abdominals: Do the Level 1 program's abdominals with the following changes: Add Exercises 56.4 or 56.5, 60, 63 (with a pack on), 64 (balancing on one foot), and 68.

Lower body: Do the Level 1 program above and add Exercises 26.2 or 26.3, 27, 31.1, 31.3, 75.1, and 76.1. Substitute Exercise 70.2 for 70.1. Do your step-ups with high steps, working up to a step on a chair, a step over 3 steps, or a high step onto a boulder or bleacher, etc.

TIMING AND PERIODIZATION

In general, begin a climbing-specific conditioning program at least 8 weeks prior to your first scramble or climb. If your first climb requires a great deal of finger, forearm, and general strength training, it is better to start 10–12 weeks before your climbing season.

For serious climbers, a year-round strategy is ultimately the best. In the late fall, begin basic overall training that includes strengthening exercises with 3 sets of 15–25 reps to build an endurance strength base, and do more climbing-specific aerobic training. The goal is to build a fitness base of aerobic and strength endurance. If you have access to a climbing gym or bouldering area, you can start some light climbing (especially traversing) after 4 weeks of your basic strengthening program. You can also start some basic weight-shifting exercises. It is good to begin some relaxation work early so that you can learn to calm yourself down in tense situations.

After 2 months, increase climbing volume (time on the wall or hanging on fingers) and do some of your strength training (1–2 sets) with reps of 8–12 to build more strength.

After a couple more months, build specific climbing strength by working harder on finger and forearm strength and consider some redpoint training (see Exercise 120).

During this period you may do 1–2 strength training sets with 6–8 reps in a set for maximum strength development. This period before your active climbing season should also be a time to increase the duration of a 1-day-a-week, lower-intensity, longer-duration (LILD) distance if you will be training for climbs that involve an approach of more than a few miles.

During the climbing season have a 2- to 3-day break between a strength training day and a climb. Take a month off of climbing at the end of the season to rest, and continue a base of aerobic and strength training to keep in shape.

BALANCE AND AGILITY

Level 1 climbers and scramblers should do Exercises 36.5, 38.1, 39.1, and 40.

Level 2 climbers should do the above program, but substitute Exercise 38.3 for 38.1.

CLIMBING-SPECIFIC EXERCISES

These exercises are to be used on climbing walls. Do them in conjunction with the strength training program earlier in this chapter.

113 | Climbing Rest Position for Your Fingers and Body

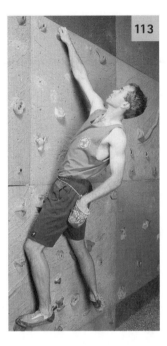

113

Equipment: Climbing wall (indoor or outdoor) or fingerboard; chalk, tape (to reinforce fingers), rock shoes (slippers are actually best because they help strengthen and train your feet and legs).
Purpose: Warming up your fingers is an essential start to any climbing-specific workout. Initially this exercise is the first step in building fundamental finger strength, weight-shifting skills, and climbing technique. Eventually it becomes a quick prelude to a full workout.

Technique: On a large handhold or the biggest hold on a finger-board, hang comfortably off of a single, straight arm. This is the rest position and is a fundamental technique to any type of climbing. Your feet should also be on good holds (or on the ground). Your legs should be straight and relaxed, hips pressed in, and your back arched. Do 5 seconds on one arm, then switch hands and hang 5 seconds on the other. This position should become second nature. As a warm-up, repeat this process 3 times, resting 20–30 seconds between exercises.

114 | Traversing

Equipment: Climbing wall, rock climbing shoes.
Purpose: Do easy climbing sideways back and forth across the wall to practice technique, train the forearms, and begin to develop climbing-specific muscle endurance.

Technique: Traversing can be done solo. You never need to get more than 1 foot off the ground. Begin climbing for 10-minute sessions. Rest 10 minutes, and then climb continuously for another 5 minutes. Build up to 10 minutes climbing, 10 minutes resting, then repeat. With good traversing technique, the climber moves with hips parallel to the wall, shuffling the hands and feet in one direction or the other. Try not to cross hands or feet, and stay on the inside edges of your rock shoes. Imagine Spiderman moving sideways across a wall.

WEIGHT-SHIFTING EXERCISES

The purpose of good weight-shifting is to coordinate the movement of the core of your body to your extremity motions so that you are balanced and move with the least muscular effort. The following exercises will help you to develop skill in moving your center of gravity and extremities while maintaining your balance on a wall.

115 Five Moving Parts

Equipment: Climbing wall, rock climbing shoes.
Purpose: Weight-shifting skills can be developed while traversing.

Technique: Imagine that you have five body parts that move when you climb: two hands, two feet, and one torso. Start in a rest position, and then try to climb by moving each part separately and distinctly from the others. Start in the crunch position (115a). Move your left

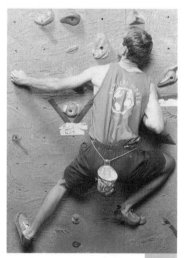

115a

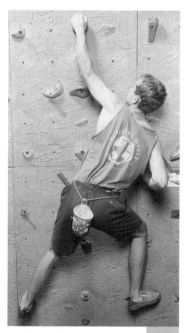

115b

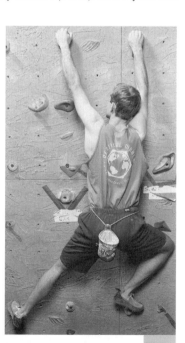

115c

hand to a hold (115b). Then move your right hand to a hold (115c). Then move your left foot up (115d). Then move your right foot up (115e). Then move your core/torso (115f). Have a friend watch you and announce which body part should move, i.e., "hand, hand, foot, body . . . " Never move any two parts at once.

Variations: 115.1 Try moving your core (back, abdomen, and chest) before you move your legs or your arms. Try to do this smoothly and move a foot or hand when you have first shifted your weight to get yourself in an ideal position for the next move. 115.2 Next, try moving your core *while* you initiate an arm or leg motion, to determine the best combination of movements.

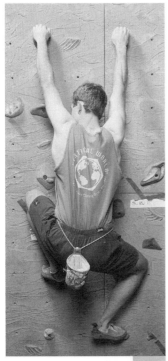

115d

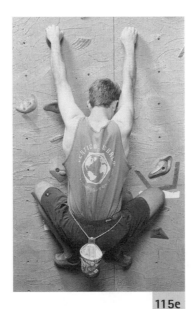

115e

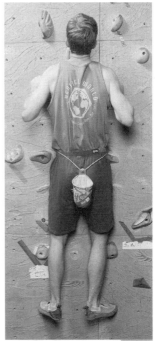

115f

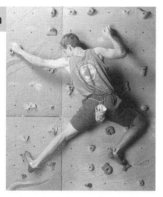

116a

116 Round-the-Clock Weight-shifting

Equipment: Climbing wall, rock climbing shoes.
Purpose: Improve your balance abilities and efficiency of motion on a climbing wall.

Technique: Locate four suitable holds in a square configuration (two handholds and two footholds). Have both hands and feet on the holds, with hips parallel to the wall. Now move your body around in a circle: Shift your weight to the right (116a), then down, then across to the left (116b), up, then back to the middle. Never remove a hand or foot. Feel how shifting your hip and torso positions weights or unweights certain areas. Gradually enlarge your range of motion as you feel more comfortable.

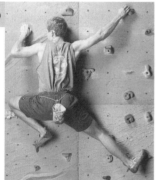

116b

117 Flagging

Equipment: Climbing wall, rock climbing shoes.
Purpose: Further improve your balance and weight-shifting on a wall.

Technique: To try flagging out, reach up and to the right with your right hand while lifting your left foot as a counterweight, so you can lean and reach farther to the right. Only your left hand and right foot have weight-bearing contact with the wall (see 117a). Then, to flag in, shift your weight to the left foot and cross the right leg behind the left leg as a counterweight that balances you so you can reach with the right hand up and over the left hand (see 117b). The only two points of contact at this point are the left hand and the left foot. You can try alternating between these positions as you warm up.
Variations: Incorporate other combinations of handhold and footholds.

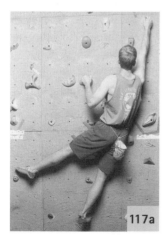

117a

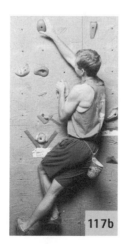

117b

118 Fingerboards

Equipment: Fingerboard.
Purpose: Fingerboards are very effective tools for climbing-specific upper-body strength training. Novice climbers are advised to build a base of strength training before starting fingerboard exercises.

Technique: On a fingerboard, position yourself with an open grip, with your elbows slightly flexed and your lats activated (see 118a). An endurance workout on a fingerboard consists of long, timed hangs off of large holds. Try not to hang in a "dead hang" with your weight supported by fully extended shoulders and elbows (see 118b).

Note that at this level, appropriate techniques for training will sometimes differ from what is proper technique for climbing. For example, the rest position used while climbing has the climber relaxing all body weight on a straight arm. The "dead hang" is OK while climbing. Also, don't crimp on a fingerboard; use the open grip (see 118c). If you can't hang onto a particular hold without crimping, then don't use that hold. Wait until you have built up sufficient strength to use an open grip.

Variations: 118.1. Time yourself for your maximum hang time on a large hold. Rest for at least 2 minutes and repeat your maximum hang. Try to get through the routine 3 times. 118.2. Try the "20/20": Hang for 20 seconds, then rest for 20 seconds. Repeat 10 times. Always begin a fingerboard workout with a warm-up consisting of 5–10 minutes of easy hanging off of big holds. Hang long enough to get your forearms warmed up, but not pumped. Then start the endurance workout on the largest hold. When you can accomplish the 20/20 on the biggest hold, move to smaller and/or sloping holds. 118.3. Power workouts demand maximum effort of a short duration. Longer rests between sets are necessary. Working on smaller holds is one way to increase power. Time yourself for maximum hang time on progressively smaller holds. Record the number of pull-ups you can do on the smallest hold. If the hang time exceeds 10 seconds, or you can do more than 5 pull-ups, move to smaller holds. Or add resistance (in 2-pound increments) by hanging weight off of your chalk bag belt. Adding weight to yourself and then performing pull-ups on a fingerboard is one of the most effective means of increasing finger power for extreme sport climbing. Only attempt this after a very good base of finger strength has been developed.

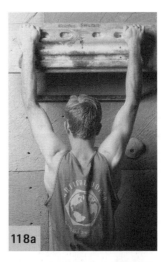

118a

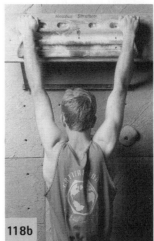

118b

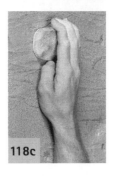

118c

Endurance Climbing

Equipment: Climbing wall, rock climbing shoes.
Purpose: Build climbing-specific endurance by using high repetitions with low resistance.

Technique: Choose a relatively easy climb and do "laps" on it. The goal is to climb until you are pumped due to muscle failure. Technical difficulty is not an issue, but the climbing surface must be at least vertical. An excellent goal in a bouldering situation is 30 minutes of continuous climbing, either traversing back and forth, climbing up then down (don't touch the ground), or some creative combination. Try to simulate a long pitch, where you've got to take advantage of rests, move through cruxes, and sometimes do down climbing to figure out a problem. If you are top-roping with a partner, take turns climbing several laps in a row on a single climb. Climb to the top, get lowered back to the ground, and then immediately begin climbing again. Build to 5 laps on a typical half-rope-length top-rope climb. In either scenario, the ideal wall is difficult enough that you can just complete the task. If you can't get pumped on a vertical wall, move to progressively steeper and steeper terrain.

Red Pointing

Equipment: Climbing wall, rock climbing shoes.

Purpose: In red pointing, you spend numerous attempts working each section of a specific route. Figure out individual moves by resting on the rope (or "hang dogging") to relax between attempts. The goal is to link each section together without falling on the red-point attempt. Red pointing generally refers to leading a route without falling, but the concept of working a route to build power can be applied to top roping or bouldering. It is climbing at, or attempting to push, your limit.

Technique: Pick a hard route, and begin breaking it down in to manageable sections. Figuring out each move, and then linking them all, can be a process that takes hours, days, weeks, even months. With each hard move accomplished, you get a little better. Warm up well before a hard session. Use the rating system to keep track of your progress. Breaking through the threshold of each higher grade is one of the more rewarding moments for every climber. The 5.10 level is traditionally a major step for a recreational climber. There are several excellent resources to learn about the complexities of hard red-point climbing (see *Flash Training* and *Performance Rock Climbing* in Selected References).

GOAL PROGRAMS

A MINIMUM CLIMBING OR SCRAMBLING PROGRAM

This is a combination of a Level 1 climbing or scrambling strength training program with traverses (see Exercise 114) and the aerobic program recommended earlier in this chapter for your activity. With this program you can create a base of strength endurance and technique that will enable you to participate in a full day of climbing, i.e., a moderate/novice climb or a strenuous, all-day scramble.

At the end of Week 8 you should be ready for some easy climbs. Follow the aerobic guidelines earlier in this chapter. Do flexibility work with each training session. Weeks 1–8 consist of building the base.

Weeks 1–2: Start very lightly and increase gradually until you can do a set of 15–20 reps before you fatigue. Do 2–3 sets of each strength training exercise for Level 1. Do Exercises 113 and 114.

Weeks 3–4: Strength workout: Two times per week, 2–3 sets each exercise, 12–15 reps of each exercise, gradually increasing the resistance or degree of difficulty of the exercises. Do 30 minutes of climbing 2 times per week. Do climbing-specific Exercises 113 and 114.

Weeks 5–8: Strength workout: Decrease reps to 8–12 per set and do 2–3 sets of each exercise. Do climbing exercises same as for Week 4, but add Exercises 115, 116, and 119. Gradually increase the difficulty of the Endurance Climbing exercise (Exercise 119).

ADVANCED CLIMBING GOAL PERIODIZATION PROGRAMS

This program trains for techniques and additional strength required in steep, technical climbing. One basic goal for the activity is to accomplish a multipitch Grade III or IV rock climb and/or increase your rock climbing standard by two number grades. Two or three months in a goal program should get you ready for all but the most demanding climbing. Remember: Your ability to accomplish a climb successfully is related to many factors besides your conditioning program, including your age, frame size, amount of muscle mass, preexisting injuries, arm and leg lengths, and technique. There is no guarantee that every person completing a goal program will be able to safely complete a climb.

Incorporate a goal program schedule after 8 weeks of the minimum program above, or the equivalent if you are already doing a part of the minimum program. Do flexibility work with each training session. Follow the aerobic guidelines earlier in this chapter.

Weeks 9–15: Do a weight workout 2 times per week. During this time you may want to do a weight workout with 1 set of 15–20 for endurance and 2 sets of 8–10 for strength. Add specific forearm and finger exercises in this period as listed in the Level 2 strength program earlier in this chapter. Do climbing-specific exercises 2 times per week. Warm up and divide your workout between Exercises 114, 115, 116, 119, and 120.

Weeks 16–24: Sport-specific. Do a weight workout (same as for Weeks 9–15, above) and consider increasing the finger/forearm strengthening exercises with more emphasis on fingerboards (Exercise 118). Do climbing exercises 2 times a week: Exercises 114, 115, 116, 117, 119, and 120.

Weeks 25–41: Climbing season maintenance. Do a weight workout 2 times per week. Leave 2–3 days between a weight workout and a climb. Do 30 minutes of aerobic exercise 3 times per week and 1 hour of climbing twice per week (warm up, and do Exercises 113, 114, 117, and 120).

19

Conditioning for Mountaineering

By David Musnick, M.D.

▶ **THIS CHAPTER WILL HELP YOU:**
- Understand the aerobic and strength demands of mountaineering.
- Plan an exercise program to train to climb a mountain or do significant trekking.

Climbing a mountain with rock, snow, and glacier terrain requires significant aerobic endurance, strength, and balance abilities. Your goal is to get to the top, injury free, with the least amount of fatigue. The combination of altitude, heavy loads, difficult and steep terrain, and exposure make it mandatory to modify your conditioning program. Plan a minimum of 12 weeks to train for most mountaineering activities.

MUSCULOSKELETAL DEMANDS

The movement demands of mountaineering are similar to those for climbing (see chapter 18). In addition, there may be more demands on your lower body to take high or long steps without the use of your arms; to do this, it is important to maximize your body positioning.

This can be done by weight-shifting (see chapter 6 for more information on weight-shifting). Practice taking progressively higher steps with Exercises 48 and 73 within 4–6 weeks of your first mountaineering trip. Add a moderately heavy pack to these exercises within 2–3 weeks of your first climb.

MUSCLE IMBALANCES

Muscle imbalances become apparent as physical demands become greater. Muscle weakness or tightness affects your ability to reach or step in a particular range or direction. Characteristic lower-body muscle imbalances of mountaineer athletes include weak gluteals and quadriceps in association with tight hamstrings. This affects your ability to negotiate a steep climb while in a precarious position. This type of muscle imbalance also decreases your ability to decelerate and control your upper body and pack descending a steep slope.

Upper-body muscle imbalances include weakness of the upper and lower back muscles in comparison to tight and strong chest muscles. Other imbalances may include stronger biceps in comparison to weakened shoulders and latissimus dorsi muscles. The brachioradialis may be weak and make it difficult to do a pull-up in a hand pronated position (see chapter 16 and Exercise 99.1). These muscle imbalances can prohibit you from performing repetitive pulling and climbing tasks associated with mountaineering.

WARM-UP

An appropriate warm-up is important for mountaineers due to the significant demands placed upon all body regions. A minimum warm-up should consist of 5–10 minutes of vigorous walking incorporating repetitive shoulder and arm motions in all directions, simulating climbing motions. Consider performing all or parts of the Dynamic Warm-up (chapter 4), excluding moves that are unsafe depending on the terrain and weather conditions. Modify the stretches to use rocks and snow to support your feet.

STRETCHING

Good flexibility of your spine, legs, hips, and ankles as well as chest and shoulders is important. You can do the following exercises during the week or after a warm-up before your climb begins.

Exercises 1, 3.1, 3.3, 5, 7, 8, 9, 11, 13, 16, 17, and 19.

AEROBIC CONDITIONING

Mountaineering requires a significant amount of aerobic endurance. You will need to improve your maximal aerobic capacity and your ability to work near your lactate threshold, because you will walk on steep slopes at higher altitude. Develop this by doing specific aerobic activities 5 times a week for 30–50 minutes and a longer-duration training activity once every week. Mountaineering-specific training includes:

Outside: running, cross-country skiing, snowshoeing, hiking, scrambling, and stair climbing. Stair climbing should be a part of your in-city training within 6 weeks of your first climb. Vary your stair climbing workouts with running single or double stairs and walking double and triple stairs. Do descents of single and double stairs.

Inside: cross-country ski machines, step aerobics, EFX cross trainer, and stair climbing (especially on real stairs or on a revolving stair machine).

Cross training: cycling and rowing.

STRENGTH TRAINING

Strength training is very important for mountain climbers and should emphasize functional exercises of your whole lower body (buttocks, hips, thighs, etc.), upper body, and lower/upper body combination. Abdominal exercises are important for balance and for back support.

Refer to chapter 18 for more information on strength training if you are going to be doing any significant rock or ice climbing.

BEGINNING

Lower body: Exercises 23, 24, 31.1, 31.3, 70.1, 70.2, 70.3, 73, 74, 76, and 76.1.

Abdominals: Exercises 50, 56.3, 61, 62, 63, 64 (with both feet on the floor), and 67.

Upper body: Exercises 20, 31.1, 31.3, 86, 88.4, 91, 92.1, 93, 94, 98, 99, and 102. Note: Do Exercise 98 and 99 on assisted machines and work up to at least half to three-quarters of your body weight.

INTERMEDIATE/ADVANCED

Lower body: Do the Beginning program above for 4 weeks, then omit Exercises 24 and 73, and add Exercises 26, 27, 32, 75.1, 76.2, and 76.3.

Abdominals: Do the Beginning program above, and add Exercises 51, 56.4 or 56.5, 60, 63 (with a pack on), 64 (balancing on one foot), and 68.

Upper body: Do the Beginning program above for 4 weeks, then add Exercises 30, 30.1, 85 (decline press), 89, 98, 99.1, 99.2 (as close to unassisted as possible), and 107; substitute 101 for 86 and 104 for 102.

THE DESCENT

Descending from a climb requires a high degree of strength and control. There are significant forces on the knees and ankles to control the pace of the descent and keep you from falling. Often a climber grows fatigued because of awakening early and spending many arduous hours on the ascent. It is important to stay well fueled with food and fluids and take breaks on the descent.

Training for the descent can be done in town by doing stepping exercises off a step—Exercises 74.1, 74.2, and 74.3—by doing walking lunges—Exercises 72.5 or 72.6 on level ground and downhill surfaces—and by descending stairs 2–3 at a time in a controlled manner. Ideally these should be done with a pack on within 4 weeks of your first climb. On weekend hikes, choose steeper terrain and snow as you near your first climb.

BALANCE AND AGILITY

Mountaineering terrain is often unstable (scree, snow, and ice slopes), which challenges your balance while you are under significant loads with a pack. When you are on snow or ice, you must be very stable, balancing on one leg while you are cutting or finding the next step. It is important to be able to balance on one leg with a heavy pack with your legs in variable positions (different amounts of knee bending) and in different planes of motion (front, side, and diagonal).

Start balance exercises within 4–6 weeks of your first climb and do them twice a week. In town, you can do some of these on a hill or a sloped driveway, as well as on a flat surface in your home or in a gym. Practice with a pack once you feel fairly confident without one. You can also practice some of the balance exercises on snow slopes or non-snow terrain that is not subject to dangerous exposure.

Do Exercises 27.1, 27.2, 37.1, 37.2 (especially), 37.3, 38.1, 38.3, 39.1, 40, 40.1, 63.1, and 63.2.

PACK POSITIONING AND LIFTING

Positioning and safe lifting of your pack is described in chapters 14 and 17. Make sure ropes and other gear are packed so your neck and head are not pushed forward. These safe lifting and movement techniques are extremely important on mountaineering trips and should be practiced at all times during the trip to avoid injuries.

A GOAL-SPECIFIC MOUNTAINEERING PROGRAM

Make sure your goal is both realistic and that you have enough time to achieve it. For significant aerobic activity goals such as climbing a very high mountain, approximately 5–6 training days a week for 10–12 weeks is usually necessary. Remember that it takes a certain amount of time for physiological adaptation to take place in your cardiovascular, respiratory, and musculoskeletal systems.

Devote approximately 90–120 minutes to strength and balance training per week (with 2 sessions per week).

Break up your available training time by quarters into the aerobic training levels listed below. The percentages listed are related to your in-city aerobic training time. In addition, do a general strength-training program 2 days per week. One day a week, do a hike of gradually increasing distance and elevation gain.

Within 10–12 weeks of your first climb, start increasing the duration of 2 of your in-town aerobic sessions from 30 minutes to 50 minutes (by 2 minutes each session).

Within 3–4 weeks of a major climb, try stair climbing with a pack on (on a machine or on stairs). Revolving climbing walls are good for cross training. Your intensity on these activities should be in a range of 60%–85% maximum heart rate (max HR). Add interval training to your program if you are healthy (see chapter 2). You can do this with intervals of 15–240 seconds on a stair-climber, on stairs, during running, or while on your training hikes as in Fartlek training.

Within 8–12 weeks of your first mountaineering trip, start your longer, lower-intensity day trips with a hike or, if there is too much snow, a snowshoe or cross-country ski trip. Start with a round trip of 4–6 miles and a 2,000- to 2,500-foot elevation gain. Gradually work your way up each week in length and elevation gain. Within 4 weeks choose trips with steep and difficult terrain, and with some snow if possible. Gradually increase the weight in your pack as you get closer to your climb. Try to have finished a 1-day trip (and ideally a 2-day trip) of at least 8 hours of difficult hiking with a heavy pack, with some snow and with at least 4,000 feet elevation gain before you attempt your mountaineering climb. Remember that altitude problems can result if you are training above 8,000 feet (see chapter 1 and additional altitude references in Selected References).

Below is a sample training program based on a heart-rate training zone approach as presented in chapter 2. This is just one example of a training program. You can achieve a reasonable level of fitness without doing the interval training outlined below. The main difference may be that you perceive less stamina when brief spurts of high intensity are required on steep or challenging sections of your climb.

A SAMPLE WEEKLY PLAN FOR HEART-RATE ZONE TRAINING

Total planned aerobic training time is 5 hours a week in the city and 1 long day of increasing duration (4–8 hours) in an outdoor setting. Spend 45–60 minutes 2 times per week in strength and balance training.

For example, when you are in the increasing endurance level (second month), the amount of

time you spend per week is:

20% = 60 minutes in zones 1 and 2
70% = 210 minutes in zone 3
10% = 30 minutes in zone 4

Log your activities to keep on track. An example of a week in the increasing endurance level:

Monday: 8-minute warm-up and 4-minute cool-down (zone 1, 2); 50 minutes (zone 3) preferably on a stair-climber. Strength and balance training 30–45 minutes.

Tuesday: 8-minute warm-up; 30 minutes interval training on the treadmill (50% in zone 4, 50% in zone 3), 4-minute cool-down.

Wednesday: Same as Monday, or substitute another specific aerobic activity.

Thursday: 8-minute warm-up and 30 minutes of intervals, 4-minute cool-down.

Friday: 30 minutes (zone 3) cross training. Strength training 30–45 minutes.

Saturday: Hike in the mountains (including snow walking as the season and weather permit), carry a pack of gradually increasing weight, and gradually increase the distance, slope, and elevation gain to simulate the climb (zones 1, 2). A few weeks before the climb, you should be up to an 8- to 12-mile hike with 4,000 feet elevation gain if possible. If you do not live in an area where this is possible, spend extended periods of time doing stair running and climbing in a tall building and outside.

Sunday: Same as Monday, except omit strength training.

This schedule can be altered in the third training month by increasing interval training as well as the difficulty of your strength training. At this stage you would add some strength sets of higher resistance, lower reps, and some hops and jumps for power.

Plan a reduced volume of training 1 week before your event so your body can rest and not be overtaxed before your climb. The day before should either be without exercise or no more than light activity.

SNOWBOARD- AND SKI-SPECIFIC CONDITIONING
Alpine, Telemark, Cross-Country, and Skate Skiing

BY CARL PETERSON, P.T., RICH HARRINGTON, AND MARK PIERCE, A.T.C.

▶ **THIS CHAPTER WILL HELP YOU:**
- Ski an 8-mile cross-country course with some elevation gain.
- Telemark a course with 3,000-foot elevation gain and loss.
- Ski a full day of advanced alpine skiing.
- Snowboard a moderately difficult slope.

All snowboard and skiing activities are demanding sports that require some form of pre-season preparation and training in all areas of fitness. Adequate pre-activity preparation not only enhances your enjoyment and performance but minimizes the risk of injury.

MUSCULOSKELETAL DEMANDS
The musculoskeletal demands for skiing and snowboarding are very similar. Your lower body, abdominals, and back muscles are required to initially decelerate your body against gravity and the terrain to prevent falling. The velocities are high in downhill skiing and snowboarding, requiring very rapid muscular contractions in squatting, lunging, and jumping motions.

Next, these muscles are required to accelerate your body in a chosen direction or pattern of movement. These musculoskeletal demands occur simultaneously in three planes of motion (see chapter 5 for a description of the planes of motion). Alpine, cross-country, and telemark skiing are sagittal plane (forward progression or

movement)–dominant sports. When moving in a forward direction, your muscles are required to control joint motion continuously in the other two planes. Skiers may want to pay more attention to the sagittal (forward) and transverse (rotational) planes.

The same applies to snowboarding; however, the dominant plane of motion is the frontal plane (sideways). While progressing in a relative forward direction, the transverse plane (rotation) becomes very important for changes in direction. Snowboarders should emphasize exercise in the frontal (side-to-side) and transverse (rotational) planes.

MUSCLE IMBALANCES
Common muscle imbalances that emerge in skiing and snowboarding are weak gluteals, adductors (including the medial quadriceps), abdominals, hamstrings, and interscapular muscles opposed by the typically stronger and tighter quadriceps, hip flexors, iliotibial band, heel cord, and upper chest muscles. If these

imbalances are not corrected they can contribute to numerous snow-sport injuries.

WARM-UP

A morning warm-up should be done prior to hitting the slopes or trails. In cold conditions it is vital. A proper warm-up prepares your muscles for skiing and snowboarding and also prepares your joints for movement and stability. Start slowly, and progressively increase the intensity of your warm-up. By using ski-specific activities, you will help improve the coordination of your muscles and joints, leading to more efficient movement and performance.

A dynamic warm-up can include an agility drill and is important before performing agility circuits or your snow activity. The Dynamic Warm-up in chapter 4, Warm-up and Stretching, could be used as your core dynamic warm-up prior to activity. Modify this routine depending on the safety of the surface available, or include one or two other functional exercises specific to your sport. Other dynamic warm-ups are listed below.

DYNAMIC WARM-UP 1

This is an easy, quick warm-up before exercise or an activity. It is appropriate for cross-country skiing or any other activity on a cold day. Start with a skipping routine or a light 5-minute jog. Then perform the Dynamic Warm-up exercises and Exercises 7 and 25.

DYNAMIC WARM-UP 2

This is appropriate for snowboarders and downhill and telemark skiers.

Do 5 fast hops to your right with your left leg; 5 fast hops to your left with your right leg; 5 vertical jumps; 10 walking lunges; 5 fast hops at 45 degrees to the right with your left leg; 5 fast hops at 45 degrees to the left with your right leg; and 5 continuous jumps—long-high-long-high.

STRETCHING

Flexibility is important for technique and minimizing injury potential. You need to be able to bend your knees at least into a half squat and to extend your hips. Ankle flexibility is important for all snow activities.

AEROBIC CONDITIONING

Aerobic and anaerobic conditioning are both important for snowboarding and skiing. Aerobic conditioning is important for telemark, cross-country, and skate skiing. Anaerobic conditioning is important for brief spurts of high-intensity effort such as climbing a hill, skiing a mogul field, or cross-country sprinting.

STRENGTH TRAINING

Strength and power enable you to negotiate turns and terrain. Plan your strength training for each body region 2 times per week. Incorporate your agility and balance training (see below) 2 times a week within 6–8 weeks of your activity season.

Skiing and snowboarding require significant abdominal and lower body strength. The chest, shoulders, and arms are most used in telemark, skate, and cross-country skiing. They are also used in snowboarding for balance and catching falls. Some exercises should be done on slopes, outdoors on a downhill or traverse pitch, to simulate actual conditions.

Torso (core) strength is very important in skiing and snowboarding. Do the majority of your leg, thigh, and abdominal exercises on your feet so that strength gains will mimic the demands of your activity. Standing positions allow you to perform rotational or side-to-side challenges with your torso and use your abdominal muscles as controllers of motion. Just doing an abdominal crunch will not prepare your abdominal muscles for skiing or snowboarding.

BALANCE AND AGILITY

Moving dynamic balance is critical for snowboarding and all types of skiing, which require a high level of agility, balance, and coordination. Agility is the ability to move quickly and change your body position in a coordinated, controlled fashion. Dynamic balance improves your ability to control rapid changes in direction and adapt to changing snow conditions and terrain. The agility circuits at the end of this chapter are designed to improve your moving dynamic balance.

You can use machines to develop speed and balance. The "fitter" (see the balance exercises at the end of this chapter) is a standing balance machine best for training for snowboarding and downhill skiing with a rapid side-to-side challenge.

See Figure 28 for a brief look at the training components of snowboarding and each type of skiing.

CONDITIONING FOR ALPINE (DOWNHILL) SKIING

DYNAMIC WARM-UP

Perform 5 minutes of walking, skipping, or jogging; then do the Dynamic Warm-up exercises in chapter 4, and add all or part of Dynamic Warm-up 2, above.

STRETCHING

Adequate hip, knee, and ankle mobility is required to attain a full squat position. Try Exercises 1–10. For your upper body do Exercises 21, 30, and 33.

AEROBIC CONDITIONING

Do any continuous standing aerobic activity of 30 minutes or more, including step aerobics and/or "slide" activities. Other aerobic activities are running, using a stair-climber, and using cross-country ski machines.

ANAEROBIC CONDITIONING

Do short intervals of a higher intensity. A ski training device ("the fitter") can be used for interval training. Hopping or jumping on a slope can also be an alternative; see Exercises 49, 50, 75, and 76.

STRENGTH TRAINING

Beginning
Upper body: Exercises 22, 85, 98, and 104.
Abdominals: Exercises 58.1, 62, and 63.
Lower body: Exercises 25, 26, 27, 40, 70, and 72.

Intermediate
Upper body: Exercises 21, 22, 25, 95, 98, 103, and 104.
Abdominals: Exercises 59, 61, 62, and 63.
Lower body: Exercises 25, 26, 38, 40, 70, 72, 72.3, 72.4, 72.7, 75, 96, 104, and 106.

Advanced
Upper body: Exercises 21, 22, 25, 98, 101, 103, and 104.
Abdominals: Exercises 60, 64, 65, 66, and 68.

FIGURE 28. TRAINING COMPONENTS

	FLEXIBILITY	ANAEROBIC STAMINA	AEROBIC STAMINA	STRENGTH	AGILITY & BALANCE
Alpine	med	high	low	high	med-high
Telemark	high	med-high	med-high	high	med-high
Cross-Country	med	low	high	low-med	low-med
Skate Skiing	high	high	high	med	low-med
Snowboarding	high	high	low	high	high

Lower body: Exercises 28, 39.4, 49, 70, 72, 72.3, 72.4, 72.7, 75.3, 100, and 106.

SPEED/POWER

For alpine skiing, you need to be able to hop repeatedly, side to side, for 30 seconds to 2 minutes.

Beginning: Exercises 75.1, 75.4, 75.5, 75.6, and 75.7.

Intermediate/Advanced: Exercises 75.1, 75.7, 128, 130, 132, 134, 135 or 136, and 137.

BALANCE AND AGILITY

Beginning: Exercise 124.

Intermediate: Exercise 124. Include abdominal challenge stations such as Exercises 58 and 62.

Advanced: Exercises 124, 136, and 137. Have a downhill component with some traverse sections if available.

CONDITIONING FOR SNOWBOARDING
DYNAMIC WARM-UP

Perform 5 minutes of walking, skipping, or jogging; then do the Dynamic Warm-up exercises in chapter 4 and add all or part of the dynamic warm-up.

STRETCHING

Adequate flexibility and mobility of your legs and hips is necessary for snowboarding in order to assume a prolonged and balanced "squat" position. To improve your flexibility in these areas try exercises 110 and 21.

AEROBIC CONDITIONING

Any continuous standing activity of 30 minutes or more that allows you to maintain your target heart rate (see chapter 2) is recommended. Step aerobics as well as the use of a slide board, stair-climber, or treadmill are all aerobic conditioning activities suitable for snowboarding.

STRENGTH TRAINING
Beginning

Upper body: Exercises 82, 102, and 104.
Abdominals: Exercises 58 or 59, 61, and 63.
Lower body: Exercises 24, 27, 36, 38, 70.1, and 104.2.

Intermediate

Upper body: Exercises 100, 101, 102, 104, and 106.
Abdominals: Exercises 58, 59, 61, 62, and 63.
Lower body: Exercises 24, 27, 30, 37.3, 37.4, 40, 70.2, 70.3, 72, 72.3, 72.4, 72.7, 75, 75.4a, 96, 104, and 106.

Advanced

Upper body: Exercises 75.4b and 75.4c.
Abdominals: Exercises 60, 64, 65, 66, and 68.
Lower body: Exercises 26, 27, 30.1, 49, 70, 72, 72.4, 75.3, 75.4d, 100, 101.4, 102, 104, and 106.

BALANCE AND AGILITY

Beginning: See Exercise 125, Snowboard Circuit, and build yourself a 6- to 10-station circuit that includes Exercises 39, 40, 59, 122, and 127. Perform each exercise for 20–30 seconds then jog, skip, or hop to the next station.

Intermediate/Advanced: See Exercise 125, snowboard circuit, and build an 8- to 12-station circuit that includes Exercises 39, 40, 59, 75.5, 75.6, 76.2, 76.4, 122, 127, and 128. Perform each exercise for 20–30 seconds then jog, skip, or hop to the next station.

CONDITIONING FOR TELEMARK SKIING
DYNAMIC WARM-UP

Perform 5 minutes of walking, skipping, or jogging; then do the Dynamic Warm-up exercises in chapter 4 and Exercise 24 as a walking lunge.

STRETCHING

Adequate hip, knee, and ankle mobility are needed to be able to attain a full squat and split squat or lunge position. Do the stretches listed for alpine skiing, above, but also do Exercises 3, 6, and 8–10 and spend extra time on the adductor and achilles stretches.

AEROBIC CONDITIONING

Do any continuous activity for 30–40 minutes. If you are planning to do backcountry touring, train to sustain your activity for a period of up to 2–3 hours at an intensity zone of 50%–70% maximum heart rate (max HR). Do a low-intensity, longer-duration (LILD) day and gradually increase the duration and slope to approximate two-thirds to three-fourths of your expected telemark trip. The best activities would be using a cross-country ski machine with a sloped angle, in-line skating, doing an uphill run or treadmill workout, using a stair-climber (especially the revolving stairs), using the Precor EFX elliptical machine, and using the slide board. Outside, snowshoeing and regular cross-country skiing are also excellent alternatives.

ANAEROBIC CONDITIONING

Do repeated bursts of activity for 20 seconds–3 minutes. Do intervals in the 80%–100% max HR range.

STRENGTH TRAINING

Telemark turns require you to be in a modified lunge position, which exerts a significant amount of internal force on the forward leg. This requires significant strength of the ankle, quad, hamstring, groin, hip, abdominal, and buttock muscles. This force can be simulated with rotational lunges in which a weight is brought toward the front leg and across the midline of your body. Doing these on a hill, in a traverse, or on a downhill pitch is helpful. Start slowly and then increase the speed.

Beginning
Upper body: Exercises 21, 22, 25, and 104.

Abdominals: Exercises 58, 59, and 61.
Lower body: Exercise 25–27, 70, and 72.

Intermediate
Upper body: Exercises 21, 22, 25, 34, 95, 99, 103, and 104.
Abdominals: Exercises 58, 59, 61, and 62.
Lower body: Exercise 25, 26, 34, 38, 39.3, 96, 104, and 106.

Advanced
Upper body: Exercises 21, 22, 25, 34, 99, 100, 101, 103, and 104.
Abdominals: Exercises 60, 64–66, and 68.
Lower body: Exercises 26, 28, 34, 38, 39, 48, and 106.

SPEED/POWER

You need to be able to do fast rotational or side-to-side lunges (mimicking telemark turns) for 30 seconds. Do Exercises 130, 133, 135, and 136.

BALANCE AND AGILITY

You must have adequate balance and coordination to allow total body control with rapid changes of direction over rough terrain.

Beginning/Intermediate: Do Exercise 126, telemark circuit, with the following modifications: Omit Exercises 27, 37.4, and 38.3.

Advanced: Do Exercise 126, telemark circuit.

CONDITIONING FOR CROSS-COUNTRY SKIING

DYNAMIC WARM-UP

Do Exercise 141.

STRETCHING

You need adequate hip, knee, and ankle mobility to be able to attain a stride lunge position. Pay special attention to Exercises 3, 4, and 6–8.

AEROBIC CONDITIONING

You must be able to perform continuous activity for 2–3 hours at 50%–70% max HR. Some work on an uphill slope is important if you wish to climb hills. Performing side stepping and V-shaped uphill walking or lunges can help your uphill abilities. Increase your aerobic duration each week. Good activities are a cross-country ski machine, especially with some time spent going up a slope, a slide routine, or in-line skating. Alternatives are any standing aerobic activity such as hiking, snowshoeing, or running on a hill. Your routines should be 30–50 minutes long with some cross training to prevent overuse injuries. If you intend to race, perform some ski interval training (see Fartlek interval training in chapter 2). Your low-intensity, longer-duration (LILD) activities should ideally start on a weekly basis 4–6 weeks before your first full day of skiing.

ANAEROBIC CONDITIONING

You must be able to perform occasional bursts of activity for 20 seconds. If you wish to enhance your anaerobic abilities, do some interval training.

STRENGTH TRAINING

Do continuous weight-bearing exercises repeated on either both or a single leg for 20–30 reps. Do the skate-ski strength and balance programs, below.

Beginning
Upper body: Exercises 21, 52, 97, and 98.
Abdominals: Exercises 58 and 62.
Lower body: Exercises 25, 70, and 72.

Intermediate/Advanced
Upper body: Exercises 21, 25, 34, 91, 98, 103, 104, and 107.
   Abdominals: Exercises 59, 60, and 62–64.
   Lower body: Exercises 24, 26, 28, 34, 76, 76.2, 89, and 106.

SPEED

You should be able to accelerate on an uphill grade.

BALANCE AND AGILITY

Beginning/Intermediate: Make a cross-country obstacle course. You can do fast walking or running, and make quick turns (or do Exercise 24) between obstacles that simulate the distance between turns. Incorporate lunge stations in Exercise 72.5 and step-up stations as in Exercise 73. Use abdominal challenge stations such as in Exercises 58 and 62. Incorporate balance stations such as in Exercises 37.1, 37.2, 38.1, and 40. Link stations with a fast walk, a run, the Dynamic Warm-up exercises in chapter 4 or do Dynamic Warm-up 2 earlier in this chapter. You can add a daypack and speed up the pace to make it more challenging.

Advanced: Do Exercise 126, telemark circuit, with the following modifications: Omit Exercises 27, 37.4, 38.3, and 76.

CONDITIONING FOR SKATE-SKIING
DYNAMIC WARM-UP

Perform Exercise 141 along with Exercise 76.2.

STRETCHING

Perform all of the stretches for cross-country skiing, above, especially Exercises 7 and 8.

ANAEROBIC/AEROBIC CONDITIONING

Using slide boards or cross-country ski machines, or running, are the most sport-specific activities. Make two of your off-snow (gym) sessions last 40–50 minutes. Incorporate 5- to 10-minute intervals of slide board training at the beginning and end of your aerobic session. Consider doing some aerobic and anaerobic intervals 2 times per week within 6 weeks of the ski season (see chapter 2).

STRENGTH TRAINING

This is similar to the program for cross-country skiing, above, with extra work needed for your groin and hip muscles. Skate-skiers should work up to the cross-country advanced program for strength, and add the exercises listed under the advanced program for strength, below.

Beginning
Upper body: Exercise 21, 52, 82, 97, and 98.

Abdominals: Exercises 58 and 62.
Lower body: Exercise 25, 40, 70, and 72.

Intermediate/Advanced
Upper body: Exercises 21, 25, 34, 89.2, 91, 98, 102, 103, 104, and 107.
  Abdominals: Exercises 59–62.
  Lower body: Exercises 26–28, 70.2, 72.3, 76.2, 76.5 (uphill hopping), 106, 122, 130, and 139.

EXERCISES

If you are planning to alpine ski, telemark ski, or snowboard, consider adding agility and balance drills to your routine within 6 weeks of your first trip. It is important to have a good aerobic and strength base before adding agility circuits. If you are planning on only cross-country skiing, fine-tune your stamina and strength, and then add balance activities when time permits.

Try to sequence your training and do your agility and coordination drills prior to other types of training, to derive optimum benefit. Also include some agility work as part of your warm-up or during a Fartlek interval aerobic session. In designing balance and agility circuits, make use of natural obstacles for balance and coordination, such as balancing on or jumping back and forth over logs, steps, rocks, or snow slopes.

SNOW ACTIVITY–SPECIFIC BALANCE EXERCISES

121 Balance Boards

Equipment: Balance board.
Purpose: Improve your ability to balance side to side.
Technique: There are two varieties of ski balance boards. The basic board is a flat surface with a track that sits in a groove on a roller. The side-to-side rocking motion develops awareness of your body position during motion. The more advanced board has an elevated platform, and the ends of the roller are beveled to allow rocking forward and back, as on a snowboard. As you get comfortable with the

balance required, increase the difficulty by holding a tuck position, balancing on one foot, or adding a pack. You can also do this with ski poles to provide added stability.

122 Shuffle Lunge with Reach

Equipment: None.
Purpose: Improve your ability to balance and recover from a side-to-side and rotational challenge.
Technique: Perform a lateral lunge step to the right, with a left arm reach, as in Exercise 139.1. After reaching in one direction, sidestep to the left for a couple steps, moving back into a lateral lunge, and reach across your body with the right hand at knee height. For lateral lunge technique, see chapter 11.

123 "The Fitter Machine"

Equipment: Fitter machine, ski poles.
Purpose: Develop your balance and coordination during side-to-side motions used in snowboarding and alpine skiing.
Technique: While holding your ski poles (or two 4-foot lengths of doweling), stand on the fitter platform. This platform is very wobbly, so allow your knees to slightly bend and find a secure, balanced position. Once you feel balanced, slowly shift your weight to either the right or the left. The stance platform will yield and move sideways in the direction you choose. When you have reached the end point of your initial side, shift your weight and balance while you travel across the fitter in the opposite direction. This exercise simulates the gliding motion common to alpine skiing. Snowboarders should assume a foot position similar to what you use on your snowboard. The fitter can be adjusted with changes in resistance by changing the variable-tension cords on the rollers on the undersurface of the machine.

AGILITY EXERCISES AND CIRCUITS

You can practice dynamic moving balance and coordination by creating your own agility obstacle course with cones, poles, trees, balls, and other objects. Place 8–12 obstacles 10–20 feet apart in a Z-shaped pattern to simulate ski or snowboard turns. In an alpine skier or snowboarder course, your stations should be close enough to require you to react quickly from one station to the next. Jog or run between the obstacles. When you reach an obstacle, make a quick change in direction and proceed to the next obstacle. This direction change can proceed from a beginning level of a running cut to more advanced jumps and hops. This will improve your ability to make quick changes in body position.

In ski and snowboard agility and balance circuits, you can work through 8–12 stations (with one station being the obstacle course) 1–2 times. Work hard for 30–45 seconds at each station, then move to the next station. If you are in a gym and are unable to do an obstacle course, perform the balance exercises as indicated.

124 | Alpine Ski Circuit

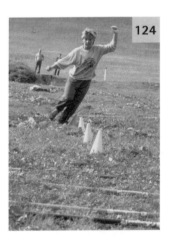

124

Equipment: Circuit of 8–12 stations, including obstacle course; have a downhill component with some traverse sections if available.
Purpose: Improve your agility and ability to react to changes in direction and various degrees of terrain.
Technique: Include stations such as Exercises 127, 128, 130, and 132. For other stations, use Exercise 122 as well as Exercises 37–40. Use a walking lunge (Exercises 72.4 and 72.5) on a slope if available. See photo 124 for an example of a downhill or snowboard agility course.

125 | Snowboard Circuit

Equipment: Circuit with poles, rope, and steps marking areas for jumping drills.
Purpose: Improve your ability to meet the various sudden directional challenges of snowboarding.
Technique: Jump in patterns to simulate snowboarding. Try putting some of the circuit stations on uneven surfaces such as steps, hills, snowpiles, and logs if your circuit is outside, and on steps or platforms if indoors. Include stations with lateral shuffles (Exercise 122), lateral hopping (76.2), and rotational jumps of 90–180 degrees (75.4). Consider jumping Exercises 136 and 137.

126 Telemark Circuit

Equipment: Telemark agility course with stations and an obstacle course.

Purpose: Improve your ability to change directions and meet the physical demands of telemark skiing.

Technique: You can do fast walking or running and make quick turns between stations. Consider performing Exercise 24 on a downhill obstacle course. When you have reached your obstacle, perform the telemark lunge, then quickly jump into an inward quarter turn and proceed to the next obstacle, simulating the distance between telemark turns. Incorporate lunge stations (Exercise 72.5), hop stations (Exercise 76 and 76.1), and step-up stations (Exercise 74). Use abdominal challenge stations such as Exercises 58 and 62. Incorporate balance stations such as Exercises 27, 37.1–37.4, 38.1–38.3, and 40. Link stations with a fast walk, a run, the Dynamic Warm-up exercises in chapter 4, or Dynamic Warm-up 2 earlier in this chapter. You can add a daypack and speed up the pace to make it more challenging.

RUNNING AGILITY CIRCUITS

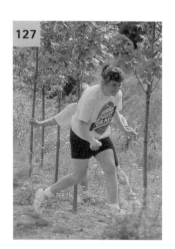

127 Pole-running Agility Circuit

Equipment: Ski or garden poles, gentle hill.

Purpose: Develop your lateral agility.

Technique: Set up ski or garden poles along a gentle hill, traverse, or downhill course. Position your poles closely enough so that you have to make quick changes in direction as you run through the course. (Always face forward.)

128 | The "Z" Agility Course

Equipment: Cones or markers.

Purpose: Improve your ability to decelerate and change directions while improving your anaerobic strength.

Technique: Arrange cones or markers as shown in illustration 128, placing a cone at the end of each arrow. If you have a workout partner, use a stopwatch to time each other. On "Go," sprint from point A to point B and quickly change directions, then proceed on to the next cone.

Variations: 128.1. When you reach each cone, perform a jump turn, then proceed on to the next cone. 128.2. Reach across your body and touch the base of the cone with your opposite-side hand. Always face front. This simulates a body position similar to skiing. Set as many cones as you would like. Complete two trials and record your best time.

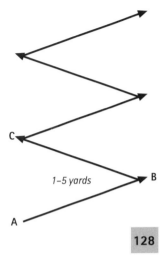

1–5 yards

128

PLYOMETRIC (POWER) EXERCISES (HOPPING AND JUMPING)

Plyometrics train your muscles to reach maximal force in the shortest time possible. Plyometrics are useful for sports that require explosive power, including high-level downhill skiing, snowboarding, and telemark skiing. The U.S. Ski Team uses plyometrics for both pre-season training and in-season maintenance. Level A is easier than Level B.

Level A

Progression of hops and jumps should follow the rules of easy-to-hard and simple-to-complex. These exercises are most appropriate for downhill skiers, snowboarders, and telemark skiers. Please review the basic technique of hops and jumps in Exercises 75 and 76.

129 | Dynamic Jumping Warm-up 1

Equipment: None.

Purpose: Try this before hopping and jumping routines.

Technique: Do an easy 10-minute running warm-up. Next, stretch your torso (Exercise 21 without dumbbells), shoulders (Exercise 14), and legs, particularly the groin and Achilles tendon (Exercises 1, 3, 6–8, and 10). Next perform some agility drills for 5 minutes at half to three-fourths speed (the Dynamic Warm-up exercises in chapter 4).

130 45-degree Hopping

Equipment: None.
Purpose: Improve your ability to push off of one leg.
Technique: Push off from your right foot, moving diagonally forward at a 45-degree angle, land on your left foot, and rapidly contract to push off to land on your right foot. Do 15–20 hops.

131 Simulated Ski Turns

Equipment: None.
Purpose: Practice ski turns during the pre-season.
Technique: Do quick jumping on a downhill slope (a park or snow-field) and simulate your ski style in regards to height and frequency of turns. Within 6 weeks of your first downhill trip, start this training with a few jumps and gradually progress to 20 linked jumps. If your knees hurt, perform these exercises on a level surface and take a shallower jump.

132 Slalom Jumps

Equipment: Rope.
Purpose: Simulate skiing downhill or snowboarding while connecting multiple turns.
Technique: Lay a rope down a slope that is long enough so that you can do 10–20 jumps. Practice a few jumps, then jump side to side over the rope as if you were connecting multiple turns.

Level B

The Level A workout may be adequate for most beginners. The following are intermediate and more advanced exercises.

133 Dynamic Jumping Warm-up 2

Equipment: None.
Purpose: Prepare your muscles and joints to accept increasing loads.
Technique: Do the Dynamic Warm-up exercises in chapter 4. Then do some running drills (forward sprints), and progress to dynamic

flexibility exercises such as Exercises 7 and 10; then add some lunge walks (72.5). After this warm-up, add diagonal hops and progressive power jumps, Exercise 135, or telemark jumps, Exercise 134.

134 Telemark Jump

Equipment: None.
Purpose: Condition your legs and improve your coordination for telemark skiing.
Technique: From the lunge position, jump up and bring the opposite leg forward. This is excellent training for telemark skiing. Work your way up to 10–15 reps.

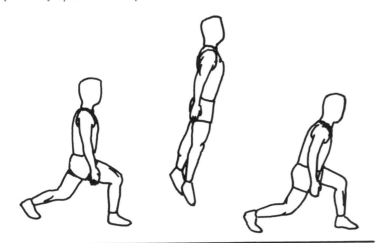

134

135 Progressive Power Jumps

Equipment: Smooth grass or dirt surface or gym floor.
Purpose: Strengthen your legs and gluteals to accelerate out of a turn and increase your vertical leap.
Technique: Do 3 sets of regular, vertical, or rotational jumps (Exercise 75 or 75.1, or 75.4 for snowboarders) First do 3 at 30% maximum height, then do 3 at 60% maximum height, and end with 3 at 90% maximum height. Be careful and progress gradually with these.

136   Single-leg Lateral Jumps

Equipment: Smooth grass or dirt surface or gym floor.
Purpose: Snowboarders and alpine skiers.
Technique: Jump high and far to your right, recover to ski or snowboarder position, then push off your right foot and jump high and far to your left. Repeat this maneuver for 4–6 times in each direction.

137   Crossover Bench Jumps

Equipment: Sturdy bench or wooden box.
Purpose: Closely approximate the side-to-side requirements of skiing or snowboarding.
Technique: Position yourself to the left side of a box or platform and place your right foot on the box. Push off with your right foot (assisting with your left foot) and jump up for maximum height, moving sideways. End up with your left foot on the box and your right foot on the ground. Repeat to the opposite direction as soon as your outside foot touches the ground. Do 8–10 jumps to each side.

137

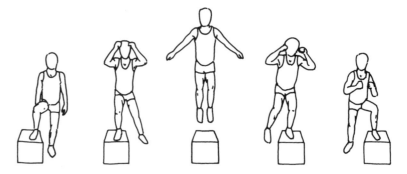

138   The Hex Circuit

Equipment: 3 hurdles 8 inches high; 1 each of hurdles 10 inches, 12 inches, and 14 inches high.
Purpose: Improve coordination, strength, and agility to make lateral movements with precise foot placement.

Technique: You can make the hurdles from 1½-inch-diameter PVC pipe and elbows available at hardware stores (138a). Hurdles can also be purchased from athletic equipment suppliers. Set up the six hurdles in the pattern shown in illustration 138b. Begin inside the Hex. On "Go," jump to the outside laterally over the first 8-inch hurdle, then immediately back into the center of the Hex. Continue around clockwise, jumping out of the Hex and back in until you have completed all six hurdles. Turn around and return counterclockwise without stopping.

Variations: 138.1. Set up the hurdles in a spoke pattern. Jump over the hurdles, either facing toward or away from the hub. Move clockwise and counterclockwise. 138.2. Hop on one leg and have your training partner call out when to switch legs or directions. 138.3. If you have a beach or playground with loose sand available, do the Hex and hurdle variations on sand. This requires more power, and teaches you awareness of your foot and ankle position.

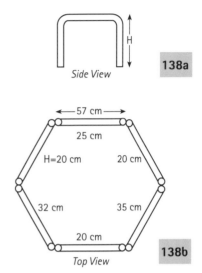

Side View **138a**

Top View **138b**

LOWER-BODY ANAEROBIC POWER (SPEED) EXERCISES

The following drills can be used separately or in conjunction with the jumping routines above to add interval training and power to your workout.

139 | Acceleration Sprints

Equipment: Field or gymnasium.

Purpose: Prepare your musculoskeletal system and coordination centers for sustained quick movements.

Technique: This is a forward sprint. Start with two 30-meter runs at 65% maximum speed. Then progress to one 30-meter sprint at 80% of your maximum speed by the 30-meter mark. Progress to two 30-meter sprints at 85% of your maximum speed and then three sprints at 90% of your maximum speed.

Precautions: Slow down gradually to avoid excessive strain on your knees. You must be in excellent aerobic shape and meet the interval requirements in chapter 2, Aerobic Conditioning and Interval Training, to do this.

140 Slide Boards

Equipment: Smooth surface, fabric shoe covers.
Purpose: Develop both endurance and power in lateral movement patterns. This is very useful in the skating technique of Nordic skiing, giant slalom racing, and any sport requiring lateral agility and power.
Technique: Slide to the right. When you reach a barrier, reach across your body with your left hand at knee height, approximately 1 foot past your body. Repeat this to the left. For strength training, perform this exercise for 45 seconds–1 minute at a higher intensity. For aerobic training, do it for 5–15 minutes at lower intensities.

141 Tuck Drills

Equipment: None.
Purpose: Train your muscles and joints to accept quick and constant loads in a tuck position, common to skiing.
Technique: Assume a low tuck position as used in downhill ski racing. Position your back parallel to floor, arms forward, eyes looking ahead. Hop up and down as fast as possible, with your feet clearing the floor by at least 3 inches. Try to keep your body parallel to the floor, and build up to 2 minutes.
Variation: 141.1. From the low tuck position, step to the right, bring your left leg in next to your right leg, and immediately spring straight up for maximum height as in rebounding a basketball; then drop back to the low tuck and step to the left. Repeat for 10 reps on each side.

Conditioning for Canoeing, Kayaking, and Rowing

BY SHERRI CASSUTO, CERTIFIED ROLFER,® AND DAN NELSON, D.C.

▶ **THIS CHAPTER WILL HELP YOU:**
- Become aware of the basic muscle groups used in propelling boats.
- Understand the musculoskeletal demands of these boating activities.
- Identify areas of the body that commonly exhibit muscle imbalances.
- Be aware of areas of the body that are susceptible to injury.
- Be able to implement appropriate water- and land-based training methods for each sport.

Human-propelled oar and paddle craft rely on an unstable and constantly shifting surface (the hull) from which to exert a driving force through the face of the paddle/oar blade to the water. There is no real substitute for time on the water in variable conditions. This book assumes that you either have the necessary skill base and are preparing for your season, or you are enrolled in a skill development course. This is especially important for whitewater boating and sea kayaking. This chapter includes suggestions for both water-based and land-based training to help improve your performance and reduce the likelihood of injury. Training information is designed for the recreational boater, although the stretching, agility, and resistance training programs are also applicable to racers.

MUSCULOSKELETAL DEMANDS

Canoeing, kayaking, and rowing are total body exercises. All involve translation of power from the feet/knees through the body and hands to the paddle/oar. All involve significant load to the muscles of the back, torso, shoulders, and arms.

In canoeing and kayaking, the legs provide a stable connection to the boat, and are used to initiate the stroke and rotation of the pelvis and torso. Sidebending of the spine is a necessary and integral part of paddle sports, because hull placement in the water is variable. The torso is used as a lever both in a front-to-back and a side-to-side plane, with all intermediate positions possible.

In rowing, the use of the legs is more propulsive and the torso undergoes very little sidebending. The torso is primarily used as a lever in a front-to-back plane of motion. The rowing shell is designed to ride on a stable hull surface. Sweep rowing involves some rotation.

BACK POSITION

A proper neutral low-back position can be achieved by putting your low back through a range of motion from full extension to full flexion, as outlined in Exercise 43, Sitting Arcing. This neutral position is just slightly off full extension. You can practice it by pushing upon the boat slightly to unweight your spine. Finding your neutral position intermittently throughout the day is important to protect your low back from excessive strain.

If you have very tight hamstrings, stretching them is necessary to enable you to sit in the boat with your spine in good position, avoiding the compensation of excessively flexing (or forward slumping) your low back. You need to be able to tolerate sitting in this position for at least 3–4 hours consecutively to be able to tolerate a full day of boating. For rowing, the same flexibility requirements are necessary for less time on the water.

Rounding of the midback or excessive forward head and neck positions can lead to shoulder fatigue and injury as well as neck pain. Accomplishing the stroke by excessive use of the upper trapezius instead of allowing the shoulder to drop, relax, and reach forward also leads to neck pain.

MUSCLE IMBALANCES

The following recommendations are for the average recreational boater. If you have been very active in your sport over a number of years, it is likely that your body has changed to accommodate it. The major muscle groups used repetitively will become hypertrophied compared to the rest of your body. For this reason, strength training should be used to have a general and balanced effect. As your body becomes adapted to your sport, the goal of strength training shifts to create more balance in the underdeveloped body regions. Boaters involved in asymmetrical sports (whitewater canoeing and sweep rowing) will find themselves more developed on one side than the other. More important is the effect of overdevelopment and repetitive motion on flexibility. As time goes by, continue to evaluate your flexibility.

SHOULDER, CHEST, AND UPPER BACK (UPPER TORSO) REGION

In many individuals the shoulder and upper back muscles are less developed and less coordinated than the muscles of the chest and lower extremity, due to less awareness of the need for a balanced strengthening program. Any or all of these may be poorly conditioned, but a very common pattern is for the chest muscles to be significantly stronger than the upper back. Most shoulder injuries in water sports are the result of relative weakness in the upper back and in the rotator cuff muscles. The prevalence of rib injuries is largely due to muscle imbalances as well as the significant repetitive load experienced in this region. To prepare for these activities, spend time strengthening this region, especially emphasizing the rotator cuff, middle and lower trapezius, serratus anterior, latissimus, teres, and rhomboids (see chapter 15 and the strength recommendations in this chapter for further details on these muscles).

HIP, ABDOMINAL, LOW BACK, AND BUTTOCK (LOWER TORSO) REGION

Another common problem is weakness in the torso stabilizing muscles. These include the abdominal muscles; muscles associated with extension, lateral flexion, and rotation of the back; hip flexors; and muscles associated with the ribs and chest. All boating activities rely heavily on the torso/buttocks/hips region for stability of the boat and placement of the hull. The torso region is used as a lever for transferring force from the powerful lower extremity to the upper extremity and ultimately to the paddle/oar.

WRIST, FOREARM, AND ELBOW REGION

This is a relatively weak link in the musculoskeletal system because most of us do not significantly use these muscles in our daily lives. All water sports use the forearm for strength, endurance, and agility. Keeping this area stretched and limber is extremely important. When it is poorly prepared to absorb the large forces and repetitive motion of paddling or rowing, this region may become susceptible to a variety of forearm/elbow tendon inflammation syndromes and/or carpal-tunnel (nerve) problems.

WARM-UP

You can do all or part of the following warm-up before boating or working out: Do a short aerobic period (5–10 minutes) of fast walking or jogging. Before your on-land training, perform 5–10 minutes on a rowing ergometer. After that, stretch (you can do Exercise 14 with your paddle). Before beginning your paddle do Exercise 18 in the boat in calm water. Include Exercises 19 and 101.1 (push-ups against a wall). Once on the water, begin with 10–15 minutes of paddling at low intensity. Concentrate on form and gradually build intensity, as you feel ready.

STRETCHING

Flexibility of the hamstrings is vital to maintain a safe and effective body position in all three types of boating. In whitewater boating especially, the quadriceps and hip flexors need to be very limber. Other muscles in the lower body benefit from stretching in order to meet the inherent balance challenges in these sports. This can be accomplished by doing stretching

Exercises 1, 2, 3, 5, 6, 8, and 9.

Flexibility in the upper/lower back, chest, and shoulders is important in all of these activities. It becomes especially important for boaters who have been very active in their sport over a number of years. This can be accomplished by doing Exercises 11, 12, 14, 15, 16, 17, and 18.

AEROBIC CONDITIONING

In this chapter, the aerobic training intensities are defined as follows:

Low intensity: Any level of effort below medium intensity.

Medium intensity: 70%–85% maximum heart rate for the duration of the training interval. This type of training is not an all-out sprint, but is a fast enough pace to make you feel like you are working harder than normal.

High Intensity: Above 85% maximum heart rate for the duration of the training interval.

STRENGTH TRAINING

See the strength training programs for the various types of boating, later in this chapter.

BALANCE AND AGILITY
ON THE WATER

Try these training drills for canoe and kayak. For whitewater boating, do drills 1–3 with more sudden, higher-amplitude motions.

1. In a tandem canoe/kayak, have one person make sudden side-to-side movements requiring a bracing response from the other paddler.
2. If the water is warm enough (or you have a wet suit on), have a friend suddenly grab at the sides of the canoe/kayak, requiring a bracing response. If you are a whitewater kayaker, challenge yourself further by having someone straddle your bow or stern while making sudden movements.

3. Using obstacle courses (abrupt turns, etc.) helps develop coordination and balance for sudden changes in attitude of the boat due to outside forces. Set up a course by throwing oranges (or tennis balls, buoys, or life preservers) into the water, creating the obstacles to turn around. Alternatively, make abrupt turns randomly. Random turns can be done in response to a countdown timer or to a friend yelling out, "Turn to the right," etc.
4. Consider canoeing/kayaking a safe distance from motorboat wakes, but paddling through them or riding them at various angles.

ON LAND

It is important to utilize exercises to enhance sitting balance. These are best done within 4–6 weeks of starting your sea kayak or whitewater training. You can expect to spend 5–10 minutes per session twice a week on balance training. Do the following: Exercises 41 and 69. Secondarily, choose from Exercises 34 and 35.

TOURING OR FLATWATER CANOEING

Flatwater canoeing is a repetitive motion that involves rotation and flexion of the torso (initiated with the legs) in concert with pulling of the paddle-side arm and shoulder (and to a much lesser degree, pushing of the opposite side). It is symmetrical in that the paddler switches sides regularly.

The primary propulsive muscles are those of the hips, thighs, torso, and large muscles of the shoulder girdle. The paddler's feet or knees are linked to the boat and provide a base to utilize the power of the lower body. The drive phase of the stroke involves a rotation of the torso, followed by a slight flexion of the elbow, resulting in the draw of the blade against the water. In performance flatwater paddling, the leg on the same side of the paddle extends, initiating the drive. All of these muscles must function as a linked system to yield efficient power. The scapular stabilizer (upper back) and serratus anterior muscles are extremely important in providing a base to transfer the forces from the large torso muscles through the shoulder and arm to the paddle. Significant weakness or imbalance in these chains of muscles may compromise performance and lead to injury. Areas that are particularly susceptible to injury include the back, shoulder, forearm, and wrist.

AEROBIC CONDITIONING

Flatwater canoeing depends on muscular and aerobic endurance. There are occasional periods when high-intensity activity prevails (inclement weather, exposed open-water conditions). Most training should focus on longer sustained efforts at lower to moderate intensities.

On-the-water training should involve variety, with time devoted to both technique training and progressively longer cardiovascular exercise. Most training days on the water should be 45–90 minutes. If you are preparing for an extended trip on exposed water, spend 1 longer water training day per week, gradually building up to a full day of paddling. Occasionally load your boat up with weight to approximate the gear you will be carrying. Try to do some paddling in challenging water conditions. On land, aerobic training could consist of the use of a rowing ergometer (including Exercise 33), cross-country ski machine, aerodyne bike, or swimming.

Interval training can be helpful to improve your general aerobic endurance, as well as to prepare for unexpected high-intensity paddling efforts. Consider starting your interval training after you have established an aerobic base (about 4 weeks into your paddling training). Once a week, work toward moderate-intensity intervals of 10–20 minutes. Return to low-intensity paddling for 1–2 times the duration of the interval. Alternatively, rest only as long as you need to and start the next interval when you feel ready. Try to do 2–3 intervals per interval training session. As your conditioning level improves, the duration of each work interval is increased and the time for rest is decreased. The duration of training should not increase more than 15–25% per week. If a long trip is planned during the season, adjust training to prepare for it. This is done by gradually increasing the duration of low- to moderate-intensity paddling until 4 hours of Fartlek-type paddling is comfortable. When this level is reached, you are ready for a full day of paddling. This can usually be done within 8 weeks of beginning training.

STRENGTH TRAINING

In addition to aerobic training, your time on the land should be a time to work on stretching and strengthening any deficiencies you may have in your musculoskeletal system as appropriate to canoeing. Common areas of strength deficiency include the torso, upper back, (scapular stabilizers), and forearm muscles. Appropriate exercises are rows, lat pulls, biceps curls, triceps extensions, pull-ups, dips, and sitting balance exercises on a gym ball. Several of these exercises should include a trunk rotational component. A basic strength training program can be done twice a week and would include:

Upper body: Exercise 35, 86, 88.4, 89 (with a parallel hand grip), 91, 91.3, 92.1, 95, 96 (done with a parallel grip), 98, 102, and 105. If you will be on a multiday trip doing portages, add Exercises 20 and 93.

Abdominals: Do Exercises 56.1, 56.2, 62, and 67. Add a rotary torso machine exercise if you have access to one in your gym. Alternatively, do Exercise 80.

Lower body: If you will be on a trip involving portages, add squats and lunges to your program: Exercises 24, 26, 70, and 72.

WHITEWATER CANOEING

Whitewater canoeing in anything above Class II water is classically done with the body positioned differently than for flatwater. The boater assumes a kneeling position with both knees apart and braced into the bottom of the boat. This keeps the center of mass lower and adds to hull stability. The sitting balance challenges in whitewater boating are among the most significant of any sitting activity, and the speed demands of intermediate and above levels of whitewater canoeing require that the paddler not switch paddle grip while in a drop. Because of this, more load (often in unexpected and awkward positions) is placed on rotational muscles of the torso as well as shoulder stabilizers. In addition, aggressive use of the hip flexors, quadriceps, gluteus, and hamstrings in concert with rotation of the trunk provides the base to paddle from. Therefore, trunk strength, flexibility, and shoulder stability are primary requirements. Due to the potential for asymmetry in whitewater canoeing as opposed to flatwater, pay particular attention to equal development and flexibility on both sides of the body.

If you are an advanced whitewater canoeist, the strength demands increase, especially due to the addition of rolling and extreme bracing.

AEROBIC CONDITIONING

Whitewater boating is not as demanding aerobically, but is very skill dependent. Spend at least 30 minutes 2 times per week paddling on flat water. On land, aerobic training uses the same equipment suggested for flatwater boating for 30-minute sessions. After 3–4 weeks of base-level aerobic training, add high-intensity intervals (15- to 90-second bursts) once or twice a week. Have some of your aerobic training be interval-free.

STRENGTH TRAINING

Strength training is similar to that for flat water, but should include some advanced strengthening exercises for your upper body to improve bracing strength and to protect against dislocations.

Upper body: Do Exercises 82, 86, 87.1, 88.4, 89 (parallel grip), 90, 91.2. 91.3, 92, 92.1, 94, 95, 96 (parallel grip), 97, 98, 101, 102, 104, 105, 110, and 111. To help simplify this program, choose two from the rowing exercises (89, 90, 102, 104, and 105); choose one from each of the following groups: 94 or 95, 97 or 98, and 82, 86, or 101; and do Exercises 110 and 111. After 6 weeks of gradually increasing the resistance, add one set of higher resistance, with lower reps per set (4–6 reps per set), except for Exercises 88, 91, 91.2, 92, 104, and 105.

Abdominals: For whitewater boating, abdominal development is especially necessary. Do the following: Exercises 56.5, 57.2 or 67, 60, 62, 66, and 68. Add a rotary torso machine exercise if you have access to one. Alternatively, do Exercise 80.

Lower body: Do Exercises 24, 70, and 72.

BALANCE AND AGILITY

Spend at least 30 minutes 2 times per week on agility and balance practice. Gradually intensify these sessions to quick and higher-amplitude balance and agility challenges. Particularly focus on doing agility drill 3, earlier in this chapter, at high-speed intervals. Work toward doing a 2-minute obstacle course 8–10 times. Once this fitness base has been established (about 4–6 weeks), start on easy rivers. Continue the agility training and roll practice throughout the season (see the rolling section in Whitewater Kayaking,

later in this chapter). For balance, see the general dry-land balance drills listed earlier in this chapter.

SEA OR LAKE KAYAKING

Kayakers should read the Touring or Flatwater Canoeing section, which contains basic information for both canoeing and kayaking.

Kayaking, like canoeing, uses symmetrical, repetitive, linked motion that involves same-side leg and paddle drive. The hips are flexed and knees nearly extended, which places a continuous load on the low back. The drive phase is accomplished through leg extension and rotation of the torso, followed by elbow bending. The kayaking stroke involves a significant degree of torso rotation and sidebending, which requires a high level of torso strength and endurance. The hip flexors are used for control of hull position as well as for maintaining slight forward flexion of the torso during the stroke. This makes flexibility in the hamstrings, hip flexors, and low back very important. In kayaking, the chest and back need to be equally well developed. The major muscles of the upper body listed for flatwater canoeing also apply to kayaking.

ROLLING

Rolling is considered an advanced skill for sea kayakers and a necessary skill for whitewater kayakers. Rolling the kayak requires a very rapid, powerful combination of hip, back, abdominal, shoulder, chest, and arm muscles. The movement is primarily initiated from the hips, then progressively with the back, abdomen, and shoulders. It is best to practice this in a class or pool with other people around who can assist before trying it in cold water or with a loaded kayak. You should have good flexibility and torso strength before trying your first roll. Do not practice rolling if you have active shoulder or back problems, as they might be significantly exacerbated by it.

STRETCHING

Do the stretching exercises outlined in the Stretching section earlier in this chapter, paying particular attention to the hamstrings (Exercises 1 and 2).

AEROBIC CONDITIONING

Your aerobic training is best done on the water in a kayak with a program similar to the one suggested for flatwater canoeing earlier in this chapter. Start in calm waters with 30–60 minutes of low-intensity kayaking. Once weekly, do a long paddle, increasing the duration by 20 minutes per week up to one half day. By week 3–4, include 1–2 sessions of moderate-intensity intervals of 10 minutes (initially) and gradually work up to 60 minutes. After increasing the duration of your moderate-intensity training to 30 minutes, take your kayak out during windy conditions on a lake to practice your higher-intensity kayaking under rougher conditions. After 4–6 weeks, consider adding some high-intensity interval training.

Off-the-water training emphasizes aerobic base training with rowing ergometers (or use Exercise 33), cross-country ski machines, or other equipment that combines upper- and lower-body training. Use the same principles outlined for on-the-water training.

Interval Training for Rough or Windy Conditions

Sea or rough-water lake kayaking demands the stamina and skill level to do long-term, high-intensity paddling in order to get through windy or rough water. Training for this should include higher-intensity intervals, and should incorporate training time in challenging sea conditions. Start this type of interval training after you have been able to do approximately 45 minutes of on-water medium-intensity training (as outlined for flatwater canoeing earlier in this chapter).

Get comfortable with 1–2 hours of moderate-to high-intensity paddling if you would like to handle rough, windy conditions in sea kayaking, common during full-day or multiple-day sea kayaking trips. For high-intensity training, start with intervals of 1–2 minutes. Alternate this with periods of low-intensity paddling of double the duration of the high-intensity interval, to have some relative rest. Start with a few intervals mixed in with your regular paddling practice, and work up to 4–6 intervals. Gradually add some longer intervals. Intervals can also be done as Fartlek training (see chapter 2).

STRENGTH TRAINING

Upper body: Do the flatwater canoeing program earlier in this chapter, with the following modifications: Exercises 91.2, 91.3, 92.

Abdominals: Do the exercises outlined for whitewater canoeing earlier in this chapter.

Lower body: Do Exercises 24 and 70.

BALANCE AND AGILITY

Dynamic sitting balance and agility are particularly important for rough, exposed water conditions. If you are training for difficult conditions, do the strength training outlined for whitewater kayaking, below.

GOAL PROGRAM FOR A FULL-DAY OR A MULTIDAY SEA KAYAK TRIP

For this goal, begin approximately 8–10 weeks before your expected first day trip. You can feel reasonably prepared to embark on a 1-day or multiday sea kayak trip when you are able to sit comfortably for 4 hours and kayak at low intensity, do 30–45 minutes of moderate-intensity kayaking on smooth and rough water, do six 2- to

4-minute intervals of very high-intensity paddling, and handle capsizes.

Within 4–6 weeks of your sea kayak trip, practice some rolling or wet exits/re-entries in a swimming pool with a partner or preferably in a class, especially if you do not have any active injuries in your back and shoulder. Make sure you feel comfortable tipping and exiting the kayak in open water and getting back in with or without the assistance of another boater. If you will be boating in cold water, make sure you have tried your roll/wet exit in cold water before going on your trip.

WHITEWATER KAYAKING

The paddle stroke is much the same in whitewater kayaking as in sea kayaking; however, the boat is normally fit snugly to the paddler in order to make immediate use of hip movements for boat placement. Hamstring stretching is even more important for proper spine position, as the kayaker's lower body position varies little over the course of the day.

The sitting balance challenges in whitewater boating are among the most significant of any sitting activity. The speed demands of intermediate and above levels of white water require that the paddler often perform in highly loaded, awkward positions. This places tremendous demands on the muscles of the torso as well as shoulder stabilizers. Shoulder injuries are not uncommon. In addition, aggressive use of the hip flexors, quadriceps, gluteus, and hamstrings in concert with rotation of the trunk and pelvis provide the base to paddle from. Therefore, trunk strength, flexibility, and shoulder stability are primary requirements.

AEROBIC CONDITIONING

Follow the whitewater canoeing program discussed earlier in this chapter.

STRENGTH TRAINING

Your time on the land should be a time not only to train aerobically, but also to work on stretching and strengthening any deficiencies you may have in your musculoskeletal system as appropriate to kayaking. Common areas of strength deficiency include the torso, upper back (scapular stabilizers), and forearm muscles. Appropriate exercises are rows, lat pulls, biceps curls, triceps extensions, pull-ups, and sitting balance exercises on a gym ball. Several of these exercises should include a trunk rotational component.

See the Whitewater Canoeing section earlier in this chapter for a good basic strength training program.

BALANCE AND AGILITY

Follow the whitewater canoeing program described earlier in this chapter.

GOAL PROGRAM FOR A FULL DAY OF WHITEWATER KAYAKING

You should be ready for your full-day trip when you can spend 3–4 hours in your kayak, do 8–12 intervals on an obstacle course, roll, and feel comfortable bracing and turning in rough water. You should have mastered the strength and balance training program. This includes doing some sets of the upper-body exercises at higher speed and some sets at higher resistance.

ROWING (SCULLING AND SWEEP)

Sport rowing involves mechanics that are in many ways very different from canoeing and kayaking. Rowing shells have extremely little side-to-side stability and are generally designed to run on a stable hull surface on calm waters; therefore, the rowing motion involves very little sidebending of the trunk. The plane of travel of the oar handle remains fairly constant, and the body is required to adjust to it around the shoulder joint. A rower's feet are secured to the bottom of the boat, and the rower moves forward and back on a rolling seat positioned just slightly higher than the feet. This allows the legs to become the primary propulsive element in the stroke. Rather than the alternating right/left cycles of canoe or kayak paddling, rowing involves simultaneous extension of both knees with contraction of both arms.

The propulsive phase of the stroke is initiated with a powerful contraction of the gluteal and quadriceps muscles. This power is transferred through a neutral spine through the shoulders and arms to the face of the blade. This is accomplished by rolling on the sit bones (ischial tuberosities of the pelvis), rather than dramatically flexing and extending the low back. The power generated by the lower body is sudden and considerable. The support structure of the shoulders and arms must be strong enough to absorb the load, and to transfer those forces to the oars.

Sculling, in which the rower grasps two oars, is a symmetrical activity. Unless the sculler is in rough, open conditions in an appropriate open-water boat, there is negligible torso side-bending or torso rotation. The spine has a high requirement for flexibility in flexion and extension and, as mentioned above, hamstring flexibility is quite necessary to attain proper positioning. Scullers may race or tour on flat or open water.

Sweep rowers (*crew*) grasp a single oar. It is unlikely that sweep rowers will be touring. Generally, sweep is a specifically competitive activity. It involves a rotational component to the torso, and, most important, the torso is rotated and slightly sidebent when the legs impose their greatest load. Sweep rowers row on one side

only, at least during any given workout, so their potential for asymmetrical body development is quite high. It is therefore important to understand the high level of flexibility necessary in this activity.

AEROBIC CONDITIONING

It is beyond the scope of this book to design appropriate training programs for sprint and distance rowing races. The rower with those intentions has adequate other published materials to draw upon and is likely involved in a coached competitive program. The stretching, resistance, and balance training aspects of this book, however, are certainly applicable to the competitive rower. The focus here is to enable the recreational touring rower to be adequately prepared. Because rowing shells are particularly unstable, it is also assumed that the rower attempting to follow this program has the necessary skills to handle the boat during periods of hard work.

On-the-water training: Rowing is very aerobically demanding, as it engages an enormous number of muscles and is done in an explosive manner. It is also highly skill-dependent. Although some of each training time should be used to focus particularly on skill development, it is important to maintain good body mechanics by remaining aware of them with every stroke. Otherwise, the potential to injure oneself increases greatly.

Begin with sessions of 30–60 minutes of low-intensity training while focusing on balance and technical skills. Once a week, take a longer row, increasing the duration by 15–30 minutes. Your regular training sessions should build to 45–90 minutes, and your longer row to 2 hours. If you are training for a long rowing trip, adjust the maximums accordingly. Remember that the load on the extensor muscles of the spine is great in rowing, and that the increases in time should be made only if they can be done comfortably.

By week 3–4, include 10-minute intervals of moderate intensity, working toward 2–3 in a session. Gradually increase the proportion of medium-intensity work until you are able to spend your whole row (excepting warm-up) at medium intensity.

After increasing your medium-intensity interval to 30 minutes and doing so with good, relaxed control, begin adding high-intensity bursts of anywhere from 30 seconds to 2 minutes at a higher stroke rate. This is necessary to develop the boat handling skills needed when encountering foul weather, boat wakes, or even other boats. Do this in a Fartlek-type format (see chapter 2).

Off the water: A rowing ergometer is a good tool for aerobic training. It is widely available in health clubs and closely mimics the actual rowing motion. If being on the water is not an option, use an erg to do the aerobic training outlined above. Consider varying your stroke rate to music as you keep at a moderate intensity. The different beat of different tunes will vary the workout and the aerobic demand. Try to make it fun.

If an ergometer is unavailable, a cross-country ski machine is the next best option. If you choose running for your aerobic cross training, use hills and/or stair running (not stair-climbers) as part of your training, but remember that running does little for the upper body.

STRENGTH TRAINING

Your time on land should be used not only to train aerobically, but also to work on stretching and strengthening any deficiencies you may have in your musculoskeletal system as appropriate to rowing. Common areas of strength deficiency include the legs, back, abdomen, and upper back (scapular stabilizers). In sweep rowing, trunk rotation is also necessary to prepare for load. Flexibility deficiencies are common in the hamstrings and muscles of the forearm.

Upper body: Exercises 87, 88.4, 89, 91 or 99.1, 92, 95, 96, 98, 102, and 105 (sweep only).

Abdominals: Exercises 56.4, 57 (or, better, 67), 65 (sweep only), 80 (sweep only). Sweep rowers add a rotary torso machine if you have access to one in your gym.

Lower body: Exercises 27, 28, 70, 70.2, 70.5, and 72 (with weights).

Conditioning for Road and Mountain Bicycling

By Erik Moen, P.T.

▶ **THIS CHAPTER WILL HELP YOU:**
- Appreciate the physiological demands on the cyclist.
- Create a basic mileage plan for a known ride.
- Establish a functional strengthening program specific for bicycling.
- Successfully perform coordination drills to enhance confidence on the bicycle.

The first objective of anyone who is interested in bicycling should be proper equipment fit and then development of an aerobic base. Following this you can add interval, strength, balance, and agility training depending on the demands of your activity. Mountain cyclists should spend extra time on strength and agility training.

MUSCULOSKELETAL DEMANDS
The quadriceps, hamstrings, and gluteals play a big role in the propulsion of a cyclist. The hamstrings should be strengthened to approximately four-fifths the strength of the quadriceps. The shoulders and arms are used for pulling but are primarily used in the maintenance of torso posture and the absorption of shock from the terrain. More upper-body, balance, and agility training are required for mountain bikers.

MUSCLE IMBALANCES
Muscle imbalances commonly associated with cycling are mid- and upper-back weakness contrasted with tight pectorals (chest). This can lead to other upper-body imbalances, which can affect the neck and front of shoulders. In the lower body, inadequate hamstring-to-quadriceps strength can lead to early leg fatigue during a cycling trip.

WARM-UP
Warm up for cycling by performing 5–10 minutes of low-resistance pedaling.

STRETCHING
Follow the warm-up with stretching Exercises 1, 2, 3, 6, 9, 11–13, 17, and 19.

AEROBIC CONDITIONING
Effective training for a selected bicycling event requires answers to two questions:

What is the goal riding volume (as defined by distance or time)?

How much time prior to the event do you have to achieve your goals?

Phasic training and preparation time for different bicycling events are suggested in Figure 29. Each event is listed by distance or time and has a minimum preparation time suggested in

FIGURE 29. PHASIC TRAINING FOR BICYCLE EVENTS

Weeks Prior to Event	Typical Event	Phase 1 (weeks)	Phase 2 (weeks)	Phase 3 (weeks)	Suggested Weekly Training Plan
14	2 days of 100 miles each on road	6 weeks	5 weeks	3 weeks	2D
13		5	5	3	
12	150 miles on road in 1 day	5	4	3	2D
11		5	4	2	
10		4	4	2	
9	100 miles on road or 5 hours on MTB	3	4	2	1D or MTB
8		3	3	2	
7		3	2	2	
6	50 miles on road or 3 hours on MTB	2	2	2	1D or MTB

Abbreviations: D = day, MTB = mountain bike, 2D or 1D = mileage covered in 1 or 2 days

weeks prior to that event. Your total preparation time is broken into three phases of training: phase 1, base mileage; phase 2, strength and aerobic capacity; and phase 3, specific preparation for the event. Each typical event has a suggested weekly training plan, outlined in Figure 29, to help create weekly training specific for your goals. There is room for individual variation of basic training. Please be aware that rushing preparation time may lead to an overuse injury. The following training programs assume that your bicycle is properly fit and that you are not adjusting to new equipment.

CALCULATING WEEKLY GOAL MILEAGE

The next step of planning is to define weekly mileage goals as a function of how many weeks you need to prepare for an event. One must always count *backward* from the event date in determining mileage goals. A reasonable peak mileage goal (PMG) for whatever event you pick is the distance of the event. In the example of a 2-day event, a reasonable PMG would be the most miles expected in 1 day. Each phase of training has a reasonable percentage of volume change (VC) per week to ensure progression of mileage. Net VC per week is discussed in each phase below. Weekly mileage goals (WMG) are calculated as a function of PMG, and calculations are given for each phase:

Note: Y equals the number of weeks from completion of the phase.

Phase 3, or the specific preparation phase, allows a rider to adapt to the basic mileage/time volumes required for successful completion of a goal. The VC for Phase 3 is 10% of PMG, so the generic formula is: WMG = PMG − (0.10 x PMG x 4).

Example: Lance chooses to train 12 weeks for a 150-mile 1-day ride. Phase 3 of a 12-week plan has 3 weeks. Lance's PMG should equal 150 miles, thus WMG for weeks 10–12 are as follows:

Week 12 150 miles – (0.10 x 150 x 1) = 135 miles

Week 11 150 miles – (0.10 x 150 x 2) = 120 miles

Week 10 150 miles – (0.10 x 150 x 3) = 105 miles

Phase 2 is designed to increase a rider's bicycle-specific strength and aerobic capacity. Peak mileage goals will be no more than 70% of PMG. The VC for Phase 2 is 5% of PMG and the generic formula is: WMG = PMG x 0.7 – (0.05 x PMG x 4). Continuing with the example begun above:

Week 9   150 miles x 0.7 – (0.05 x 150 x 1) = 98 miles

Week 8   150 miles x 0.7 – (0.05 x 150 x 2) = 90 miles

Week 7   150 miles x 0.7 – (0.05 x 150 x 3) = 83 miles

Week 6   150 miles x 0.7 – (0.05 x 150 x 4) = 75 miles

Phase 1 is designed for your body's adaptation to basic miles on the bicycle. Peak mileage goals will be no more than 60% of PMG. The VC for Phase 1 is 8% of PMG and the generic formula is: WMG = PMG x 0.6 – (0.08 x PMG x 4). Continuing with the example begun above:

Week 5   150 miles x 0.6 – (0.08 x 150 x 1) = 78 miles

Week 4   150 miles x 0.6 – (0.08 x 150 x 2) = 66 miles

Week 3   150 miles x 0.6 – (0.08 x 150 x 3) = 54 miles

Week 2   150 miles x 0.6 – (0.08 x 150 x 4) = 42 miles

Week 1   150 miles x 0.6 – (0.08 x 150 x 5) = 30 miles

Thus 14 weeks prior to the event, the highlight of Lance's first week of training will be a 30-mile ride. Mileage overlap between Phases 1 and 2 is designed to allow your body to compensate for Phase 2's added intensity as described in Weekly Training Plans, below.

WEEKLY TRAINING PLANS

Figure 30 shows suggested weekly training plans for ride distances given in Figure 29. These are suggested weekly plans as a function of phase and WMG to create a sufficient aerobic base to achieve your goals. Please note the inclusion of physiological intervals and skill drills. These are described later in this chapter.

Five to seven days prior to your goal event should be a period of relative rest. Relative rest includes activities of minimal intensity and significantly reduced mileage. Volumes are not to exceed 30% of your most recent WMG.

PEDALING CADENCE

Basic pedaling mechanics are of high priority for efficiency, aerobic conditioning, and avoiding overuse injury. These pedaling drills do not have to be performed exactly as described here. They may be altered to suit your level.

Optimal pedaling cadence for the cyclist is largely individual and dependent on terrain, but generally should be 70–90 revolutions per minute (rpm). Maintenance of this relatively quick pace allows you to ride more efficiently and thus decreasing the opportunity for injury or fatigue. If you don't have a bicycle computer with cadence, don't worry. Monitoring cadence is as simple as taking a heart rate.

This self-test should be done on a quiet, uncrowded stretch of road. Simply monitor your watch as you pedal. Count the number of pedal strokes in a 15-second period and then multiply that number by 4. This will give you an rpm value. Now that you have an appreciation for rpm, practice maintaining your goal.

Work your way through the progression of pedal cadences found in Figure 31. Practice your ability to determine approximate levels of cadence. This is easiest when using an indoor trainer or exercise bike. This may and should also be done outdoors. Pay attention to your path of travel to avoid obstacles. Note: Although the word *interval* is used, these drills should be done in an aerobic level below 75% maximum heart rate.

When the more difficult interval becomes easy, maintain your 90 rpm value for the duration.

High-cadence intervals are performed to overload your body's ability to perform pedaling at levels greater than 90 rpm. The ability to pedal greater than 90 rpm for short periods of

FIGURE 30. WEEKLY TRAINING PLANS

2D: 2 DAYS OF LONG ROAD RIDING

	PHASE 1	PHASE 2	PHASE 3
M	off	off	off
Tu	30% WGM	35% WGM	30% WGM
W	off	off	off
Th	40% WGM	30% WGM Lactate threshold*	35% WGM
F	off	off	off
Sat	100% WGM	100% WGM	100% WGM
Sun	55% WGM	65% WGM	85% WGM

1D: 1 DAY OF LONG ROAD RIDING

	PHASE 1	PHASE 2	PHASE 3
M	off	off	off
Tu	45% WGM	30% WGM	30% WGM
W	off	off	off
Th	20% WGM	30% WGM Lactate threshold*	30% WGM
F	off	off	off
Sat	100% WGM	100% WGM	100% WGM
Sun	20% WGM	25% WGM	25% WGM

MTB: MOUNTAIN BIKE RIDING

	PHASE 1	PHASE 2	PHASE 3
M	off	off	off
Tu	30% WGM	40% WGM	45% WGM
W	off	off	off
Th	50% WGM on road	Lactate threshold interval*	Anaerobic power interval
F	off	off	off
Sat	0.5 hour of skill and agility	0.5 hour of skill and agility	0.5 hour of skill and agility
Sun	100% WGM	100% WGM	100% WGM

*Lactate threshold interval should be performed and included as part of the daily volume.

FIGURE 31. BASIC PEDAL CADENCE DRILLS

	BEGINNER	INTERMEDIATE	ADVANCED
Total number of efforts	3	4	8
Sets	1	2	2
Repetitions in a set	3	2	4
Duration	3 minutes	5 minutes	2 minutes
Rest between reps	5 minutes	3 minutes	1 minutes
Rest between sets	–	10 minutes	3 minutes
Cadence for efforts	70–90 rpm	70–90 rpm	70–90 rpm

FIGURE 32. HIGH-CADENCE INTERVALS

	BEGINNER	INTERMEDIATE	ADVANCED
Total number of efforts	6	4	8
Sets	2	2	2
Repetitions in a set	3	2	4
Duration	30 seconds	3 minutes	45 seconds
Rest between reps	1 minute	2 minutes	1 minute
Rest between sets	5 minutes	5 minutes	5 minutes
Cadence for efforts	100 rpm	110 rpm	120 rpm
Cadence during rest	70 rpm	70 rpm	70 rpm

time is important in both road and mountain bicycling. It is often difficult for individuals to perform this task efficiently. You frequently see inefficient pedalers bounce on their saddles when attempting high-cadence efforts. Bouncing compromises your ability to control the bicycle, steering, braking, shifting, and traction.

The intervals shown in Figure 32 should be performed so you do not bounce on the seat or create excessive motion in your upper body. Using an indoor trainer or stationary bike in front of a mirror is an excellent way to monitor your progress.

INTERVAL TRAINING

The following intervals are included to enhance your efficiency in pedaling. See chapter 2, Aerobic Conditioning and Interval Training,

regarding precautions and other information on interval training.

Intervals can be done on level surfaces and hills. The mountain bicyclist should do some intervals on trails and off-road terrain. All interval training requires a warm-up that includes 10–15 minutes of low-intensity, easy riding, stretching, and surveying the interval course for possible hazards. All intervals should be ended with a cooldown period of 10–15 minutes of easy, low-intensity riding and stretching.

Anaerobic Power Intervals

These are short, all-out intervals of 20 seconds or less.

Terrain: Section of uninterrupted hill approximately 2–3 blocks long. May be either dirt or pavement. Dirt better simulates real mountain biking terrain and requires attention to proper weight-shifting in order to maintain traction. Pavement allows you to focus clearly on the pure physiological effort.

Required time: Approximately 30–45 minutes.

High-intensity effort: Should last 10–20 seconds.

Cadence: 60–70 rpm.

Recovery: 3–5 minutes of easy, low-intensity pedaling to regain normal breathing.

Total number: Start with 4 and work up to 8 intervals.

Moderate-Duration Intervals

Terrain: Long, straight roads, hills, or trails with long straight sections

Required time: 40–60 minutes.

High-intensity effort: 20 seconds–4 minutes, with the majority at 3 minutes.

Cadence: 70–90 rpm.

Recovery: 5 minutes of easy, low-intensity pedaling to regain normal breathing.

Total number: 4–8 intervals.

Lactate-Threshold Longer Intervals

These build fitness for sustained efforts such as long hill climbs. These efforts are aerobic in nature, less intense than the above intervals, and sustained for 5–10 minutes. You should be in a heart rate zone of 75%–85% maximum heart rate.

Terrain: 2–4 miles of flat or rolling uninterrupted terrain, or a 1- to 3-mile section of gradual climbing.

Required time: 40–60 minutes.

Interval: 5–10 minutes of sustained heavy breathing while maintaining your pedal cadence.

Cadence: 70–90 rpm.

Recovery: 5 minutes of easy, low-intensity pedaling to regain normal breathing.

Total number: Start with 2 and work up to 4.

STRENGTH TRAINING

The following exercise recommendations can help the cyclist improve performance and balance. Exercise each body region 2 times per week.

ROAD CYCLING

Lower body: Exercises 23 and 36.6, or Exercises 70.1, 70.2, 70.4, 71 (hamstring curls done with a single leg, sitting if possible), and 72 (basic lunge).

Abdominals: The road cyclist should do these if riding hills, doing fast cornering, etc. Do Exercises 59.4, 61, 62, and 69.

Upper body: Exercises 82, 84 or 86, 88, 89, 91.1, 92, 98, and 102.

MOUNTAIN BIKING

Lower body: Do the road cyclist program above, adding the following: Exercises 72.10, 75, 75.1, 75.3 (advanced cyclists can try 75.4), 76, and 76.1.

Abdominals: Mountain cyclists have a significant demand on their arms, legs, torso, and abdominal muscles to maintain balance. Do the road cyclist program above, adding Exercises 41 and 69. See the agility exercises below.

Upper body: Do the road cyclist program above, adding Exercise 99, and substituting 101 for 86 and 104 for 102.

FUNCTIONAL AGILITY EXERCISES

The development of agility takes practice. The following exercises are considered dynamic and functional exercises. They challenge your moving balance in simulated environments. Effective practice means calculated risk. Please be aware that bicycling in general, and possibly these exercises, can be dangerous. The successful practice of the following exercises will help to decrease the potential danger of bicycling. Please use common sense and a properly fitted helmet when on your bike.

GENERAL ROAD AND MOUNTAIN BICYCLE SKILLS

148 Balance-ready Position

Equipment: Bicycle, curb.
Purpose: The balance-ready position is your most effective posture on the bike for meeting challenging situations. This position should be learned and readily accessible for both road and mountain biking.
Technique: The balance-ready position maintains the center of mass over the bottom bracket of the bicycle. This exercise takes the rider down off the curb. You should be off the saddle with your cranks horizontal, knees and elbows slightly bent, head upright, vision forward, with a firm grasp on the handlebars. Approach the curb in an easy gear while on the saddle. As you approach the curb perpendicularly, control your speed with your rear brake as you attain the balance-ready position. Roll off the edge of the curb, landing the front wheel as softly as possible; continue to control your speed as you slowly roll the back wheel off the curb. Repeat until you are able to roll your bike off the curb as smoothly and quietly as possible.

149 Maintaining a Straight Line

Equipment: Bicycle, quiet road.
Purpose: The maintenance of a straight line while riding your bicycle is important for injury prevention. It requires balance and concentration.
Technique: Find a line on a quiet road that you can ride along for 30–120 seconds. Concentrate on your pedal speed and rhythm. Try not to pedal off the line.

150 Slalom

Equipment: Uninterrupted level surface approximately 30–100 feet long; objects such as cones, water bottles, hats, etc., set up in a slalom course.

Purpose: Steering through challenging surfaces such as hills takes concentration, coordination, balance, steering, speed control, and vision (picking a line) to put together a clean ride. It is important that you be able to avoid consecutive objects.

Technique: Place the objects 4–6 feet apart, with an exit gate 2 feet wide. Start with a short course with objects at 6-foot distances and gradually progress to shorter object-to-object distances and more challenging courses. Enter the course traveling slalom-style around the objects. Control your speed as you travel through the challenge so that you exit through the gate without knocking over any obstacles.

Variation: 150.1. You may include shorter distances between objects, or see how quickly or slowly you can do the course. Mountain bikers should set up obstacle courses on hills (uphill and downhill sections).

MOUNTAIN BIKE–SPECIFIC DRILLS

151 Downhill

Equipment: Slalom course setup for Exercise 150, on a downhill grade 100–300 feet.

Purpose: Control your speed and maintain your balance on downhill trails.

Technique: Start at the top of a downhill grade. You don't have to pedal much for this exercise, but an appropriate (easy-to-pedal) gear should be predetermined in the event that you have to regain balance. Enter the course with your weight slightly behind the saddle in a balance-ready position. Control your speed with the rear brake as you navigate the slalom course. Remember to keep your weight over the bike rather than leaning out to the side.

Variation: 151.1. You can make this exercise more difficult by increasing the pitch of the slope.

152 | Ride the 2-by-4 Line

Equipment: 3- to 10-foot-long 2-by-4.
Purpose: Challenge your ability to maintain a narrow path and refine ability to balance on the bike in tricky off-road areas.
Technique: Set the 2-by-4 down flat, 4-inch side down, on a quiet lot. Approach the 2-by-4 with enough speed to carry yourself 10 feet along its length. As you near the board, assume the balance-ready position. Control your speed with your rear brake. Lightly lift, or unweight, the front wheel by leaning slightly back on the bike. Move back to the balance-ready position as you traverse the wood. Pay attention to keeping your head up and forward. Focus on where you are going rather than your immediate front wheel; you should have already seen that territory.

BUNNY HOP

Mastering the bunny hop and its components takes skill, agility, and coordination. This is an important survival skill for both the off-road and road cyclist. It allows you to avoid objects such as potholes without swerving into traffic or other riders, and to avoid objects that would otherwise cause a flat tire.

153 | Lifting the Front Wheel

Equipment: 3- to 5-foot-long 2-by-4.
Purpose: The first component of the bunny hop is helpful in activities such as going up a curb.
Technique: Pick a gear that can be easily pedaled. Make a slow, perpendicular approach to the board. Attain the balance-ready position. Just before you get to the wood: a) crouch down, loading your weight over the pedals; b) spring up and back, unloading the pedals (feet continue their contact with the pedals), and lift up on the handlebars; c) let your rear wheel roll over the 2-by-4. Use caution to not make the lifting up and back too ballistic, as you may fall over backward. The 2-by-4 is an excellent object to work with, as you can easily roll over it if you do not adequately lift your front wheel. Try many times until you have a sense of control and are able to quietly clear the 2-by-4 with your front wheel.
Variation: 153.1. You can increase the difficulty by using a curb or larger piece of wood.

154 | Lifting the Back Wheel

Equipment: 3- to 5-foot-long 2-by-4.
Purpose: The second component of the bunny hop is a handy skill to master for off-road survival.
Technique: Make a perpendicular approach to the 2-by-4 with controlled speed. Hop the front wheel over the board and then: a) shift your weight forward so your center of mass is in front of the bottom bracket of the bicycle; b) simultaneously push down on the handlebars and lift up on the pedals. You will notice a hop of the rear wheel. Again, use caution to not make too large a leap when trying to hop the rear wheel, as there is potential to go over the handlebars onto your head. Lifting up on the pedals can be done without toe straps. This is achieved by pointing your toes slightly down prior to lifting up. The combination of this with leaning slightly forward creates the lift. Try this exercise repeatedly, with a goal of control and ease.
Variation: 154.1. You can increase the difficulty by using a curb or larger piece of wood.

155 | Bunny Hop

Equipment: 3- to 5-foot-long 2-by-4.
Purpose: The intentional full clearance of bike and rider off the ground incorporates the skills of front and rear wheel hops.
Technique: The 2-by-4 is an excellent practice piece, as you will know if you don't clear it, since 99% of the time it will not cause you to crash. Make the usual perpendicular approach to the board. Making a faster approach will not necessarily ensure that you will clear the board with greater success; therefore, maintain a controlled speed. Attain the balance-ready position as you approach the 2-by-4: a) crouch down, loading your weight over the pedals; b) spring up, lifting the front wheel up via the handlebars; c) quickly shift your weight forward, pushing the handlebars forward to help lift the rear wheel up and over the object. It helps to use the same foot lift in the last part of the hop as you used in Exercise 154, Lifting the Back Wheel. As you can see, the bunny hop is a combination of the two single-wheel hops.
Variation: 155.1. If you are a little tentative about using a 2-by-4 to start with, establish a line in the dirt as your first practice setup. You might become proficient at hopping a line in the sand prior to moving to a 2-by-4.

CONDITIONING FOR RUNNING

BY LISA FOX, P.T., AND DAVID MUSNICK, M.D.

▶ **THIS CHAPTER WILL HELP YOU:**
- Put together a comprehensive conditioning program to meet distance goals from a 5K run through a marathon.
- Use running as a part of your outdoor fitness program.

Running can be used for general fitness, to train for other activities, or as a goal in itself. From the information in this chapter, you can develop a conditioning program to improve your running. In this chapter, most distances are listed in miles, except for some shorter distances and marathon distances, which are in meters or kilometers (abbreviated as K). Appendix A at the back of this book gives conversions for standard and metric units of measurement.

MUSCULOSKELETAL DEMANDS

Running is primarily a forward-motion activity that also involves side-to-side and rotational forces. It generates an impact of two to four times your own body weight and is thus considered a high-impact and repetitive activity. Running involves alternating deceleration forces by pronation (foot flattening, internal rotation of the leg, and flexing and sidebending of the hip and spine), followed by propulsion or supination (foot arching, external rotation of the leg, and extending of the hip and spine). Because of the forces involved, it makes sense to follow an aerobic and strength training program to avoid injuries of the foot, knee, and hip.

MUSCLES USED IN RUNNING

All of the muscles from your buttock to your feet are used in running. They work to push you off of the ground and to decelerate you. Leg, thigh, and buttock muscles are stressed the most when they slow down your knee, hip, and ankle from bending excessively and your foot from pronating. They are functionally strengthened during squats, lunges, and hops. Step-ups and step-downs are important if you are planning to run on hilly terrain. You may improve your running speed and endurance by doing functional strength training.

RISK FACTORS THAT MAY LEAD TO AN INJURY

Overuse injuries can occur in running as a result of foot problems, muscle imbalances, and low-back problems as well as from common training errors, including:
- excessive mileage (especially when easy days are not incorporated into the program)
- excessive interval or hill training
- running on improper terrain (including running on canted or very uneven surfaces and excessive downhill running)

Build your weekly mileage slowly, and vary the routes and the terrain. For example, don't always run the same route that requires you to face traffic on the left side of a canted road. Also, don't run the same hilly route each time you go out for a run.

MUSCLE IMBALANCES

The most common areas of imbalance that become apparent in runners are tighter heel cords in comparison to the weaker tibialis anterior; tighter iliotibial bands compared to their counterparts, the adductors and medial quadriceps; and gluteal weakness and tight quadriceps in relation to the hamstrings and hip flexors. These common areas of imbalance can be addressed with exercises to enhance flexibility, such as Exercises 1, 3, 5, 6–11, and strength, Exercises 26 and 73.

WARM-UP

You can warm up for running with a fast walk for 5 minutes followed by 1–3 minutes of skipping, or a jog of increasing intensity until you get up to your running pace. After your aerobic warm-up, you could do some functional exercises, such as Exercises 21.1 and 72.5. Do a few stretching exercises, including Exercises 1, 3, and 7–9.

STRETCHING

Running predominantly strengthens the calves, hamstrings, lower back, and front hip muscles. Over time, as these muscles become stronger, they will also become tighter. Do the following stretches after a warm-up or after your run: Exercises 1, 3.1, 3.2, 5, 7–9, and 21.

AEROBIC TRAINING

Aerobic training for running is best done by running, with occasional cross-training sessions. Running is a high-impact activity, so be careful to increase your duration of each run by no more than 10%–15% per week. Training for races can be done by following the training tables (Figures 33–36) later in this chapter.

INTERVAL TRAINING

You can do interval training with running to enhance your general aerobic endurance and your ability to do sprints. See chapter 2, as well as the sections on the second and third pyramid levels later in this chapter, for details on interval training.

CROSS TRAINING

If running is your major activity, you can use cross-training options to use your leg muscles and decrease the impact of running. These include hiking, cross-country skiing or using cross-country ski machines, snowshoeing, using a stair-climber, using an EFX cross trainer, using a slide board or a step, or doing regular aerobics workouts. Cycling can also be used, but uses the muscles in a different way.

You can also use running as a cross-training tool for other activities. Running is an excellent form of aerobic conditioning. It is good preparation for participation in hiking, mountaineering, snowshoeing, and cross-country skiing.

STRENGTH TRAINING

Strength training should focus on higher-repetition sets rather than bulking exercises (high resistance, low repetitions) for the lower body. You can do these strengthening exercises 2–3 times per week. For the lower-body exercises, do 2–3 sets of 15–20 reps. Note: An abdominal and upper-body strength training program can enhance your running, but doesn't yield as much of a return in performance as do lower-body exercises. (For definitions of beginning and intermediate/advanced, see Developing a Training Program later in this chapter.)

BEGINNING
Lower body: Exercises 23, 23.3, 24, 70, 70.2, 71, and 73.
Abdominals: Exercises 21, 56.3, 57.1, and 58.
Upper body: Exercises 86 and 102.

INTERMEDIATE/ADVANCED
Lower body: Do the beginning program, adding Exercises 27, 76, and 76.3. Consider adding Exercise 26 and omit Exercises 23 and 24.
Abdominals: Exercises 21, 56.4, 57.2, 59, and 64.
Upper body: Exercises 20.1, 65, 86, and 104.

BALANCE AND AGILITY

Balance and agility are crucial components of function for runners. Poor balance and poor reaction to unpredictable surfaces are primary factors contributing to injury. To improve your balance and agility for running perform Exercises 37, 38, 58.1, and 76.2 twice a week.

DEVELOPING A TRAINING PROGRAM

You can train for distance running or races in many different ways. The tables at the end of this chapter (Figures 33–36) will help you gradually build up your mileage. You can also progress your training in a pyramid method (described below) that adds mileage, long runs, and then hill and speed work.

The program should look like a stack of building blocks, with each level providing the foundation for the next one. This program may take 4–6 months to safely reach the goal of a specific marathon. Training for 5K, 10K, and half-marathon runs will take less time, depending on your fitness level and running experience.

Beginning runners are those with 0–1 year of experience. Intermediate/advanced runners have more than 1 year of experience, have run races, and have been in training programs for increasing mileage or speed in the past 1–2 years. Beginning runners should start with the first pyramid level and refer to the beginning training schedule later in this chapter (see Figure 33).

The beginning runner may need at least 4 weeks to slowly introduce a running program that is injury free. At the fourth week, you will be running with alternate cross-training days. You should initially walk briskly for 30 minutes, 3 times per week, for 2 weeks. Then progress into jogging by inserting short jogging distances during the walk. An example would be to insert 400-meter (440-yard) jogs (the distance once around a standard track) repeatedly throughout the session. Initially insert 1 jog per mile, then 2 jogs, etc., until you are jogging a mile, and then gradually increase the jog until you are jogging 30–40 minutes 3 times per week.

At this point you can begin a "pyramid" training schedule, especially if you have goals for running races. The first pyramid level, called base training, develops greater endurance and aerobic capacity for distance or race running. It accounts for 50% of the training program. During the second level, add strengthening drills (with strength training and hill running), speed interval workouts, and longer runs. The third level also incorporates interval training. (See chapter 2 for information and guidelines on various types of interval training.) The beginning runner can follow the guidelines under base training and the second pyramid level, or simply follow the training tables in Figures 33–36 to achieve various race distances.

A reasonable first running goal would be a 5K–10K. See Figures 33 and 34. Beginning runners should start with the walking program described in the Warm-up section earlier in this chapter. Weekly runs should include a long run in addition to 2–3 additional easier days. Intermediate runners with 4 months of a consistent base can insert speed work once a week if they are able to tolerate 20–30 miles a week. The distance of your long run depends upon what your experience level is at the time that you begin the program. An intermediate runner can enter a training schedule in line with your present weekly mileage. Strength training can be done on your cross-training or off days.

Do long runs every 1–2 weeks to prepare your body to tolerate longer distances and prepare you for races or longer-duration outdoor activities. Advanced runners may tolerate long runs every week. Beginning runners should initially do them every other week.

The pace for a long run is 1½–2 minutes per mile slower than your current 10K race pace, or 2 minutes per mile slower than your expected marathon pace. Long runs are developed by taking the longest run in the past 2 weeks and increasing it by 1–2 miles. If you are running for fitness alone, do your long run based on time and add a 10%–15% increase in time or distance.

PRACTICAL POINT

Plan an easy activity for 1–2 days after a long run to assist in recovery.

RULES FOR TRAINING

There are a few simple rules that apply whether you are training for that first 5K run, have set a goal to break the 3-hour barrier for the marathon, or are conditioning for a weekend hike.

Rule 1: Start slow and with short distances.

Rule 2: Always incorporate a warm-up and cooldown phase into the daily program.

Rule 3: Do not increase the total exercise time or mileage by more than 10% per week.

Rule 4: Beginning and intermediate runners should take a rest week of fewer miles each third or fourth week.

Rule 5: Beginning runners should run at an intensity in which they are able to carry on a conversation while running.

Rule 6: Beginning runners should target distance before speed. The beginner will notice consistent improvements simply by adding distance.

Rule 7: Don't rigidly follow someone else's training schedule. Be flexible. If you feel tired, run easy for 1–2 days. If after 2 days of rest you are still tired, think about reducing the entire week of training and reevaluating the schedule.

Rule 8: Always follow a hard training day with an easy day of running or cross training.

Rule 9: Provide an adequate tapering-down period prior to a race.

Rule 10: Allow sufficient time to recover from a race. The recovery of muscle strength and endurance capacity are attained sooner if you rest for 6–7 days after a marathon vs. continuing to run.

Rule 11: Limit the number of races you participate in. Most runners can't tolerate more than 2 races a month.

THE FIRST PYRAMID LEVEL: BASE TRAINING

Base training consists of daily runs, long runs on alternate weeks, and occasional participation in races. The goals are to develop endurance and aerobic capacity, which will lead to improved speed and ability to run longer distances.

Pace should be a comfortable speed, and you should be able to easily talk while running (70%–80% maximum heart rate). The pace should be 1½–2 minutes per mile slower than your current 10K race pace (if known). These runs should be relatively easy and enjoyable.

Races should be of moderate pace and done no more than every other week.

Mileage: Do up to 40 miles a week if training for a half- or full marathon.

Long runs: If you are a beginning runner, take long runs on alternate weeks at a relaxed pace.

Intermediate and advanced runners can do long runs every week.

THE SECOND PYRAMID LEVEL: HILL REPEATS

Once a week, run hill repeats on a 5%–15% grade only. The distance can be from 150 yards to ½ mile. Proper form includes looking at the top of the hill and bringing your hips forward rather than slumping and leaning into the hill. Improved form on a hill allows you to propel yourself up with less effort. You should feel your hamstrings and gluteals working while your legs move behind your body. Emphasize pushing off your feet and pumping your arms.

Pace: Run uphill at an intensity of 80%–90% maximum heart rate (max. HR) and jog easily back down to recover.

Frequency: Start with two hills, and increase by one to two hills per week to build up to 6–8 repeats for the longer hills and 8–10 repeats for the shorter hills. Perform this session once or twice per week.

Duration should be once or twice a week for 4–6 weeks, and should not be performed during the third pyramid level, the speed-training phase.

Mileage remains the same as the for first pyramid level, except for adding 1–2 days of hills.

THE SECOND PYRAMID LEVEL: FARTLEK TRAINING

Fartlek training consists of interval training runs of varying speed designed to build stamina. It allows you to control the pace in different environments, on cross-country trails or on the road, with the goal of feeling challenged but not exhausted when you are done (see chapter 2 for more details on Fartlek training). Examples:

1. Run 1,200 meters moderately hard, then run at an easy pace for equal or double the time.

2. Do speed bursts (80%–90% max. HR) of 100–400 meters with short, easy jogs between each sprint.
3. Run with a moderately hard effort up hills you encounter, followed with an easy pace between each hill.
4. Run for 1-, 2-, and 3-minute intervals (at approximately 85% max. HR), with equal or double rest times of easy jogging between efforts.

Pace: During a jog, randomly mix in intervals of higher intensities (80%–85% max. HR) and distances when you feel like it. These can be done as timed segments of 30 seconds–4 minutes or as distances. Go back to a jog pace in between the interval.

Frequency is 1–2 times per week.

Duration is 20–50 minutes after a warm-up of easy jogging.

THE THIRD PYRAMID LEVEL: SPEED TRAINING

The speed-training phase is the building block preceding the targeted goal. A runner who has more than a year of experience may need to target speed work in order to reach a new plateau in performance. Speed training results in markedly improved efficiency in your cardiovascular system within the initial 7 weeks. After 7 weeks the gains are slower. This phase is shorter because of the increased risk of injury due to the greater stress placed upon the body.

The best speed work for marathon distances are long intervals of ½ mile or more. Typically, 800 meters–3 miles are utilized for 10K and half-marathon training. Shorter distances of 400 meters–1½ miles are utilized for 10K or 5K goals. Discontinue hill repeats and begin speed or interval workouts 1–2 times per week using one of several variations listed in The Third Pyramid Level: Interval Training, below.

Frequency: The intermediate runner should start speed work after 4–6 months of base training, then only once a week until the following season. During the second season, increase this to twice a week.

Duration is 4 to a maximum of 7 weeks.

Mileage: Cut total mileage by 10%.

Long runs can be continued, gradually increasing them to your goal distance.

PRACTICAL POINT

Speed training cannot be performed year-round except by experienced runners. The average runner should develop a speed program of 7 weeks to avoid injury and to take advantage of the best peaking time.

THE THIRD PYRAMID LEVEL: TEMPO RUNNING

This is fast distance training that can be performed on a road or track. For example, if your 5K pace is 7:45 minutes per mile, then practice a 5K course at an 8:15-minutes-per-mile pace.

Pace is slightly slower than race pace for the same distance. The goal is to maintain a consistent pace.

Mileage is 2 miles or more.

THE THIRD PYRAMID LEVEL: INTERVAL TRAINING

Anaerobic intervals are intervals of less than 4 minutes' duration done at anaerobic intensities of 85%–95% max. HR, with rest periods of lower-intensity running or fast walking (at 60%–70% max. HR) for 1–2 times the interval duration. Work up to 3–8 shorter anaerobic intervals of 30 seconds, 1 minute, 2 minutes, 3 minutes,

and 4 minutes, or do them as distances of 200, 400, and 800 meters.

Aerobic intervals of longer duration (greater than 4 minutes) should be done at 80%–85% max. HR. Other interval examples:

— 2 at 5 minutes
— 400 meters, 800 meters, 1,200 meters, 800 meters, 400 meters
— 4 at 400 meters
— 3 at 1,200 meters
— 3 at 1 mile

Duration is 5 to 30 minutes.

Mileage is 800 meters–3 miles for longer race distance goals (half- or full marathon).

AT THE TOP OF THE PYRAMID: THE GOAL EVENT/TAPERING

This is the 2–4 weeks before the big race or the planned climbing trip. Start about 14 days prior to a shorter event, reducing total mileage by 30%–50%; at 7 days, reduce by 70%–80%, with the final 2–3 days consisting of only 1–3 miles daily. You can continue the same speed with each run since the fewer miles will allow ample rest. Begin tapering 3–4 weeks prior to a marathon, tapering to 50% by week 3, and at 7 days reduce by 70%–80%, again with the final 2–3 days consisting of only 1–3 miles daily.

With a running training program it is easy to see that one distance goal can be the base of the next. For example, a 5K schedule in May will provide the strength and skill for a half-marathon in the fall. A half-marathon in February will provide a base for a weekend glacier climb in the late spring.

FIGURE 33. EXAMPLE TRAINING PROGRAM FOR A 5K (BEGINNING)

WK	M ~~(SAT)~~	TUE (SUN)	WED (M)	TH (TUE)	FRI (W)	SAT (TH)	SUN (FRI)	TOTAL MILEAGE
1	off	3	CT	3	off	CT	4	10
2	off	3	CT	3	off	CT	3	9
3	off	3	CT	3	off	CT	5	11
4	off	3	CT	3	off	CT	3	9
5	off	$3\frac{1}{2}$	CT	$3\frac{1}{2}$	off	CT	5	12
6	off	$3\frac{1}{2}$	CT	$3\frac{1}{2}$	off	CT	4	10
7	off	$3\frac{1}{2}$	CT	$3\frac{1}{2}$	off	CT	4	11
8	off	3	CT	3	off	CT	3	10
9	off	3	CT	3	off	CT	2	9 tapering
10	off	3	CT	2	off	CT	1	5
11	off	2	CT	1	off	CT	race	5K

CT = cross training

Distances are in miles

Races of 10K or shorter should be followed by 1 easy week.

FIGURE 34. EXAMPLE TRAINING PROGRAM FOR A 10K
(WITH A 5K AS A BUILDING BLOCK)

WK	MON	TUE	WED	TH	FRI	SAT	SUN	TOTAL MILEAGE
1	off	3	CT	3	CT	3	5	14
2	off	4	CT	4	CT	3	4	15
3	off	4	CT	3½	CT	3	6	16½
4	off	4	CT	4	CT	3	4	15
5	off	4	H + CT; 1 x ¼ mile	4	CT	3	7	18
6	off	4	H + CT; 1 x ¼ mile	5	CT	3	5	17
7	off	2	H + CT; 1 x ¼ mile	3	CT	2	3	10
8	off	3	H + CT; 1 x ¼ mile	2	CT	1	race 5K	
9	off	rest	CT	rest	CT	rest	rest	0
10	off	4	CT	5	CT	3	7	20
11	off	4	CT	5	CT	3	5	17
12	off	5	CT	6	CT	3	8	22
13	off	5	CT	6	CT	3	5	19 tapering
14	off	5	CT	6	CT	3	8	22
15	off	3	CT	3	CT	2	3	11
16	off	2	CT	2	CT	1	race 10K	
rest	rest	rest	rest	rest	rest	rest	rest	rest

CT = cross training
H = hill training
Distances are in miles. Total mileage at the beginning should be no greater than 20–30 miles per week.
Note: Hill training can be added to any of the running days at the end of a workout.
Races of 10K or shorter should be followed by 1 easy week.

FIGURE 35. EXAMPLE TRAINING PROGRAM FOR A HALF-MARATHON

WK	~~MON~~ SAT	~~TUE~~ SUN	~~WED~~ M	~~TH~~ TUE	~~FRI~~ W	SAT TH	~~SUN~~ FRI	TOTAL MILEAGE
1	off	4	CT	4	CT	3	6	17
2	off	4	CT	4	CT	3	7$^1/_2$	18$^1/_2$
3	off	5	CT	4	CT	3	4	16
4	off	5	CT	5	CT	3	7$^1/_2$	20$^1/_2$
5	off	6	CT	5	CT	3	4	18
6	off	6	CT	5	CT	3	8$^1/_2$	22$^1/_2$
7	off	6	CT	6	CT	3	5	20
8	off	6	H + CT; 1 x $^1/_4$ mile	6	CT	3	10	25
9	off	6	H + CT; 1 x $^1/_4$ mile	6	CT	3	5	20
10	off	6	H + CT; 2 x $^1/_4$ mile	6	CT	3	10	25
11	off	6	H + CT; 2 x $^1/_4$ mile	6	CT	3	5	20
12	off	2	H + CT; 3 x $^1/_4$ mile	4	CT	3	4	13
13	off	2	H + CT; 3 x $^1/_4$ mile	2	CT	1	3	8
14 tapering	off	3	H + CT; 3 x $^1/_4$ mile	2	CT	1	race 10K	
15	off	rest	CT	rest	CT	rest	rest	0
16	off	6	CT	6	CT	3	10	25
17	off	6	CT	6	CT	3	6	21
18	off	6	CT	6	CT	3	12$^1/_2$	27$^1/_2$
19	off	6	CT	6	CT	3	8	23
20	off	7	CT	6	CT	3	14	30
21	off	7	CT	7	CT	3	7	24
22	off	8	CT	8	CT	3	14	33
23 tapering	off	4	CT	5	CT	3	5	17
24	off	2	CT	3	CT	1	4	10
25	off	2	CT	2	CT	1	race $^1/_2$ Marathon	

CT = cross training

H = hill training

Distances are in miles. Total mileage at the beginning should be no greater than 20–30 miles per week.

Note: Hill training can be added to any of the running days at the end of a workout.

FIGURE 36. EXAMPLE TRAINING PROGRAM FOR A MARATHON

WK	MON	TUE	WED	TH	FRI	SAT	SUN	TOTAL MILEAGE
1	off	6	CT	6	CT	3	10	25
2	off	6	CT	6	CT	3	5	20
3	off	6	CT	6	CT	3	10	25
4	off	6	CT	6	CT	3	5	20
5	off	6	CT	6	CT	3	12$\frac{1}{2}$	27$\frac{1}{2}$
6	off	6	CT	6	CT	3	8	23
7	off	7	CT	6	CT	3	14	30
8	off	7	H + CT; 1 x $\frac{1}{4}$ mile	7	CT	3	7	24
9	off	7	H + CT; 1 x $\frac{1}{4}$ mile	7	CT	3	6	33
10	off	7	H + CT; 2 x $\frac{1}{4}$ mile	7	CT	3	16	27
11	off	8	H + CT; 2 x $\frac{1}{4}$ mile	7	CT	3	10	36
12	off	8	H + CT; 3 x $\frac{1}{4}$ mile	7	CT	3	18	28
13 tapering	off	4	CT	4	CT	3	10	14
14	off	3	CT	2	CT	1	race $\frac{1}{2}$ Marathon	
15	off	rest	CT	rest	CT	rest	rest	0
16	off	8	CT	7	CT		10	28
17	off	8	CT	7$\frac{1}{2}$	CT	3	21	39$\frac{1}{2}$
18	off	8	CT	7$\frac{1}{2}$	CT	3	10	28$\frac{1}{2}$
19	off	8	CT	7$\frac{1}{2}$	CT	3	22	41$\frac{1}{2}$
20 tapering	off	8	CT	7$\frac{1}{2}$	CT	3	10	28$\frac{1}{2}$
21	off	4	CT	6	CT	3	7	20
22	off	2	CT	3	CT	1	4	10
23	off	2	CT	2	CT	1	race Marathon	

rest week

rest week

CT = cross training
H = hill training
Distances are in miles. Total mileage at the beginning should be no greater than 20–30 miles per week.
Note: Hill training can be added to any of the running days at the end of a workout.
Completely rest the first week following a marathon and allow at least 3 easy months for a full recovery, especially if you are prone to injuries.

24

CONDITIONING FOR WINDSURFING

BY MARK PIERCE, A.T.C., AND DAVID MUSNICK, M.D.

▶ **THIS CHAPTER WILL HELP YOU:**
• Develop an exercise program that will increase your balance and musculoskeletal ability to meet the rigorous demands of windsurfing.

Typically, a windsurfing run lasts between 10 and 30 minutes before a rest or fall, followed by about 2 minutes of recovery and repositioning. This requires a moderate amount of sustained and intermittent strength.

MUSCULOSKELETAL DEMANDS

Windsurfing requires significant balance and agility along with sustained whole-body strength. The typical body posture while windsurfing is hands grasping the boom; hips, knees, and ankles bent with your shoulders forward; and upper back in a flexed position. Most of your body weight is supported by a belt harness around your hips or chest and hooked to the boom. Assuming this posture allows you to change the position of your center of gravity and direct the sail for maneuverability while reacting to the constant movement of your board. Windsurfing requires significant quad, back extensor, and shoulder girdle strength in order to decelerate and respond to quick forces. Throughout this chapter, exercises preceded by an asterisk (*) are considered to be the most important for windsurfers.

MUSCLE IMBALANCES

Considering the sustained posture required to maneuver your board and boom, muscle imbalances can become apparent. Imbalances common to the sport of windsurfing are weaker hand and wrist extensors in comparison to their counterparts, the flexors; a weaker upper back as compared to the chest; and weaker gluteals and hamstrings as compared to the quadriceps. When physically preparing yourself for the challenges of windsurfing, consider training these usually weaker areas more intensely than their stronger counterparts. The functional exercises listed in this chapter will challenge your musculoskeletal system to respond with improved functional muscular balance.

WARM-UP

Before windsurfing, consider doing all or parts of the following warm-up to prepare yourself for the agility and flexibility demands. Do the Dynamic Warm-up in chapter 4. Before your in-city workouts, consider doing a modified warm-up consisting of 5 minutes of aerobic activity; the Carioca, Crazy Legs, and Shuffle Run (chapter

4); followed by stretching Exercises 7, 10, 11, 13, 15, and 16.

STRETCHING

Adequate flexibility of your ankles, knees, and hips along with spinal and shoulder mobility is essential for windsurfing. Do Exercises 1, 3, 5.1, 5.2, and 7–18, 3–4 times per week.

AEROBIC CONDITIONING

A good windsurfing run may last up to 30 minutes. This duration places a great deal of aerobic demands on your body. Do the minimum aerobic program in chapter 2, Aerobic Conditioning and Interval Training. Make sure that 2 sessions per week are 40 minutes long. Aerobic training options are running, using a stair-climber, using an EFX cross trainer, using cross-country ski machines, or using rowing ergometers.

STRENGTH TRAINING

The exercises listed below are designed to enhance your ability to meet the key physical components of windsurfing. Make sure to do the warm-up and stretching exercises described above before starting your strengthening program.

For best results, select 3–4 exercises from each category and construct a 12-station circuit. Perform each exercise for 45–60 seconds. This is a very effective way of challenging and enhancing your response to the physical demands of windsurfing. If you choose to exercise each body region individually, choose 3–4 exercises and follow the recommended number of sets and reps from the chapters indicated.

BEGINNING

Upper body: Exercises 35; 82 or 86; *89, 90, or 102; 91.1; 91.2; 92; *98; and 100.

Abdominals: Exercises 56.3, 58.1, 58.2, *60, *61, *62, 64, and 67.

Lower Body: Exercises *28, 28.1, 36.7, 70, 70.2, 72, and 72.3.

Upper/lower body: Exercises *28, *30, *104, 104.2, and 106.

INTERMEDIATE/ADVANCED

Upper body: Do the beginning program above.

Abdominals: Do the beginning program above.

Lower body: Do the beginning program above, adding Exercises 26, 27, *75.1, 75.4, and 75.5, and omitting Exercise 72.

Upper/lower body: Do the beginning program above.

BALANCE AND AGILITY

Because your board is continually moving, good balance and agility in all directions are crucial to coordinate your board and boom. Do Exercises 37, 37.1, 37.3, 37.4, *38.1, 38.2, 38.3, 40, 75.5, 75.6, and 121–123. For advanced agility training do Exercise 125.

General Aerobic Conditioning and Strength Training

BY MARK PIERCE, A.T.C., AND DAVID MUSNICK, M.D.

▶ **THIS CHAPTER WILL HELP YOU:**
• Develop a basic aerobic and functional strength and balance program for general fitness.

If you do not have specific outdoor activity goals, you can still benefit from a well-designed fitness program. Integrating functional balance and strength training can improve your ability to meet the challenges of daily activity and of many sports. This type of program could be your only strength training or it could be added to your present program to make it more functional. If you have musculoskeletal problems, you may need to modify the exercises listed in this chapter. The exercises in this chapter are designed to help you improve general muscle strength and tone, stimulate growth hormone to improve your ratio of lean body mass, and establish a base for progressing to more specific activity training.

MUSCULOSKELETAL DEMANDS
Maintaining your muscle mass and bone density is very important throughout your life. A certain amount of strength is required to conduct your daily activities and avoid repetitive stress and acute injuries. Child care, household chores, gardening, shopping and carrying luggage while traveling are all common activities that impose musculoskeletal demands on our bodies. Appropriate exercise can enable you to do such activities with a lower likelihood of injury.

MUSCLE IMBALANCES
Generally, common muscle imbalances occur because of poor posture, problems in your spine or or the joints of your extremities, or conditions resulting from previous injuries. Refer to chapter 4 for information on common patterns of tight muscles and chapter 9 for patterns of weak and inhibited muscles. You may wish to see a health professional trained in biomechanics and kinesiology as well as muscle testing and joint function to determine if you have any particular structural imbalances.

WARM-UP
A warm-up is always recommended prior to any activity that stresses your muscles, joints, or cardiovascular system. Performing these warm-up activities helps prepare your body for strenuous activities and decreases your chances of injury. Perform the Aerobic Warm-up, with or without

the Weight-lifting Warm-up, described in chapter 4 before starting your general conditioning program.

FLEXIBILITY

Consider doing Exercises 1, 3, 5, 8, 9, 17, and 19.

AEROBIC TRAINING

Do the Minimum Aerobic Program, described in chapter 2.

STRENGTH TRAINING
INTERMEDIATE

Do the following exercises 2–3 times a week for best results:

Lower body: Exercises 70, 70.4, and 71.

Abdominals: Exercises 56.3 (2–3 sets of 15 reps), 58 (2 sets of 30- to 45-second intervals), 61 (2 sets of 12–15 reps on each side), 62 (2 sets of 12–15 reps to each side of your body), and 67 (2 sets of 12–15 reps).

Upper body: Try the following exercises in the order given. All exercises can be done in 2–3 sets of 12–15 repetitions. Exercises 86, 88, 91, 92, 96, 98, and 102.

Upper/lower body: Exercises 20, 21, 23, and 31.

ADVANCED

Do the intermediate program above, plus:
Upper/lower body: Exercise 26.1.

BALANCE AND AGILITY

Balance is the most fundamental component of function. Good balance enables you to move, change direction, reach, push or pull objects, and control your body on unstable surfaces. As your balance becomes more efficient, invariably your normal activities become more efficient. Do Exercises 38, 38.1, 39, and 40.

GENERAL TRAINING PROGRAM FOR OLDER OR DECONDITIONED INDIVIDUALS

If you have arthritis or balance problems or feel generally out of condition, follow the recommendations below. Consider seeing a physical therapist or athletic trainer skilled in strength and balance training.

STRENGTH TRAINING

Lower body: Focus on regular squats, Exercise 70, before you do single-leg squats, Exercise 70.2. Do lunges, Exercise 72, with minimum knee bending at first, and progress gradually to about 60 degrees. When you feel comfortable with the basic lunge, progress to Exercise 72.3 and then add Exercises 23 and 24 to add arm work and balance challenges to the lunge. Your lunge should be done in functional motions to simulate your needs for movement in the kitchen, in the yard, and in your normal activities. If you have knee pain with a regular lunge, do Exercise 72.1. Practice Exercise 47 and apply the concepts to Exercises 73 and 74.

Abdominals: Do Exercises 56.1, 56.2, 57.1, and 62.

Upper body: Focus on biceps, Exercise 23 or 96; modified push-ups, Exercise 101.1, and knee push-ups, Exercise 86.1; and dips, Exercise 98 (with most of your weight assisted by the machine) or squat/dip chair combo: Focus on these dips for getting out of chairs etc. (Use a stable chair with sturdy armrests. In this dip, hold onto the armrests and straighten your elbows while you assist by pushing with your legs. This is similar to a simultaneous squat and dip.)

BALANCE AND AGILITY
Do Exercises 39 and 40.

Special Issues for the Conditioning Woman

By Jane A. Moore, M.D.

▶ **THIS CHAPTER WILL HELP YOU:**
- Learn about eating disorders and how they can lead to health problems in women.
- Understand menstrual disorders and the relationship to osteoporosis and injuries.
- Understand special nutritional needs of women.
- Learn about osteoporosis in younger and older women.

We are gaining information on problems specific to women athletes, including unique medical and nutrition problems and the effects of training on the menstrual cycle. Can women be as good as men in outdoor activities such as kayaking, hiking, rock climbing, and glacial mountaineering? Absolutely! In these activities, there are no significant limiting factors based on male vs. female physiology and structure.

WEIGHT CONTROL AND DISORDERED EATING

Attempts to control weight in order to improve performance are very common in women athletes. One study found that 32% of collegiate women athletes used vomiting, laxatives, diuretics, or diet pills on a regular basis. Such behavior is more common in women involved in endurance sports, sports with weight classes, and sports where judging can be influenced by appearance, but may be seen in athletes in any sport.

Eating disorders that lead to decreased calorie intake are more common in women than men because of cultural patterns in regard to appearance and self-esteem and expected norms for female athletes. The spectrum of disordered eating behaviors ranges from mild to severe. Behavior may progress from mild disturbances to the severe, clinically defined disorders of anorexia or bulimia.

Anorexia nervosa is a medical syndrome in which the individual consumes an inadequate number of food calories compared to the amount they need to maintain their body weight at a reasonable level for their age, height, build, etc. Characteristics of anorexia nervosa include:

1. refusal to maintain body weight at or above 85% of that expected for age and height
2. intense fear of gaining weight or becoming fat, even when very thin
3. disturbance in the way one's body weight

or shape is perceived, or seeing oneself as fat even when one is very thin

4. undue influence of body weight or shape on self-evaluation
5. denial of the seriousness of a low body weight
6. amenorrhea, or the absence of at least three consecutive menstrual cycles after periods have become established

Bulimia is a medical problem in which a person may take in adequate calories but will try to decrease the amount their body retains by vomiting or using laxatives. Characteristics include:

1. recurrent episodes of binge eating (at least twice a week for 3 months)
2. recurrent inappropriate compensatory behavior or purging (at least twice a week for 3 months)
3. self-evaluation unduly influenced by body shape and weight

Personality traits such as compulsiveness, perfectionism, and high achievement expectations may help a high-level athlete but may also be associated with the development of disturbed eating patterns. Low self-esteem is common in those with disordered eating, and there may be a history of previous sexual or physical abuse. A woman may also lack a sense of identity other than being an athlete.

An athlete suspected of disordered eating should be approached thoughtfully about the problem. It is appropriate to see a medical professional when this problem is recognized.

DISORDERS OF MENSTRUAL FUNCTION

Disorders of menstrual function can occur in women as a result of an intense conditioning program in relation to inadequate calories consumed. These include changes in the cycle length, lack of ovulation, and lack of periods (amenorrhea). Secondary amenorrhea is the absence of 3–6 consecutive menstrual cycles in a woman who has already been menstruating. Exercise-associated amenorrhea may be related to vigorous/high-volume exercise and to inadequate calorie intake to meet energy balance. Athletic women with amenorrhea or infrequent periods are at risk for early osteoporosis because of low female hormone (especially estrogen) levels. A very low level of estrogen can lead to calcium and bone density losses.

PRACTICAL POINT
If you have stopped menstruating for more than 2 cycles, seek a medical evaluation. It could help prevent serious medical problems.

OSTEOPOROSIS AND CALCIUM AND OTHER NUTRIENT SUPPLEMENTATION

Osteoporosis is a disease associated with extensive bone density loss. This results in low bone mass and changes in bony architecture that can lead to fragile bones and an increased risk of stress and regular fractures. It is most common in women after menopause. It may occur at any age when bone mass falls below a critical threshold. Women with absent or infrequent periods might have hormonal levels similar to those of post-menopausal women and so may develop premature osteoporosis.

Exercise, calcium intake, and reproductive hormone status are major factors in controling bone density. Bone mass declines with age because the remodeling (rebuilding) process is inefficient and results in a small deficit at the end of each cycle of remodeling. These deficits gradually accumulate, resulting in the decline in bone mass. Peak bone mass is a factor in protection from osteoporotic fractures. Peak bone mass is reached in the early to mid 20s in women. After this, women lose up to 1% per year until menopause. They may lose 4%–6% per year for the first 4–5 years after menopause. Men maintain bone mass until about age 50, after which they lose about 0.4%–0.5% per year.

PRACTICAL POINT

To decrease the risks of osteoporosis, consider combining:

- strength training, especially of the arms
- low- to moderate-impact aerobic exercise of the legs
- calcium with vitamin D (from the sun, or supplemented in foods or a multiple vitamin of 100–400 units per day)
- minimal soft drink consumption
- other minerals, including magnesium, zinc, copper, manganese, boron, and silicon
- hormone replacement, especially in the post-menopausal woman
- treatment for menstrual disorders if you are a premenopausal female

---

Calcium is stored in the skeleton. Adequate amounts of calcium and other minerals in the diet are required to maintain healthy bones. Dietary calcium is most critical during the adolescent growth spurt and into the 30s, so that peak bone mass can reach its full potential. Large amounts of caffeine, phosphorous, and protein in the diet may increase calcium loss. Exercise is an important component in maintaining bone mass. Physical activity provides mechanical stress to bone, which stimulates bone formation. It is important to do strength training such as bicep curls and modified dips so as to put forces through the forearm to help prevent significant declines in arm bone density. Aerobic exercise that involves moderate-impact loading through the feet and legs (see chapter 2) can help slow bone loss in the hips and spine. Women should do impact-loaded aerobic exercise 3–5 times per week as part of their conditioning program.

RECOMMENDED DAILY AMOUNTS OF CALCIUM

Adolescence and up to age 24:
1,200 mg per day
Post-adolescence and premenopause:
800–1,200 mg per day
Pregnancy and menopause:
1,500 mg per day

Sources of calcium include milk products (about 300 mg per 8 ounces), broccoli, canned salmon, soy products, and calcium supplements. In general, calcium bound to amino acids (calcium citrate, etc.) is more absorbable than the calcium carbonate and calcium oxide forms. Calcium in the form of hydroxapatite is also a highly beneficial form.

THE FEMALE ATHLETE TRIAD

The female athlete triad refers to the combination of amenorrhea, osteoporosis, and disordered eating. If a female athlete has disordered eating and a high training volume, she is more likely to develop amenorrhea. If she develops both of these conditions, she is more likely to develop early osteoporosis and possibly stress fractures. If a woman with the triad doesn't receive early medical attention, she can have serious medical problems.

HORMONES AND BIRTH CONTROL PILLS

Birth control pills can have numerous side effects, including a risk of thrombosis (excessive clotting) in the deep veins of the legs, pelvis, etc. This may manifest with calf swelling or pain in the leg, thigh, or chest. Chest pain and shortness of breath at rest, or markedly decreased stamina, are more serious symptoms. Women on climbing expeditions or other prolonged outdoor trips should be aware of this risk. Consider going off of the medication approximately 2–4 weeks before the trip and using another form of birth control. If you experience any of the above symptoms while on or off birth control pills, seek medical attention promptly.

MENOPAUSE

Exercise is extremely important for the post-menopausal woman because it can help decrease risks of cardiovascular disease, maintain a good body image, slow down osteoporosis, and maintain good strength and balance. Low- to moderate-impact aerobic exercise and strength training can have a role in decreasing the decline of bone density. Balance training and functional strength training exercises, such as lunges and mini-squats, can be helpful to prevent falls that could lead to hip, spine, and wrist fractures.

APPENDIX

U.S.-METRIC CONVERSIONS

	U.S.	*METRIC*
WEIGHT		
	1 ounce	28.35 grams (g)
	1 pound	453.59 grams (g)
	1 pound	0.454 kilograms (kg)
LENGTH		
	1 inch	2.54 centimeters (cm)
	1 foot	30.48 centimeters (cm)
	1 yard	9.1 meters (m)
	1 mile	1600 meters (m)
	1 mile	1.6 kilometers (km)

METRIC-U.S. CONVERSIONS

	METRIC	*U.S.*
WEIGHT		
	1 gram (g)	0.035274 ounces
	1 kilogram (kg)	35.274 ounces
	1 kilogram (kg)	2.2046 pounds
LENGTH		
	1 centimeter (cm)	0.3937 inches
	1 meter (m)	39.37 inches
	1 meter (m)	3.281 feet
	1 meter (m)	1.0936 yards
	1 kilometer (km)	0.6 mile

Selected References

CHAPTER 1

Adams, J. Crawford. *Outline of Orthopedics*. 10th ed. New York: Longman Group, 1986.

Ainsworth, B. E., et al. "The Compendium of Physical Activities; Classification of Energy Costs of Human Physical Activities." *Medicine and Science in Sports and Exercise* Vol. 25, No. 1 (Jan. 1993).

Graydon, Don, ed. *Mountaineering: The Freedom of the Hills*. Seattle: The Mountaineers, 1997.

McArdle, William D., Frank I. Katch, and Victor L. Katch. *Exercise Physiology*. Baltimore: Williamson Wilkins, 1996.

CHAPTER 2

Bakoulisbloch, Gordon. *Cross Training*. New York: Simon and Schuster, 1992.

Edwards, Sally. *The Heart Rate Monitor Book*. Sacramento, Calif.: Heart Zones Co., 1993.

————. *Exercise Smart, Stay Fit and Live Longer*. Holbrook, Mass.: Adams Publishing, 1996.

Paffenbarger, Ralph F. Jr., M.D., and Eric Olson. *Life Fit*. Champaign, Ill.: Human Kinetics Publishing, 1996.

Shephard, Roy. *Aerobic Fitness and Health*. Champaign, Ill.: Human Kinetics Publishing, 1994.

CHAPTER 3

Ainsworth, B. E., et al. "Compendium . . . " (see under Chapter 1)

American Dietetics and American Diabetes Associations. *The Exchange Lists for Meal Planning*. 1995.

Foster-Powell, Kaye, and J. Branch-Miller. "International Table of Glycemic Index." *The American Journal of Clinical Nutrition* Vol. 62, supplement (1995): 871-8930

Berning, S., and S. N. Steen. *Nutrition for Sport and Exercise*. Gaithersburg, Md.: Aspen Publishing, 1998.

Bland, Jeffrey, Ph.D. *20-Day Rejuvenation Diet Program*. New Canaan, Conn.: Keats Publishing, 1997.

Broun, Fred. *Nutritional Needs of Athletes*. New York: John Wiley and Sons, 1995.

Clark, Nancy, M.S., R.D. *First Nutrition Guidebook*. 2d ed. Champaign, Ill.: Human Kinetics Publishing, 1997.

Gaby, Allan R., M.D. *Preventing and Reversing Osteoporosis*. Rocklin, Calif.: Prima Publishing, 1994.

Kleiner, Susan M., Ph.D., R.D. *High-Performance Nutrition*. New York: John Wiley and Sons, 1996.

Lukaczer, Dan. *Functional Medicine: Adjunctive Nutritional Support for Syndrome X*. Gig Harbor, Wash.: Health Comm International, Inc., 1998.

Sears, Barry, Ph.D. *Enter the Zone*. New York: Regan Books, 1995.

Wolinksy, Ira, ed. *Nutrition in Exercise and Sport*. Boca Raton, Fla.: CRC Press LLC, 1998.

CHAPTER 4

Anderson, B., and E. R. Burke. "Scientific, Medical and Practical Aspects of Stretching." *Sports Medicine* Vol. 10 No. 1 (1991).

Anderson, R. A. *Stretching*. Bolinas, Calif.: Shelter Publications, 1980.

Janda, Vladimir, and Gwendolen A. Jull. "Muscles and Motor Control in Low Back Pain: Assessment and Management," in *Physical Therapy of the Low Back*. Lantz K. Twomey and James R. Taylor, eds. New York: Churchill Livingstone, 1987.

McAtee, R. *Facilitated Stretching*. Champaign, Ill.: Human Kinetics Publishing, 1993.

Powers, S. K., and E. T. Howley. *Exercise Physiology*. Madison, Wis.: Brown and Benchmark, 1994.

Smith, C. A. "The Warm Up Procedure: To Stretch or Not to Stretch." Review, *Journal of Orthopaedic and Sports Physical Therapy*, Vol. 19, No. 1 (1994): 12–17.

CHAPTER 5

Anderson, Bob. *Getting in Shape*. Bolinas, Calif.: Shelter Publications, 1994.

Baechle, Thomas R., ed. *Essentials of Strength Training and Conditioning*. Champaign, Ill.: National Strength and Conditioning Association and Human Kinetics Publishing, 1994.

Fleck, Steven J., and W. J. Kraemer. *Designing Resistance Training Programs*. Champaign, Ill.: Human Kinetics Publishing, 1997.

Gray, Gary. *Chain Reaction Festival*. Adrian, Mich.: Wynn Marketing, 1996.

————. *Lower Extremity Functional Profile*. Adrian, Mich.: Wynn Marketing, 1995.

White, Thomas P. *The Wellness Guide to Lifelong Fitness*. New York: Rebus, 1993.

CHAPTER 6

Physical Therapy Today. Summer 1991.

Physical Therapy Today. Fall 1993.

CHAPTER 7

Galloway, Jeff. *Galloway's Book of Running*. Bolinas, Calif.: Shelter Publications, 1984.

Gambetta, Vern. "Building the Complete Athlete," in *Optimum Sports Training*. 4th ed. Performance Conditioning, Inc., 1997.

Gray, Gary W. *Chain Reaction Festival*. Adrian, Mich.: Wynn Marketing, 1996.

Sleamaker, Ross. *Serious Training for Serious Athletes*. Champaign, Ill.: Leisure Press, 1989.

CHAPTER 9

Hall, Carrie F., and Lori Theim-Brody, eds. *Therapeutic Exercise: Moving Toward Function*. Philadelphia: Lippincott, Williamson Wilkins, 1999.

Kendall, Florence. *Muscles: Testing and Function*. 4th ed. Philadelphia: Williamson Wilkins, 1993.

Renstrom, P. *Sports Injuries, Basic Principles of Prevention and Care*. London: Blackwell Scientific Publications, 1993.

Zachazewski, James E., David J. McGee, and William F. Quill. *Athletic Injuries and Rehabilitation*. Philadelphia: W. B. Saunders Co., 1996.

CHAPTER 10

Gray, Gary. 1995 (see under Chapter 5).

Hall, Carrie F. (see under Chapter 9).

Hall, Carrie M. *Fitness in Balance*. Unpublished handbook. St. Louis, Mo.: Professional Physical Therapy, 1989.

Kendall, Florence (see under Chapter 9).

Sahrmann, S. A., et al. "Diagnosis and Treatment of Muscle Imbalances and Musculoskeletal Pain Syndromes." Course notes presented at a seminar in Seattle, 1995.

CHAPTER 11

Gray, Gary. 1995 (see under Chapter 5).

Hall, Carrie F. (see under Chapter 9).

Kendall, Florence (see under Chapter 9).

Mangine, R. E. *Physical Therapy of the Knee: Anatomy and Biomechanics*. New York: Churchill Livingstone, 1988.

Marshall, J. L., F. G. Girgis, and R. R. Zelko. "The Biceps Femoris Tendon and Its Functional Significance." *Journal of Bone and Joint Surgery* Vol. 54, No. 1444 (1972).

Seebacher, J. R., A. E. Inglis, and R. F. Warren. "The Structure of the Posterolateral Aspect of the Knee." *Journal of Bone and Joint Surgery* Vol. 64A, No. 536 (1982).

Warren, L. F., and J. L. Marshall. "The Supporting Structures and Layers on the Medial Side of the Knee." *Journal of Bone and Joint Surgery* Vol. 61A, No. 56 (1979).

Williams, P. L., R. Warwick, M. Dyson, and L. H. Bannister. *Gray's Anatomy*. 37th British ed. London: Longman, 1989.

CHAPTER 12

Gray, Gary. 1995 (see under Chapter 5).

Hall, Carrie F. (see under Chapter 9).

Selected References

CHAPTER 13
Hall, Carrie F. (see under Chapter 9).
Nawoczenski, Deborah, et al. *Orthotics in Functional Rehabilitation of the Lower Limb.* Philadelphia: W. B. Saunders Co., 1997.

CHAPTER 14
Janda, Vladimir (see under Chapter 4).
Vleeming, Andry. *Movement, Stability and Low Back Pain.* New York: Churchill Livingstone, 1997.

CHAPTER 15
Baechle, Thomas R., ed. (see under Chapter 5).
Gray, Gary W. *Chain Reaction Plus.* Adrian, Mich.: Wynn Marketing, 1994.
Hall, Carrie F. (see under Chapter 9).
Hall, Carrie M. 1989 (see under Chapter 10).
Kendall, Florence (see under Chapter 9).
Keshner, E. A. "Controlling Stability of a Complex System." *Physical Therapy* Vol. 70 (1990): 854–84.
Norkin, C., et al. *Joint: Structure and Function.* Philadelphia: F. A. Davis Co., 1983.
Pearl, B., et al. *Getting Stronger.* Bolinas, Calif.: Shelter Publications, 1986.
Sahrmann, S. A., et al. "Diagnosis and Treatment of Muscle Imbalances and Musculoskeletal Pain Syndromes." Course notes presented at seminar in Seattle, 1995.

CHAPTER 16
Hall, Carrie F. (see under Chapter 9).

CHAPTER 17
Edwards, Sally. *Snowshoeing.* Champaign, Ill.: Human Kinetics Publishing, 1995.
Graydon, Don, ed. (see under Chapter 1).
Griffin, S. *Snowshoeing.* Mechanicsburg, Pa.: Stackpole Books, 1998.
Seeborg, E. *Hiking and Backpacking.* Champagne, Ill.: Human Kinetics Publishing, 1994.

CHAPTER 18
Goddard, Dale, and Uno Neumann. *Performance Rock Climbing.* Mechanicsburg, Pa.: Stackpole Books, 1993.

Graydon, Don, ed. (see under Chapter 1).
Holtzhausen, Lucy-May, and T. Noakes. " Elbow, Forearm, and Hand Injuries Among Sport Rock Climbers," in *Clinical Journal of Sport Medicine* Vol. 6, No. 3. Philadelphia: Lippincott Raven Publishing, 1996.
Horst, Eric. *How to Rock Climb Series: Flash Training.* Evergreen, Colo.: Chockstone Press, 1994.
Long, John. *How to Rock Climb Series: Gym Climb!* Evergreen, Colo.: Chockstone Press, 1994.

CHAPTER 19
Graydon, Don, ed. (see under Chapter 1).

CHAPTER 20
Gullion, Lori. *Nordic Skiing: Steps to Success.* Champaign, Ill.: Human Kinetics Publishing, 1993.
Hart, L. *The Snowboard Book.* New York: W. W. Norton Co., 1997.
Witherell, W. *The Athletic Skier.* Boulder, Colo.: Johnson Books, 1993.

CHAPTER 21
Borne, Gilbert C. *A Textbook of Oarsmanship: A Classic of Rowing Technical Literature.* Toronto: Sports Book Publishers, 1987.
Cunningham, F. *The Sculler at Ease.* Boulder, Colo.: Avery Press, 1992.
Gullion, L. *Canoeing and Kayak Instruction Manual.* Birmingham, Ala.: American Canoe Association and Menasha Ridge Press, 1987.
Heed, P., and Dick Fansfied. *Canoe Racing.* Syracuse, N.Y.: Acorn Publishing, 1992.

CHAPTER 22
Bompa, Tudor O. *Theory and Method of Training: The Key to Athletic Performance.* 3d ed. Dubuque, Iowa: Kendall/Hunt Publishing, 1994.
Broker, Jeff, Ph.D. Paper presented at the Elite Coaching Symposium/International Symposium USA Cycling 1997. Colorado Springs, Colorado.
Davis, D. *Mountain Biking.* Champaign, Ill.: Human Kinetics Publishing, 1994.
LeMond, Greg, and Kent Gordis. *Greg LeMond's*

Complete Book of Bicycling. New York: Putnam Publishing Group, 1990.

Lombardi, Blair. *Bicycling in Balance Instruction*. Paper presented at the Elite Coaching Symposium/International Symposium USA Cycling 1997. Colorado Springs, Colorado.

USA Cycling, Inc. *Training Manuals*. Colorado Springs, Colo.: USA Cycling, 1996.

CHAPTER 23

Brown, R. *Fitness Running*. Champaign, Ill.: Human Kinetics Publishing, 1994.

Burfoot, A. *Runners World Complete Book of Running*. Emmaus, Pa.: Rodale Press, 1997.

Galloway, Jeff. (see under Chapter 7).

Triathlete Magazine, Sept. 1994.

CHAPTER 24

Winner, K. *Windsurfing*. Champaign, Ill.: Human Kinetics Publishing, 1995.

CHAPTER 25

Baechle, Thomas R., ed. (see under Chapter 5).

Gray, Gary. *Chain Reaction*. Adrian, Mich.: Wynn Marketing, 1998.

Mahler, Donald A. ACSM *Guidelines for Exercise Testing and Prescription*. Philadelphia: Lippincott, Williamson Wilkins, 1995.

Roitman, Jeffrey. ACSM *Resource Manual for Guidelines for Exercise Testing and Prescription*. 3d ed. Philadelphia: Lippincott, Williamson Wilkins, 1998.

White, Timothy P. *The Wellness Guide to Lifelong Fitness*. New York: Random House, 1993.

CHAPTER 26

Agostini, Rosemary, M.D. "The Athletic Woman." *Sports Medicine* Vol. 13, No. 2 (April 1994).

———. *Medical and Orthopedic Issues of Active and Athletic Women*. Philadelphia: Hanley and Belfus, 1994.

American College of Sports Medicine. "The Female Athlete Triad." Unpublished slide set. Indianapolis: American College of Sports Medicine, n.d.

Gaby, A. *Preventing and Reversing Osteoporosis*. Rocklin, Calif.: Prima Publishing, 1994.

Haycock, Christine, M.D., ed. *Sports Medicine for the Athletic Female*. Oradell, N.J.: Medical Economics Books, 1980.

Shangold, M., and G. Mirkin. *Women and Exercise: Physiology and Medicine*. Philadelphia: F. A. Davis Co., 1988.

Walsh, W. Michael, M.D. "The Athletic Woman." *Sports Medicine* Vol. 3, No. 4 (Oct. 1984).

Index

Index

Index

Index

Exercise Index

Letters listed after exercise indicate abilities or functions improved. Agility (Ag), balance (B) and or strength or function of one or more of these body regions: abdomen (A), shoulder region (S), Buttock (Bu), Legs (L).

CHAPTER 4

CHAPTER 5

CHAPTER 6

CHAPTER 8

CHAPTER 16

CHAPTER 18

CHAPTER 20

CHAPTER 22

Acknowledgments

I would like to thank the following people: my family, for their encouragement; Gary Gray, P.T., for his excellent exercise seminars and insights in closed kinetic chain exercise; Jock Bradley for his kind donation of his photography services for many of the exercise photos in the book; Sandy Elliott, P.T., for helping out in the photography and organizational efforts; and Mark Pierce, A.T.C., for his encouragement, many hours of work, and creativity in exercise design. For further information on Dr. Musnick's practice, refer to his website:

http//www.musnick.com.

David Musnick, M.D.

My devoted thanks go to the following people for making my work on this project possible: my parents, James and Janet Pierce, for their balance of knowledge, wisdom, and understanding, from which I and my four brothers find our sense of self; David Musnick for his friendship, encouragement, and the opportunity to help write this book; Gary Gray, for his insightful seminars on biomechanics and functional exercise; my business partner, Neil Chasen, for his inspired creativity and constant support; Tim Salo, for helping with the windsurfing chapter; and to my life partner and soulmate, Janet Wong, for her inspired thoughts while tolerating the many hours spent working on the book. Thank you all.

Mark Pierce, A.T.C.

About the Contributors

Judith Aston, M.F.A., is the originator of Aston-Patterning. She teaches internationally and maintains a practice in Incline, Nevada.

Kimberly B. Bennett, Ph.D., P.T., is an orthopedic manual physical therapist at Olympic Physical Therapy in Seattle, with 18 years in practice, and is a clinical assistant professor in the physical therapy department at the University of Washington. Bennett has a Ph.D. in anatomy. Her practice emphasizes care of multisystem orthopedic problems, including acute and chronic spine and peripheral joint dysfunction, and various arthritides including fibromyalgia.

Sherri Cassuto is a Certified Rolfer® with a private practice in Seattle. She was on the 1984 U.S. Olympic Sweep Rowing Team and the 1988 U.S. Olympic Sculling Team. In the 1988 World Masters Games she won silver medals in single and double marathon canoeing. She is an avid sea kayaker and a reasonable whitewater kayaker.

Dan Cauthorn is co-founder and director of instruction at Vertical World, America's first indoor rock climbing gym, located in Seattle. A graduate of Western Washington University, he has taught, trained, and guided climbers since 1978. He is a Seattle native who began climbing in the Cascades at an early age. He has completed numerous difficult ascents in mountains from Alaska to Patagonia, including Cerro Torre and Burkett Needle.

Dorothy Sager Dolan, B.A., L.M.P., is a personal trainer and massage therapist in Seattle. She works for Technogym, an exercise equipment company in Seattle.

Sandy Elliott, P.T., is a physical therapist at Olympic Physical Therapy in Mercer Island, Washington. She assisted with photography sessions and initial organizational work on the book, especially Part II, Body Regions.

Lisa Fox, P.T., is a physical therapist in private practice in Seattle. She is an avid runner.

Joani Gelinas, P.T., is a physical therapist and certified Aston-Patterning practitioner in Seattle. She incorporates the Aston-Patterning movement principles in her treatment of patients.

Carrie Hall, M.H.S., P.T., is a physical therapist at and owner of Movement Systems Physical Therapy. She is on the clinical faculty in physical therapy at the University of Washington and a national instructor on the topic of muscle imbalances from the Shirley Sahrmann physical therapy approach. Hall is the author of *Therapeutic Exercise: Moving Toward Function,* published in 1999.

Michael Hansen, P.T., is a specialist in functional exercise at Biosports in Wenatchee, Washington.

Rich Harrington is owner of Sound Mind and Body Gyms in Seattle. He teaches ski conditioning classes at Sound Mind and Body and is an avid skier.

Craig London, P.T., is the owner of Olympic Physical Therapy in Everett, Washington. He is an avid climber.

Mark Looper, M.S., P.T., C.O.M.T., holds a master's degree in physical therapy from the University of Southern California. He is a nationally recognized speaker, instructing for the McConnell Institute, and provides therapeutic care for the Seattle Sea Dogs, a professional indoor soccer team. Mark received his certification in manual therapy (C.O.M.T.) from the North American Institute of Manual Therapy, and is the owner of Olympic Physical Therapy in Kirkland, Washington.

Bobbi Lutack, N.D., is a naturopathic physician at Evergreen Natural Health Clinic in Seattle. Her specialty is nutrition and sports medicine.

Sara Meeker, P.T., is a physical therapist at Movement Systems Physical Therapy in Seattle.

Erik Moen, P.T., is a physical therapist at and clinical director of Physiotherapy Associates, Lynnwood Orthopedic and Sports Physical Therapy Clinic. Moen is a certified strength and conditioning specialist and elite-level coach through the U.S. Cycling Federation. Moen has coached Northwest cyclists who have won Masters World Championships in mountain bike and velodrome racing, and participants in Hawaiian, German, and Canadian Ironman Triathlons. Moen competes in road and velodrome bicycle racing.

Jane A. Moore, M.D., F.A.A.F.P., F.A.C.S.M., of the Family Health Center in Tacoma, Washington, has been in private practice of family and sports medicine since 1984. She has much experience with women's health, U.S. swimming, and U.S. masters swimming sports medicine.

Leslie Moskowitz, M.S., R.D., is a registered dietician living in New Jersey. She does consulting and clinical work with sports medicine and family practice patients.

David Musnick, M.D., M.P.H., is a sports and internal medicine physician at the Sports Medicine Clinic in Seattle and at the Northwest Center for Environmental Medicine in Bellevue, Washington. In his private practice he specializes in exercise planning, nutrition, functional medicine, and nonsurgical approaches to musculoskeletal injuries and pain problems. He is an instructor in the Department of Ortho-

paedics at the University of Washington. He teaches orthopaedics and sports medicine at Bastyr University. He has contributed to two books and written numerous health education pamphlets on orthopaedic problems. He is a frequent lecturer for The Mountaineers Club on conditioning for various outdoor activities. He has taught hiking, backpacking, cross-country skiing, rock climbing, canoeing, and mountaineering. He works out regularly and is an avid hiker, backpacker, scrambler, snowshoer, and cross-country skier.

Dan Nelson, M.S., D.C., D.A.B.C.O., is clinical director and founder of Olympic Rehabilitation Specialties. He has a master of science in exercise physiology from the University of Washington, and 13 years of experience in competitive rowing. His training in biomechanics and orthopaedics has resulted in a diagnostic protocol based in identifying functional deficits. He does research with Group Health Cooperative and teaches exercise physiology and rehabilitation in the postgraduate faculties of three chiropractic colleges. He emphasizes use of osseous manipulation to enhance normal joint function coupled with exercise prescription. He is currently implementing a back fitness testing program to identify patients at risk for back problems and to help direct specific conditioning exercise programs to meet the patients' lifestyle.

Darcy Norman, A.T.C., C.S.C.S., has been a practicing certified athletic trainer and strength and conditioning specialist since 1992. He currently is working toward a physical therapy degree at the University of Washington. He is president of AdvancedFitness in Seattle. He competed internationally in all four disciplines of alpine skiing.

Carl Petersen, P.T., has worked for 12 years as a physiotherapist/fitness coordinator of the Canadian Alpine Ski Team and has recently been appointed the director of sport science for Alpine Canada. He has coached and designed recovery programs for Olympic, World Champion, and World Cup medalists as well as for weekend and recreational-level athletes. Petersen, who resides in Vancouver, British Columbia, lectures nationally and internationally and has published more than 50 articles.

Mark Pierce, A.T.C., is an owner of the Sports Reaction Center in Bellevue, Washington, a physical therapy and sports rehabilitation clinic dedicated to athletes' recovery from orthopedic injuries and physical enhancement. A sports medicine practitioner certified by the National Athletic Trainers Association, Pierce has more than 15 years of clinical and field experience in multiple settings. His unique interest in the science of biomechanics and the enhancement of human performance has enabled him to link musculoskeletal rehabilitation and sports-specific conditioning. A two-time NCAA All-American in track and field, Pierce was also the winner of top regional body-building competitions.

John Rumpeltes, P.T., is a physical therapist at Olympic Physical Therapy in Seattle. He specializes in manual therapy.

Peter Shmock, C.S.C.S., is a two-time Olympian in track and field who is nationally known for his nontraditional approach to athletic performance training. He worked as the director of strength and conditioning for the Seattle Mariners for 11 years and currently works with Pacific Northwest Ballet. He is a private fitness trainer for executives, youth, recreational athletes, and fitness professionals. Schmock specializes in outdoor and functional strength training; he was one of three top finalists for the Nike Fitness Innovation Award.

Katrina Sullivan, D.P.M., is a podiatrist at the Joslin Clinic in Seattle.

Maria Zanoni, P.T., is a physical therapist at Olympic Spinal Care in Seattle. She specializes in manual therapy and functional exercise.

Photo and Illustration Credits

Jock Bradley: Figures 3, 7a–c, 8, 22, 23a–b, 25a–b, 27 and Exercises 2.1, 3, 4, 9a–b, 29.1, 29.4, 34, 35, 37.3a–b, 39a–b, 25a–c, 56, 56.1a–b, 56.2a–b, 56.3a–b, 56.4, 56.5a–b, 57a–b, 57.1, 57.2, 74, 74.3, 77, 78, 86.1, 88, 88.1, 88.2, 88.3, 91, 91.1a–b, 93a–b, 113, 115a–f, 116a–b, 117a–b, 118a–c. 51a–b, 52.1, 52.3, 53.1, 55.2a–c, 58, 59, 60a–b, 61a–b, 62, 63.1, 63.2, 64a–b, 65a–b, 66a–b, 67.1, 68a–b, 69.1, 72, 72.3, 73a–b, 75a–c, 76a–b, 88.5a–b, 88.6a–b, 89.1a–b, 90a–b, 92a–b, 92.1a–b, 92.2a–b, 98a–b, 101a–d, 101.1a–b, 102a–b, 104, 104.2, 105a–b, 106a–b, 109, 110a–b, 112a–b.

Scott Gaudette: Exercises 75.2, 75.3a–b, 134, 137.

Michelle Lewis and Gail Smith: Figures 10, 11, 12, 13, 26a–b and Exercises 1a–b, 2, 3.1, 5, 5.2, 7a–b, 10, 14a–b, 14.1, 15.1, 16, 17a–b, 19, 20, 20.1, 23.3, 24, 26a–c, 26.1, 27, 27.2a–b, 28.1a–b, 30.1a–b, 31.1, 32a–b, 36, 36.4, 36.5, 37.4, 38.1, 40a–c, 41a–c, 48.3a–b, 49.1a–c, 49.2a–c, 50,

Carl Peterson: Exercises 49.2d, 124, 127.

Cheri Ryan: Figures 18a–c, 19a–c, 20, 21, 24.

Jennifer Shontz: Figures 6, 128, 138a–b.

Kristy Welch: Figure 43a–b

PhotoDisc, Inc.: Frontispiece, pages 15, 137, 221.

THE MOUNTAINEERS, founded in 1906, is a nonprofit outdoor activity and conservation club, whose mission is "to explore, study, preserve, and enjoy the natural beauty of the outdoors. . . . " Based in Seattle, Washington, the club is now the third-largest such organization in the United States, with 15,000 members and five branches throughout Washington State.

The Mountaineers sponsors both classes and year-round outdoor activities in the Pacific Northwest, which include hiking, mountain climbing, ski-touring, snowshoeing, bicycling, camping, kayaking and canoeing, nature study, sailing, and adventure travel. The club's conservation division supports environmental causes through educational activities, sponsoring legislation, and presenting informational programs. All club activities are led by skilled, experienced volunteers, who are dedicated to promoting safe and responsible enjoyment and preservation of the outdoors.

If you would like to participate in these organized outdoor activities or the club's programs, consider a membership in The Mountaineers. For information and an application, write or call The Mountaineers, Club Headquarters, 300 Third Avenue West, Seattle, Washington 98119; (206) 284-6310.

The Mountaineers Books, an active, nonprofit publishing program of the club, produces guidebooks, instructional texts, historical works, natural history guides, and works on environmental conservation. All books produced by The Mountaineers are aimed at fulfilling the club's mission.

Send or call for our catalog of more than 300 outdoor titles:

The Mountaineers Books
1001 SW Klickitat Way, Suite 201
Seattle, WA 98134
1-800-553-4453
e-mail: mbooks@mountaineers.org
website: www.mountaineersbooks.org

Other titles you may enjoy from The Mountaineers:

MOUNTAINEERING: The Freedom of the Hills, Sixth Edition,
Don Graydon & Kurt Hanson, Editors
The completely revised and expanded edition of the classic text on climbing and mountaineering techniques.

BICYCLING WITH CHILDREN: A Complete How-To Guide,
Trudy E. Bell with Roxana K. Bell
Everything a parent needs to know about bikes and kids, from toddlers to teens.

BACKCOUNTRY SNOWBOARDING, *Christopher Van Tilburg*, M.D.
An introduction to the concerns of backcountry snowboarding, offering safe ascent and descent techniques for beyond the mountain resorts, by an expert snowboarder and physician.

SECRETS OF WARMTH: For Comfort or Survival, *Hal Weiss*
A comprehensive guide to planning ahead, choosing the correct materials, and using common sense to prevent hypothermia, covering emergencies in the wilderness, the city, at home, or in a stalled car in a freezing climate.

BACKPACKER'S EVERYDAY WISDOM:
1001 Expert Tips for Hikers, *Karen Berger*
Expert tips and tricks for hikers and backpackers selected from one of the most popular BACKPACKER magazine columns. Covers everything from planning to emergency improvisations.

BACKPACKER'S WILDERNESS 911: A Step-by-Step Guide for Medical Emergencies and Improvised Care in the Backcountry,
Eric Weiss, M.D.
A quick-access wilderness medicine guide from the experts of BACKPACKER magazine.